KU-467-765

Cancer Pain

Magdi Hanna • Zbigniew (Ben) Zylicz

Editors

Cancer Pain

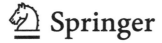

Editors
Magdi Hanna, MBBCH, FCA
Analgesics and Pain Research Unit
(APR LTD)
Beckenham
Kent
United Kingdom

Zbigniew (Ben) Zylicz, MD, PhD
Department of Research and Education
Hildegard Hospiz
Basel
Switzerland

ISBN 978-0-85729-229-2   ISBN 978-0-85729-230-8   (eBook)
DOI 10.1007/978-0-85729-230-8
Springer London Heidelberg New York Dordrecht

Library of Congress Control Number: 2013945729

© Springer-Verlag London 2013
This work is subject to copyright. All rights are reserved by the Publisher, whether the whole or part of the material is concerned, specifically the rights of translation, reprinting, reuse of illustrations, recitation, broadcasting, reproduction on microfilms or in any other physical way, and transmission or information storage and retrieval, electronic adaptation, computer software, or by similar or dissimilar methodology now known or hereafter developed. Exempted from this legal reservation are brief excerpts in connection with reviews or scholarly analysis or material supplied specifically for the purpose of being entered and executed on a computer system, for exclusive use by the purchaser of the work. Duplication of this publication or parts thereof is permitted only under the provisions of the Copyright Law of the Publisher's location, in its current version, and permission for use must always be obtained from Springer. Permissions for use may be obtained through RightsLink at the Copyright Clearance Center. Violations are liable to prosecution under the respective Copyright Law.
The use of general descriptive names, registered names, trademarks, service marks, etc. in this publication does not imply, even in the absence of a specific statement, that such names are exempt from the relevant protective laws and regulations and therefore free for general use.
While the advice and information in this book are believed to be true and accurate at the date of publication, neither the authors nor the editors nor the publisher can accept any legal responsibility for any errors or omissions that may be made. The publisher makes no warranty, express or implied, with respect to the material contained herein.

Printed on acid-free paper

Springer is part of Springer Science+Business Media (www.springer.com)

To Kate, Sam, Jonathan, and Daniel for their everlasting support.

Magdi Hanna

In memory of my Mother who died many years ago of cancer, she was my best teacher ever.

Zbigniew (Ben) Zylicz

Preface

During the professional life of the editors, and most of the authors, cancer pain management has undergone radical improvements. We have seen regular opioids adopted as the norm, and oral administration has become the preferred route of administration despite early resistance from medics and the public.

However, in spite of these improvements, recent studies demonstrate that one-third of adult patients with cancer who are in active therapy and two-thirds of patients in the advanced stages of the disease still suffer from significant pain.

To face this challenge, we have been forced to develop a fresh understanding of the dynamic pathophysiology of cancer pain, and it has become clear that a modern and more comprehensive model for cancer pain management is necessary.

Mechanism-based and multimodal combination therapies (including intervention techniques) that are tailored to the needs of the individual should prove the most efficacious techniques in the fight against cancer pain. The aim is, as ever, to optimise pain relief, minimise adverse effects of the treatment, and improve long-term outcome.

Improved survival rates among cancer sufferers, a result of enhanced anti-cancer therapy, have had the paradoxical effect of creating a significantly more complex pain syndrome. This has added a new clinical challenge for patients and physicians, and the chapters of this book are aimed squarely at confronting these issues. We have placed specific emphasis on the modern challenges that cancer care teams face in the twenty-first century and aim to provide an up-to-date outline of the current thinking in the treatment of cancer pain.

We are deeply indebted to all those who contributed to this book despite the pressure of their work and would like to acknowledge our gratitude to our publishers for their constant help and assistance.

Beckenham, Kent, UK   Magdi Hanna, MBBCH, FCA

Contents

1   **Introduction**   1
     Magdi Hanna and Zbigniew (Ben) Zylicz

2   **Epidemiology of Pain in Cancer**   5
     Irene J. Higginson, Fliss E.M. Murtagh, and Thomas R. Osborne

3   **Recent Advances in Cancer Treatment**   25
     M.J. Lind

4   **Pharmacogenetics of Pain in Cancer**   37
     Pål Klepstad

5   **Mechanisms in Cancer Pain**   47
     Jerzy Wordliczek and Renata Zajaczkowska

6   **Preclinical Cancer Pain Models**   71
     Joanna Mika, Wioletta Makuch, and Barbara Przewlocka

7   **Pain Assessment, Recognising Clinical Patterns,
     and Cancer Pain Syndromes**   95
     Malgorzata Krajnik and Zbigniew (Ben) Zylicz

8   **Opioids, Their Receptors, and Pharmacology**   109
     R.A.F.J. D'Costa and Magdi Hanna

9   **Critical Appraisal of the Breakthrough
     Pain in Cancer**   121
     Zbigniew (Ben) Zylicz

10   **Opioid-Induced Hyperalgesia**   131
     Jakob Sørensen and Per Sjøgren

11   **The Non-Pharmacological and Local Pharmacological
     Methods of Pain Control**   143
     Remigiusz Lecybyl

12   **New Drugs in Management of Pain in Cancer**   153
     Marie Fallon

13   **Neuropathic Component of Pain in Cancer**   165
     Jung Hun Kang and Eduardo Bruera

14   **Noncancer-Related Pain in Daily Practice**   191
     Zbigniew (Ben) Zylicz

ix

15 **Rehabilitation of Cancer Patients, a Forgotten Need?** 203
    Roberto Casale and Danilo Miotti

16 **Psychosocial Aspects of Cancer Pain** 211
    Marijana Braš and Veljko Đorđević

17 **Spiritual Care and Pain in Cancer** 221
    Carlo Leget

18 **Interventional Techniques in Cancer Pain:**
    Critical Appraisal 231
    Vittorio Schweiger, Enrico Polati, Antonella Paladini,
    and Giustino Varrassi

19 **Access to Opioid Analgesics: Essential**
    for Quality Cancer Care 249
    Willem Scholten

20 **Challenges for Pain Management**
    in the Twenty-First Century 263
    Mellar P. Davis

Index 279

Contributors

Marijana Braš, MD, PhD (biomedicine) Department of Psychological Medicine, University of Zagreb, School of Medicine, Centre for Palliative Medicine, Medical Ethics and Communication Skills, Zagreb 10000, Salata 4

Eduardo Bruera, MD Department of Palliative Care and Rehabilitation Medicine, University of Texas M.D. Anderson Cancer Center, Houston, TX, USA

Roberto Casale, MD, PhD Department of Clinical Neurophysiology and Pain Rehabilitation Unit, Foundation Salvatore Maugeri, Research and Care Institute, Rehabilitation Institute of Montescano, Montescano, Italy

Mellar P. Davis, MD, FCCP, FAAHPM Department of Solid Tumor, Taussig Cancer Institute, Cleveland Clinic Lerner School of Medicine, Cleveland Clinic, Cleveland, OH, USA

R.A.F.J. D'Costa, FFARCSI Department of Anaesthetics, King's College Hospital, Denmark Hill, London, UK

Veljko Đorđević, MD, PhD Department of Psychological Medicine, University of Zagreb, School of Medicine, Centre for Palliative Medicine, Medical Ethics and Communication Skills, Zagreb 10000, Salata 4

Marie Fallon, MBChB, MD, FRCP University of Edinburgh, Western General Hospital, Edinburgh, UK

Department of Palliative Medicine, Edinburgh Cancer Research Centre, Edinburgh, UK

Magdi Hanna, MBBCH, FCA Analgesics and Pain Research Unit (APR LTD), Beckenham, Kent, UK

Irene J. Higginson, BMedSci, BMBS, PhD Palliative Care, Policy and Rehabilitation, Cicely Saunders Institute, King's College London, London, UK

Jung Hun Kang, MD Division of Oncology, Department of Internal Medicine, Gyeongsang National University Hospital, Jinju, Gyeongnam, South Korea

Pål Klepstad, MD, PhD Department of Intensive Care Medicine, St. Olavs University Hospital, Trondheim, Norway

Malgorzata Krajnik, MD, PhD Palliative Care Department, Nicolaus Copernicus University, Collegium Medium in Bydgoszcz, Bydgoszcz, Poland

Remigiusz Lecybyl, MD, PhD The Pain Management Unit, University Hospital Lewisham, Lewisham, Kent, UK

Carlo Leget, PhD Ethics of Care, University of Humanistic Studies, Utrecht, The Netherlands

M.J. Lind, BSc, MD, FRCP Academic Department of Oncology, Hull York Medical School, University of Hull, Hull, Yorkshire, UK

Wioletta Makuch, MSc Department of Pain Pharmacology, Institute of Pharmacology, Polish Academy of Sciences, Krakow, Poland

Joanna Mika, PhD Department of Pain Pharmacology, Institute of Pharmacology, Polish Academy of Sciences, Krakow, Poland

Danilo Miotti, MD Palliative Care and Pain Therapy Unit, Department of Palliative Care and Pain Medicine, Fondazione Salvatore Maugeri – IRCCS, Pavia, Italy

Fliss E.M. Murtagh, PhD, MSc, MRCGP, MBBS Palliative Care, Policy and Rehabilitation, Cicely Saunders Institute, King's College London, London, UK

Thomas R. Osborne, MA, MBBS Palliative Care, Policy and Rehabilitation, Cicely Saunders Institute, King's College London, London, UK

Antonella Paladini, DR Department of Anaesthesiology, Intensive Care and Pain Medicine, Ospedale San Savatore, University of L'Aquila – Italy, Via Vetoio, 1 – Coppito, L'Aquila, Abruzzo, Italy

Enrico Polati, DR Department of Anesthesia and Intensive Care, Pain Therapy Centre, Policlinico G.B. Rossi, Verona, Italy

Barbara Przewlocka, PhD Department of Pain Pharmacology, Institute of Pharmacology, Polish Academy of Sciences, Krakow, Poland

Vittorio Schweiger, PhD Department of Anesthesia and Intensive Care, Pain Therapy Centre, Policlinico G.B. Rossi, Verona, Italy

Per Sjøgren, MDSci Section of Palliative Medicine, Department of Oncology, Rigshospitalet Hospital, Copenhagen, Denmark

Jakob Sørensen, MD Section of Palliative Care, Department of Oncology, Odense University Hospital, Odense C, Denmark

Giustino Varrassi, DR, PhD, FIPP Asl Teramo – National Health Care Service, Teramo, Abruzzo, Italy

Jerzy Wordliczek, MD, PhD Department of Pain Treatment and Palliative Care, Jagiellonian University Medical College, Krakow, Poland

Department of Anaesthesiology and Intensive Care, University Hospital, Krakow, Poland

Renata Zajaczkowska, MD, PhD Department of Anaesthesiology, Intensive Care and Pain Treatment, Province Hospital, Rzeszow, Poland

Institute of Obstetrics and Emergency Medicine, University of Rzeszow, Rzeszow, Poland

Zbigniew (Ben) Zylicz, MD, PhD Department of Research and Education, Hildegard Hospiz, Basel, Switzerland

Introduction

Magdi Hanna and Zbigniew (Ben) Zylicz

1

Abstract

Chronic pain is an extremely prevalent and complicated symptom in patients with active cancer. It is a complex and dynamic syndrome that encompasses multiple pathophysiological mechanisms and one that demands an up-to-date and flexible therapeutic toolkit.

Keywords

Cancer pain • Comprehensive strategy • Evidence-based therapy • Multidimensional • Cancer survivors

In order for physicians and cancer care teams to meet the challenges of cancer pain, a multidimensional and comprehensive strategy is required. This strategy should combine critical assessments of the pain with a balanced evaluation of the underlying disease. Treatment should be centred on an evidence-based therapy that employs specific analgesic intervention within an individualised, tailored-to-the-patient, plan of care. This plan should be "future-proofed" for any predicted progression of the disease and designed to remain appropriate throughout the course of the illness.

M. Hanna, MBBCH, FCA (✉)
Analgesics and Pain Research Unit (APR LTD),
62 Park Road, Beckenham, Kent BR3 1QH, UK
e-mail: magdihanna6262@aol.com

Z. Zylicz, MD, PhD
Department of Research and Education,
Hildegard Hospiz, St. Alban Ring 151,
Basel 4020, Switzerland
e-mail: ben.zylicz@hildegard-hospiz.ch

There have been some fundamental improvements in the field of cancer pain in the last few decades. The creation of palliative care, improved recognition of the burden on individuals and their families suffering from the syndrome, and the liberalisation of the use of opioids for management of pain by an increasing number of governments and health providers have all helped to improve our understanding and response to the problem.

Nevertheless, recent reviews state that large numbers of patients are still suffering from cancer pain, and despite rapid increases in opioid consumption (at least in the developed world [1]), the percentage of those suffering from cancer-related pain has not been reduced significantly over the course of the last 40 years [2]. On a global scale, cancer pain is barely controlled, and almost 80 % of the world cancer population receives little or no pain medication at all.

M. Hanna, Z. Zylicz (eds.), *Cancer Pain*,
DOI 10.1007/978-0-85729-230-8_1, © Springer-Verlag London 2013

Pain is not only limited to populations with active cancer but can persist in cancer survivors (patients cured of cancer or living with cancer as a chronic illness). This group of patients is increasing in numbers as a result of the significant improvements in cancer survival rates. This presents new and different challenges to physicians, and we must work to identify the appropriate therapeutic framework and best practices for this heterogeneous group [3].

In order to improve the outcome for patients suffering from chronic pain associated with cancer, it is clear that a progressive framework, one that meets the individual patient needs, as well as being fully evidence based, is required.

With this book, we hope to provide to the reader a comprehensive, up-to-date understanding of the complex demands that pain in cancer can make on a patient, their families, and the medical teams that care for them. We aim to highlight the importance of critical and continuous assessment of the many dynamic pain syndromes associated with cancer as well as providing the therapeutic modalities available. We have also aimed to highlight the necessity for psychological, emotional, and rehabilitation therapies.

In the last four decades, our understanding of pain in cancer has increased dramatically. However, the ability of the system to react to this understanding and absorb the new ideas associated with it appeared extremely limited. This seems especially so of the movement to keep patients in, or close to, their homes, and transferring this new, modern knowledge of pain to front-line treatment providers and care teams remains a significant challenge.

To many, this new knowledge may appear complicated and confusing. It may even appear that patients are suffering more pain now than they were in recent past. It is important to remember that, in the past, patients were suffering because of undertreatment and the scarcity of appropriate drugs. Now, patients are suffering because they are living longer and developing new, previously unknown pains, as well as previously undiscovered issues related to the long-term use of opioids. We hopefully address these

new pain management challenges in selected chapters of this book.

Dame Cecily Saunders, who succeeded in providing a simple scheme for the employment of morphine in the treatment of pain, also recognised the significant contribution of the psychological, social, and spiritual aspects to the intensity of a patients' suffering [4]. This is the concept known as "Total Pain." While these aspects do not fit into our pharmacological paradigm of cancer pain, they are nevertheless vital in successfully producing beneficial outcomes for patients. Although this concept was proposed by Dame Saunders, it was never fully accepted into the canon of modern medicine and, as a consequence, spiritual care workers remain the unsung heroes of the management of pain in cancer patients. It is interesting to note that in some countries spiritual care is integrated into the total and holistic care for cancer patients, with beneficial outcomes.

Ultimately, this book is created on the understanding that there is no such thing as "Cancer Pain" but rather a complex syndrome of a variety of mechanisms that contribute to "pain in cancer." As a consequence of this, we cannot approach treatment with one modality.

While opioids remain the mainstay of pain treatment, they should never be employed alone. Each pain, and a single patient may experience a number of pains, should be addressed separately [5]. The idea of this being that in the employment of pharmacological (that includes adjuvant drugs) as well as non-pharmacological treatments (that includes interventional techniques), we may minimise the dose and therefore the long-term, adverse effects of opioids.

This approach is more complicated than the WHO analgesic ladder [6] and will lead, in most patients, to polypharmacy, but with the overall aim of optimising pain control and improving overall outcome for patients.

As a consequence of accepting that our system is now more complex, we will need to redefine the roles of specialists, supporting physicians, and nurses in primary care. We need a strong network of passionate professionals who learn from each other and, most importantly, appreciate and react to the changing medical landscape around us.

References

1. van den Beuken-van Everdingen MH, de Rijke JM, Kessels AG, Schouten HC, van Kleef M, Patijn J. Prevalence of pain in patients with cancer: a systematic review of the past 40 years. Ann Oncol. 2007;18:1437–49.
2. Silbermann M. Current trends in opioid consumption globally and in Middle Eastern countries. J Pediatr Hematol Oncol. 2011;33 Suppl 1:S1–5.
3. Portenoy RK. Treatment of cancer pain. Lancet. 2011;377:2236–47.
4. Saunders C. Tribute to Dame Cicely Saunders, First Lady of the modern hospice movement. Interview by Val J. Halamandaris. Caring. 1998;17:60–6.
5. Twycross R, Harcourt J, Bergl S. A survey of pain in patients with advanced cancer. J Pain Symptom Manage. 1996;12:273–82.
6. Twycross R, Lickiss N. Pain control and the World Health Organization analgesic ladder. JAMA. 1996; 275:835; author reply 836.

Epidemiology of Pain in Cancer

Irene J. Higginson, Fliss E.M. Murtagh,
and Thomas R. Osborne

Abstract

Pain is one of the most common and feared symptoms in patients with cancer, yet the exact number of cancer patients who experience pain is difficult to ascertain. Studies vary widely in the ways they define pain, the populations they study, and the tools they use to measure this complex symptom. These differences can make it difficult to accurately combine results across studies and to generalise their findings.

This chapter gives an overview of some of the challenges in describing the epidemiology of cancer pain and presents a systematic literature review to identify the prevalence of pain in different cancer groups. The weighted mean prevalence of pain in mixed- and early-stage cancer is reported as 45.6 % (range 21.4–84.1 %). The patient-reported weighted mean prevalence of pain in advanced or metastatic cancer is identified as 73.9 % (range 53–100 %). The prevalence across different tumour groups is also discussed.

Keywords

Cancer • Neoplasms • Palliative care • Pain • Pain measurement • Epidemiology • Review • Systematic review

Introduction

Pain is one of the most feared symptoms in those diagnosed with cancer and affects millions of people worldwide each year. Exactly how many cancer

I.J. Higginson, BMedSci, BMBS, PhD
F.E.M. Murtagh, PhD, MSc, MRCGP, MBBS
T.R. Osborne, MA, MBBS (✉)
Palliative Care, Policy and Rehabilitation,
Cicely Saunders Institute, King's College London,
London, UK
e-mail: irene.higginson@kcl.ac.uk;
fliss.murtagh@kcl.ac.uk; przebar@if-pan.krakow.pl

patients experience pain is difficult to ascertain, and the reasons for this are explored within this chapter. Thankfully, good or complete pain control can be achieved in 80–90 % of cancer patients [1–3]. Nevertheless, in spite of the major advances in pain control, cancer-related pain continues to be a major public health problem globally [4–20].

Pain is an extremely common symptom in patients with cancer, and studies to date reveal wide variations in reported prevalence [21–23]. One systematic review of 19 studies found pain reported in 35–96 % of cancer patients [24]. This wide range is due to three main factors:

M. Hanna, Z. Zylicz (eds.), *Cancer Pain*,
DOI 10.1007/978-0-85729-230-8_2, © Springer-Verlag London 2013

1. Prevalence studies are conducted in different settings and in different groups of cancer patients, making it difficult to generalise findings [25, 26].
2. There is no gold standard method to assess the presence or absence of pain or pain severity.
3. It is difficult to define the type of pain [27] – cancer pain can be directly or indirectly related to the cancer and can have features of acute or chronic pain [28, 29].

Evaluation of pain in advanced cancer is primarily clinical, based on pattern recognition, and should be based on the patient's report. Attention to detail is necessary to prevent inappropriate treatment [30]. Comprehensive pain assessment is important, but initial treatment with analgesics should not be withheld until this has been carried out [31]. There are many reasons that pain remains unrelieved, and these can be associated with the patient or family, or with the doctor or nurse. These include lack of confidence or skills by clinicians, poor assessment, and fear of opioids. Understanding the epidemiology is critical to help clinicians recognise when pain may occur and improve assessment and management.

The Definition of Pain

Pain is defined as "an unpleasant sensory and emotional experience associated with actual or potential tissue damage, or described in terms of such damage" [32]. There is no definitive way to distinguish between pain occurring in the *absence* of tissue damage and pain resulting from actual damaged tissue [33]. In addition to its physiological basis, pain is affected by psychological factors such as emotion, cognition, and motivation, as well as an individual's social context and spiritual beliefs. Mood, morale, and the meaning of pain can modulate pain perception for an individual [31]. A recent study exploring and comparing the meaning of pain in black Caribbean and white British cancer patients suggested that pain means different things to different cultural groups [34]. Pain can sometimes be seen as a test or challenge, which can change a patient's attitude toward its treatment.

Difficulties in Cancer Pain Epidemiology

There are a number of challenges in describing the epidemiology of cancer pain. Studies vary in their design and scope, making it difficult to effectively combine data or generalise findings [24]. These challenges are summarised below.

Study Population

The study of pain often takes place in healthcare settings rather than in naturally occurring populations. As such, the resulting estimates of pain prevalence reflect a group of patients referred to a specific service. For example, a study by Coyle [35] looked specifically at patients referred to the Supportive Care Program of the Pain Service at the Memorial Sloan-Kettering Cancer Center. There are obvious problems in generalising these findings to the whole population of cancer patients, since those referred to a Supportive Care Service may be more likely to suffer particularly difficult or intractable pain. Moreover, some studies are limited only to patients who have pain, giving valuable information on pain syndromes, mechanisms, and treatment but cannot provide estimates of pain prevalence.

Definitions of Cancer Pain

Cancer pain is not a well-defined entity [27] and may be defined differently across studies. An individual may have a number of different pains, each with different characteristics. Some pains may be directly due to a tumour (e.g., a fungating wound), others due to treatment (e.g., oral mucositis from chemotherapy), and others unrelated to the cancer (e.g., joint pain from osteoarthritis). All may occur in a single patient, and each may be acute or chronic. Alternatively, some may define cancer pain in terms of its pathology (e.g., nociceptive or neuropathic [28]).

Assessment Methods

The tools and methods used to assess pain are not constant across all studies. This is true when assessing both the presence or absence of pain and also the severity of pain. Pain severity is an important factor in determining the impact of pain on an individual [36, 37]. Failure to assess the severity of pain, coupled with the variety of methods used for its categorisation, often compounds to make it very difficult to combine the findings from different authors or make generalisations. Moreover, some studies use proxies to estimate the prevalence of pain (e.g., asking a family member or health-care professional if pain was present), and some may infer the presence of pain from records of analgesic use. Further work is needed to develop systematic and standardised assessments of pain, which can be used in routine care and for epidemiological monitoring. Further issues in the assessment of pain are discussed below.

Further Aspects of Pain Assessment

First of all, the physician must believe the patient's report of pain and initiate further discussions. Assessment should define the nature and extent of the underlying disease, evaluate concomitant problems (physical, psychological, and social) that may contribute to patient distress and clarify the goals of care [38]. The assessment should thereby clarify the pain characteristics and syndrome, infer the putative mechanisms that may underlie the pain, and determine the impact of the pain on function and psychological well-being [38]. If necessary, additional investigations should be carried out to clarify uncertainties in the assessment [39].

When selecting a mode of measuring pain severity, the response mode must be [37] (1) sufficiently graded to identify changes, (2) clear to both subjects and investigators, and (3) easy to score.

Visual analogue, verbal descriptor, and numeric rating scales have been used in the clinical setting to assess pain severity and have been shown to approach equivalency in their results [40]. Numeric rating scales have been endorsed for use in trials and practice because they are easier to understand and to score [41]. These have also been shown to be less affected by language or cultural interpretation of pain severity. A study using multidimensional scaling to compare the rating of pain's interference in four countries revealed two dimensions to the reporting of pain, irrespective of pain severity or cultural or linguistic background [42] – activity and affect. Activity was defined in terms of walking, work, general activity, and sleep. Affect is related to functions such as relationships with others, mood, and enjoyment of life [42]. The research program of the European Palliative Care Research Collaboration is studying the methods of assessment and management of three symptoms – pain, depression, and cachexia. The pain assessment work package is seeking to develop a uniform, agreed-on, and validated method to assess pain across the collaborative. It is studying pain intensity and the extent to which pain interferes with activities – although pilot work has found high correlations between these two aspects [43]. The results of this collaborative will be valuable in unifying assessment across research studies and in practice.

Some general assessment tools include evaluating pain alongside other symptoms and problems and thus can be valuable in monitoring pain. As more and more standardised assessment tools become available [44], comparisons between settings may become feasible. Such measures include the Brief Pain Inventory [45, 46], the Edmonton Symptom Assessment System [47–50], the Palliative Care Outcome Scale [51, 52], the Support Team Assessment Schedule [53], the Memorial Symptom Assessment Scale [54], and the European Organization for Research and Treatment of Cancer (EORTC) QLQ-C30 questionnaire [55] as well as standard quality of life measures such as the SF-36 and the EQ-5D used in health economic studies.

Assessment may also be carried out by interview, either with the patient or, in certain situations, with the assistance of the family. Whether an assessment is carried out by the physician, the nurse, or the patient will obviously affect the data collected. In a study validating a staff-rated outcome measure for use in palliative care, staff were found to underrate the level of pain, and family or caregivers overrated the level of pain as compared with the patient's self-report of pain [53]. However, in a recent validation of the Palliative Care Outcome Scale caregiver version, lay caregivers showed substantial agreement with patients' self-ratings [56]. The limitations of each method of measurement need to be understood and noted when reporting cancer pain prevalence data, because the methods used will affect the outcomes of the study. Another key factor in measuring the prevalence of pain is the time period of assessment. Assessments range from pain now, to pain during the past 24 h, to pain in the past 1, 2, or even 6 months. Any binary scale of pain present/absent will lead to a higher prevalence if a longer time period of assessment is included. (Compare responses to "Have you had pain in the past 24 h?" with those to "Have you had pain in the past month?"). Graded scales (such as a 0–4 scale) do not have as many problems in interpretation as a result of changes in the period of assessment, because patients tend to average their experience over time.

The classification of cancer pain is a controversial issue. Ventafridda and Caraceni [57] suggest the following:

1. Every study involving patients with cancer pain and analgesic treatments should provide a precise description of the symptoms, including details of all clinical and instrumental diagnostic criteria.
2. A classification of pain according to the definition of somatic, visceral, and nerve pains should separate differentiation, neuropathic, or dysesthetic pain from nerve trunk pains.
3. Temporary patterns of pain and their precipitating factors should always be specified.

This classification reflects an ideal situation and would overcome many of the problems encountered when reviewing the prevalence estimates in this area. Simple clinical tools are now available to help in the classification of neuropathic pain, which is one of the key pains to differentiate because of the different outcomes and

management. For example, the Leeds Assessment of Neuropathic Symptoms and Signs [58] has now been validated for use in cancer [59]. Unfortunately, the primary data do not allow us to classify the studies of cancer pain in this way; therefore, we are restricted to making generalisations from studies, with caveats attached.

Prevalence of Cancer Pain

To identify the prevalence of cancer pain, Higginson and Murtagh carried out a systematic literature review including studies from 1979 to 2006 [60]. This review has been further updated for this chapter to include studies up to September 2011.

Literature Search

To identify any new articles published from 2006 to 2011, citation searching was carried out on all 64 included articles identified in the original review [60]. The citation search was run using Scopus in September 2011 and limited to studies published from 2006 to 2011.

Inclusion/Exclusion Criteria

Criteria were based on the work of Portenoy [23] who proposed using two related sets of survey data to provide epidemiological estimates of cancer pain prevalence. A study was included if it reported the prevalence of cancer pain in a clearly defined cancer population, which was derived from:

1. A survey on the natural history of the neoplasm that included information on pain.
2. The preliminary stage of a broader study on pain management or service evaluation.

A seminal review by Bonica [61] was included because the original studies in this review were especially difficult to locate (because of the age and location mainly of the unpublished grey literature) and the data from some would not have been included otherwise. With this exception, articles were excluded if they were reviews, letters, case studies, and personal opinions or if they selected only patients who had pain.

Study Identification

The citation search yielded 1,504 articles published between 2006 and 2011. Thirty-one of these met the inclusion and exclusion criteria. There were 64 articles published between 1979 and 2006 identified in the earlier version of this review [60] although nine of these were excluded here because they sampled only patients with pain and so could not be used to estimate pain prevalence. This gave a total of 86 included articles [22, 26, 36, 61–143].

Data Synthesis

Because of the problems of varied measurement, a meta-analysis of the data could not be carried out. Data extracted from the published studies (Tables 2.1 and 2.2) are synthesised in the text. Although cancer pain is prevalent at all stages of the disease, it is more common in advanced and terminal cancer. For this reason, studies focusing on people with cancer at early or mixed stages (Table 2.1) are considered separately from those concentrating on patients with advanced or terminal disease (Table 2.2).

The Prevalence of Pain at All Stages and in Early Disease

Forty-nine studies reported the prevalence of cancer pain in samples of mixed or early-stage disease (Table 2.1). One study by Yamagishi et al. [131] reported only the prevalence of moderate or severe pain, but not overall pain prevalence. The remaining 48 studies gave a weighted mean prevalence of pain of 40.4 % (range 21.4–84.1 %). Note, however, that this estimate includes three low estimates determined from the use of analgesics alone as a measure of pain prevalence (Foley [22] 29 and 38 %; Hiraga et al. [75] 33 %). Excluding these studies provides a weighted mean pain prevalence of 45.6 % (range 21.4–84.1 %).

There is little evidence on the prevalence of pain at or around the time of diagnosis. Vuorinen [78] reported 35 % of newly diagnosed patients had experienced pain in the past 2 weeks; Ger et al. [92] found that 38 % of newly diagnosed cancer patients had pain; Yamagishi et al. [131] reported that 14 % of newly diagnosed patients starting chemotherapy had moderate to severe pain, but did not report overall pain prevalence in this group.

Prevalence of Pain in Advanced Cancer

Thirty-seven studies reported data on pain prevalence in the advanced or terminal cancer population (Table 2.2). Excluding two studies that did not report the overall pain prevalence [63, 69], this gives a weighted mean prevalence of 76.1 % (range 53–100 %). However, six studies used retrospective data collected from caregivers of patients with cancer or from other informants who could provide information on particular patients [62, 63, 72, 82, 96, 128]. Reports from the Regional Studies for the Care of the Dying [72, 82] provided period prevalence estimates of pain in the last year of life at three time points: 87 % in 1969, 84 % in 1987, and 88 % in 1995. The study by Ward [62] considered pain in the "period of terminal illness" and gave a pain prevalence of 62 %. Bucher et al. [96] reported that 86 % of patients had a problem with pain in the last 4 weeks of life, and Costantini et al. [128] reported pain prevalence of 82.3 % in the last 3 months of life. These data from informants are subject to recall bias, as well as being subjective assessments. Overall, these estimates were slightly higher than those for patient reports, possibly because of the longer periods included (e.g., last year of life), because bereaved caregivers overestimate pain or because samples were biased by nonresponse from patients with the most severe pain. Excluding studies using informant data provides a weighted mean prevalence of 73.9 % (range 53–100 %).

The Prevalence of Pain by Primary Tumour Site

Table 2.3 combines all studies that report prevalence data separately in a given tumour type. These generally show wide ranges for reported

Table 2.1 The prevalence of cancer pain in early- or mixed-stage cancer

Study type[a]	Population	Sample size	Prevalence[b]	Reference (date order)
Prospective survey	General cancer population	540	29 %	Foley (1979) [22]
		397	38 %	
Prospective survey	General cancer population	237	72 %	Trotter et al. (1981) [64]
Prospective survey	Breast, prostate, colon, or rectum and three gynaecological tumours	667	48 % Mean score worst pain: 4.0 (SD 3.6) to 6.7 (SD 7.1)[c] Mean score average pain: 2.5 (SD 3.5) to 5.7 (SD 2.1)[c]	Daut and Cleeland (1982) [36]
Prospective survey	Lung, pancreas, prostate, and uterine cervix	536	64 % 30 % slight pain, 30 % moderate pain, 4 % very bad pain, 19 % had worst pain possible	Greenwald et al. (1987) [66]
Prospective survey	General cancer population	240	45 % Mean score most severe pain past week: 7.2 (SD 2.4)[c] Mean score present intensity: 2.9 (SD 2.5)[c]	Dorrepaal et al. (1989) [67]
Quasi meta-analysis	General cancer population	14,417	51 % 74 % in those with advanced/terminal disease	Bonica (1990) [61]
Retrospective patient record survey	General cancer population	35,683	32.6 % 11.4 % before treatment, 24.9 % in curative stage, 48.7 % in conservative stage, 71.3 % in terminal stage	Hiraga et al. (1991) [75]
Prospective survey	Newly diagnosed general cancer population	240	35 % 46 % pain related to cancer, 67 % pain secondary to cancer or its treatment, 18 % unrelated pain	Vuorinen (1993) [78]
Prospective study	Prostate, colon, breast, or ovarian cancer patients	243	64 %	Portenoy et al. (1994) [81]
Prospective survey	Ovarian cancer patients	151	42 % 40 % experienced any pain almost constantly, 21 % experienced worst pain almost constantly. Mean severity was moderate; mean severity for worst pain was severe	Portenoy et al. (1994) [80]
Prospective survey	General cancer population	369	54 % Mean score for average daily pain: 3.6 (SD 2.2) (between mild and moderate)	Glover et al. (1995) [85]
Prospective cross-sectional multicentre survey	General cancer population	605	57 % 69 % rated pain as significant (score of 5 or more on a 10-point scale)	Larue et al. (1995) [86]

Study type	Population	N	Results	Reference
Descriptive survey	Ambulatory patients with breast cancer	97	64 % / Mean score for average daily pain: 3.4 (SD 2.3) (mild to moderate)	Miaskowski and Dibble (1995) [87]
Randomised controlled trial	General cancer population	438	39 % (treatment and control groups posttest)	Elliott et al. (1997) [90]
Retrospective cross-sectional study	General cancer population	13,625	29 %	Bernabei et al. (1998) [91]
Prospective survey	Patients with recurrent breast or gynaecological cancers	64 (breast) 53 (gyne)	70 % (breast) 63 % (gyne) 51 % had mild to moderate pain	Rummans et al. (1998) [93]
Prospective study	Newly diagnosed general cancer population	296	38 % / 65 % of those in pain had worst pain scores at least 5 on a 10-point scale. 31 % of those in pain had average pain scores at least 5 on a 10-point scale	Ger et al. (1998) [92]
Cross-sectional study	General cancer population	217	64 %	Wells et al. (1998) [94]
Prospective longitudinal study	Patients with cancers of the head and neck	93	48 % at baseline, 8 % severe / 25 % had pain at 12 months, 3 % severe / 26 % had pain at 24 months, 3 % severe	Chaplin and Morton (1999) [97]
Secondary analysis of prospective data	Patients with primary lung cancer or cancer metastatic to bone	125	72 %	Berry et al. (1999) [95]
Prospective survey	General cancer population (in- and outpatients)	240	59 % / 67 % of inpatients, 47 % of outpatients / 64 % of inpatients with pain had malignant pain, 23 % nonmalignant pain, 11 % mixed	Chang et al. (2000) [101]
Prospective survey	General cancer population hospitalised for at least 24 h	258	51.5 % / 29.3 % of those in pain had pain related to the tumour	Ripamonti et al. (2000) [103]
Prospective survey	General cancer population	263	35.7 %	Beck and Falkson (2001) [104]
Population-based survey	Randomly selected patients from the cancer population	1,555	61.6 %	Liu et al. (2001) [105]
Prospective survey	General cancer population attending oncology outpatients	480	53 % / 22 % had pain reported as "quite a bit" or "very much"	Lidstone et al. (2003) [106]
Prospective survey	Hospitalised cancer patients	1,392	61 % / 30 % reporting moderate or severe pain	Rustoen et al. (2003) [108]

(continued)

Table 2.1 (continued)

Study type[a]	Population	Sample size	Prevalence[b]	Reference (date order)
Prospective survey	General cancer population attending oncology outpatients	480	54 % Severe pain was reported by 35 % and moderate pain by 35.4 % of patients	Hsieh (2005) [111]
Cross-sectional survey	General cancer population, including oncology in- and outpatients	178	50 % Moderate to severe pain in 50 % of patients surveyed, with 23 % reporting severe pain	Reyes-Gibby et al. (2006) [115]
Prospective study	General cancer population	151	72.8 %	Chen and Tseng (2006) [112]
Prospective study	Cancer patients with bone metastases	504	84.1 %	Chow et al. (2007) [118]
Prospective survey	General cancer population	1,429	55 % 44 % moderate to severe	Van den Beuken-van Everdingen (2007) [119]
Prospective study	Breast, colorectal, ovarian, lung, and prostate cancer patients	125	48 %	Collins et al. (2008) [121]
Prospective survey	Hospital inpatients with localised prostate cancer	115	69.9 %	Gerbershagen et al. (2008) [122]
Prospective longitudinal study	Inoperable lung cancer	70 (women) 89 (men)	Women: 55 % had pain at baseline and 55 % at 3 months Men: 60 % had pain at baseline and 59 % at 3 months	Lovgren et al. 2008 [123]
Cross-sectional survey	General cancer population	2,653	34.0 % 12.6 % mild pain, 15.0 % moderate, 6.4 % severe	Mercadante et al. (2008) [124]
Prospective survey	General oncology outpatients	1,549	21.4 %	Valeberg et al. (2008) [125]
Cross-sectional study	Breast cancer patients	200	42 %	Wang et al. (2008) [126]
Prospective survey	General cancer population	5,084	72 % 56 % rated pain at least 5 on a 10-point rating scale	Breivik et al. (2009) [127]
Retrospective study	Nursing home residents with cancer	1,022	49.4 % 25.8 % mild, 20.6 % moderate, 4.1 % excruciating	Duncan et al. (2009) [129]
Prospective longitudinal survey[d]	General oncology outpatients starting chemotherapy	462	14 % moderate to severe pain	Yamagishi et al. (2009) [131]
Retrospective study	Hepatocellular cancer at diagnosis	3,417	28.6 %	Carr and Pujol (2010) [132]
Prospective longitudinal study	General cancer population	304	39.3 %	Mercadante et al. (2010) [133]

Study type	Population	N	Results	Reference
Prospective longitudinal study	General cancer within 1 year of diagnosis	84	46.7 % at baseline 35.4 % at 3 months, 34.2 % at 6 months, 31.1 % at 12 months	Molssiotis et al. (2010) [134]
Cross-sectional survey	Previously treated for breast cancer	240	45 %	Reyes-Gibby et al. (2010) [135]
Prospective survey	Head and neck cancer outpatients	70	34 %	Williams et al. 2010 [136]
Prospective survey	Community-dwelling general cancer patients	312	57.1 %	Dhingra et al. (2011) [137]
Cross-sectional survey	Breast cancer patients	182	47.2 % 19.8 % mild pain, 27.5 % moderate or intense pain	Lamino et al. (2011) [140]
Cross-sectional survey	Haematological cancer patients	180	39 % 28 % Not at all/a little, 21 % somewhat, 51 % quite a bit/very much	Manitta et al. (2011) [141]
Cross-sectional survey	Sarcoma outpatients	149	53 %	Williams et al. (2011) [143]

[a]Survey = the primary aim of the study was to survey pain or symptom prevalence; Study = there was a different primary aim to the study, e.g., service evaluation

[b]Percentages for severity breakdowns may not equal overall percentages due to missing data

[c]0 = no pain; 10 = worst pain as assessed by pain rating scale

[d]Not included in weighted mean prevalence because overall prevalence not given

Table 2.2 The prevalence of cancer pain in patients with advanced disease or at the end of life

Study type[a]	Population	Sample size	Prevalence[b]	Reference (date order)
Retrospective record review and interview study	GPs and bereaved carers of those with pharyngeal, breast, bronchial, stomach, colon, and rectal cancers	279	62 %	Ward (1974) [62]
Retrospective interview study[c]	Bereaved carers of advanced general cancer population	165	36 % none to mild pain, 31 % moderate, 33 % severe to very severe	Parkes (1978) [63]
Prospective study	Terminal general cancer population or primary carers	1,754	69 % 19 % mild, 21 % discomfort, 16 % distressing, 7 % horrible, 5 % excruciating	Morris et al. (1986) [65]
Prospective evaluation study	Advanced general cancer population	256	53 %	McIlmurray and Warren (1989) [68]
Prospective study[c]	Terminal general cancer population	60	Mean scores 53.5 (SD 37.5) and 41.9 (SD 29.1) for home care and hospital care patients, respectively[d]	Ventafridda et al. (1989) [69]
Prospective study	Advanced general cancer population	65	68 %	Higginson et al. (1990) [70]
Prospective study	Terminal general cancer population	120	100 %	Ventafridda et al. (1990) [71]
Prospective survey	Advanced general cancer population	78	71 % 24 % mild, 40 % moderate, 36 % severe	Simpson (1991) [76]
Retrospective record review	Advanced cancer population	110	69 % 34 % related to the primary cancer, 43 % related to metastatic disease	Chan and Woodruff (1991) [73]
Retrospective record review	Advanced general cancer population	100	99 %	Fainsinger et al. (1991) [74]
Retrospective interview study	Bereaved carers/informants of people who had died from cancer	383	87 % in 1969 84 % in 1987	Cartwright (1991) [72]
Retrospective record review	Advanced general cancer population over 65	239	58 % 12 % mild, 18 % discomfort, 17 % distress, 7 % horrible, 6 % excruciating	Stein and Miech (1993) [77]
Prospective study	Advanced lung cancer patients	52	88 %	Mercadante et al. (1994) [79]
Prospective study	General advanced cancer population	1,000	83 %	Donnelly et al. (1995) [83]
Prospective survey	Advanced general cancer population	125	74 %	Ellershaw (1995) [84]
Retrospective interview study	Bereaved carers of general cancer population	2,018	88 %	Addington-Hall and McCarthy (1995) [82]

Study type	Population	N	Findings	Reference
Prospective study	Far-advanced general cancer population	98	64 % / Median score 4 for average pain, median score 6 for worst pain on a 10-point scale	Shannon et al. (1995) [88]
Prospective study	Advanced general cancer population	1,640	72 % / 24 % mild, 30 % moderate, 21 % severe	Vainio et al. (1996) [89]
Prospective study	Advanced general cancer population	695	70 % / 54 % mild or moderate, 16 % severe or overwhelming	Higginson and Hearn (1997) [26]
Retrospective study	Caregivers of general cancer population	170	86 % / 61 % a great deal or quite a bit, 25 % some or a little	Bucher et al. (1999) [96]
Retrospective cross-sectional survey	Advanced general cancer population	100	77 % / Majority had mild pain	Chung et al. (1999) [98]
Prospective study	Advanced general cancer population	3,577	70.3 % at referral / Mean score visual analogue scale (max score 10) was 4.4 at referral, 2.5 at 1 week, 2.3 in the last week of life	Mercadente (1999) [99]
Retrospective cohort study	Advanced cancer patients who subsequently died	223	66 % / 19 % had pain complaints documented at each visit, 13.2 % of patients never had documented pain	Nowels and Lee (1999) [100]
Prospective study	Advanced cancer patients admitted to hospice	232	81 %	Chiu et al. (2000) [102]
Retrospective record review	Patients referred to palliative care services	400	64 % / 62 % in hospice setting, 56 % in community setting, 63 % in hospital, 75 % outpatients	Potter et al. (2003) [107]
Cross-sectional survey	Hospital inpatients with metastatic cancer or stage IV lymphoma	66	78 %	Tranmer et al. (2003) [109]
Prospective survey	In and outpatients with metastatic or recurrent cancer	655	70.8 % / 63.6 % scored at least 5 on 0–10 visual analogue scale	Yun et al. (2003) [110]
Cross-sectional survey	Metastatic breast, lung, stomach, prostate, or cervical cancer	114	90.4 % / 37.7 % minimal, 20.2 % moderate, 32.5 % severe	Monestel Umana et al. (2006) [113]
Retrospective record review	Advanced general cancer population	772	87 %	Peng et al. (2006) [114]
Prospective survey	Advanced cancer patients in palliative care unit	77	88.3 %	Tsai et al. (2006) [116]

(continued)

Table 2.2 (continued)

Study type[a]	Population	Sample size	Prevalence[b]	Reference (date order)
Prospective survey	Advance cancer patients referred to palliative care	922	84 %	Walsh and Rybicki (2006) [117]
Prospective study	Patients referred for palliative treatment of brain metastases	160	60.6 %	Chow et al. (2008) [120]
Retrospective survey	Carers of deceased cancer patients	1,271	82.3 % 61 % very distressing pain	Costantini et al. (2009) [128]
Prospective interview survey	Cancer patients referred to palliative care	381	70.3 % 16.3 % minimal, 20.2 % mild, 18.6 % moderate, 10.0 % strong, 3.4 % severe, 1.8 % extreme	Wilson et al. (2009) [130]
Prospective survey	Cancer patients attending palliative care service	112	87.5 %	Harding et al. (2011) [138]
Prospective survey	Advanced cancer patients referred to palliative care	777	83 %	Kirkova et al. (2011) [139]
Prospective survey	Hospital inpatients with advanced cancer	103	71.3 %	Spichiger et al. (2011) [142]

[a]Survey = the primary aim of the study was to survey pain or symptom prevalence; Study = there was a different primary aim to the study, e.g., service evaluation
[b]Percentages for severity breakdowns may not equal overall percentages due to missing data
[c]Not included in weighted mean prevalence because overall prevalence not given
[d]Scores relate to hours of pain multiplied by a severity coefficient, values range from 0 to 240

prevalence for each tumour, which probably reflects the differences in pain assessment discussed earlier in this chapter. Cancers of the blood are said to have little pain associated with the disease, particularly in the early stages. This opinion could be substantiated by the evidence from the study by Foley [22] which reported only 5 % of patients with leukaemia experiencing pain. Nevertheless, the range of pain prevalence values for lymphoma was 20–87 % and so pain in haematological cancers should not be underestimated.

The Severity of Pain

The various stages of disease considered and the methods of measurement make it difficult to summarise the data in the tables to provide valid estimates of the prevalence of severe pain or the proportion of pain affecting or dominating the daily life of patients. However, it is obvious by looking qualitatively at the data that there is a great deal of unrelieved pain at referral to all the services carrying out these studies.

High-Risk Groups

When considering risk factors for cancer pain, it is important to be clear which "type" of cancer pain is under investigation. In this section, pain associated with direct tumour involvement is discussed. Pain associated with cancer therapy, such as postoperative pain syndromes, or pain syndromes related or unrelated to the cancer itself, such as myofascial pains or constipation, are not considered here. With increases in chemotherapy in cancer, however, they are of growing prevalence and importance.

The evidence shows that the prevalence of pain varies according to the site of the cancer and the stage of the disease. Higher prevalence estimates found for patients with advanced disease indicate that these patients are more likely to be experiencing pain at referral to a service than those at earlier stages of the disease. This is reinforced by the findings of Daut and Cleeland [36], who report that more pain is usually associated with metastatic than nonmetastatic disease. For example, 64 % of patients with metastatic breast cancer had pain, compared with 40 % of patients

with nonmetastatic disease, a pattern that is consistent in cancer types (Table 2.3).

There is no evidence as to whether age is a predictor of pain in cancer patients, but there is some suggestion that pain may be lower among elderly people with advanced disease [77], but it is not clear whether this is a result of physiological changes, different cultural systems, or ageism.

There is no evidence on whether specific psychological factors predispose to the initial onset of pain. However, the effect of pain on increasing psychological distress has been well documented, and it is likely that patients with unresolved psychosocial problems will experience more frequent or more intense pain compared with those patients who are not experiencing psychological distress, according to the models of "suffering" and "total pain."

The severity of pain is determined by the previously mentioned factors combined with the method of pain control therapy administered and whether it has been appropriate to the needs of the individual patient. The continued reports of high levels of pain prevalence on referral to cancer services suggest that pain is important and in some instances not being managed as well as it should be [26, 84, 86]. Health professionals should not assume that patients previously receiving care elsewhere have adequate pain control.

Challenges for the Future in the Epidemiology of Cancer Pain

The reality of addressing cancer pain control, coupled with the increasing number of people living to older ages and living longer with cancer, makes reducing the prevalence of pain at any stage of the disease process of paramount importance. Collaboration is needed with the nonmedical sectors of society to ensure that palliative care becomes an integral part of patient care [144]. Just as important as research in the purely medical aspects of pain and palliative care are the social, economic, and cultural attitudes toward pain, suffering, and the terminally ill [66, 145–150]. This is especially true as the proportion of

Table 2.3 The prevalence of cancer pain by primary tumour site

Study	Breast	Lung/respiratory	Head and neck	Genitourinary	Prostate	Colorectal	Gastrointestinal	Lymphoma	Pancreas	Sarcoma	Uterine/general gynaecological	Central nervous system	Cervix/vagina	Ovary	Bladder/kidney	Hepatobiliary	Leukaemia	Melanoma	Aesophagus	Bone	Multiple myeloma	Oral cavity	Stomach
Foley (1979) [22]	52 %	45 %		70–75 %			40 %	20 %									5 %			85 %		80 %	
Daut (1982) [36] – Metastatic	64 %		75 %			47 %					40 %		0 %	59 %									
Daut (1982) [36] – Nonmetastatic	40 %				30 %	40 %					14 %		35 %	39 %									
Greenwald et al. (1987) [66]		71 %			56 %				72 %				56 %										
Simpson (1991) [76]a	50 %	17 %		88 %			50–71 %	50 %		100 %		50 %						20 %					
Mercadante et al. (1994) [79]a		88 %																					
Portenoy et al. (1994) [81]	60 %				68 %	62 %								67 %									
Portenoy et al. (1994) [80]														42 %									
Donnelly et al. (1995) [83]a	89 %		91 %	94 %		79 %			85 %		90 %		87 %	71 %	83–85 %			100 %	77 %				
Larue et al. (1995) [86]	56 %	58 %	67 %	58 %			56 %	35 %															
Miaskowski and Dibble (1995) [87]	64 %																						
Vainio et al. (1996) [89]a	78 %	74 %	83 %	90 %	83 %	79 %		87 %											71 %				74 %
Higginson and Hearn (1997) [26]a	76 %	71 %	74 %	74 %		68 %		74 %															
Runmans et al. (1998) [93]	70 %										64 %												
Chaplin and Morton (1999) [97]			48 %																				
Chiu et al. (2000) [102]a	70 %	78 %	87 %			79 %			100 %	91 %			60 %										

Study	Breast	Lung/respiratory	Head and neck	Genitourinary	Prostate	Colorectal	Gastrointestinal	Lymphoma	Pancreas	Sarcoma	Uterine/general gynaecological	Central nervous system	Cervix/vagina	Ovary	Bladder/kidney	Hepatobiliary	Leukaemia	Melanoma	Aesophagus	Bone	Multiple myeloma	Oral cavity	Stomach
Lidstone et al. (2003) [106]	62 %	68 %	52 %	40 %			58 %	38 %				53 %											
Peng et al. (2006) [114]a	92 %	80 %		90 %			87 %			96 %													
Gerbershagen et al. (2008) [122]					70 %																		
Lovgren et al. (2008) [123]		55–60 %																					
Valeberg et al. (2008) [125]	23 %		25 %		13 %	31 %				39 %	29 %												
Breivik et al. (2009) [127]	62 %		86 %	82 %	53 %	82 %		75–87 %	93 %		77 %						66 %						
Costantini et al. (2009) [128]a	76 %	83 %	85 %	90 %	91 %	85 %	88 %		80 %			52 %			89 %	74 %					86 %		
Carr and Pujol (2010) [132]																29 %							
Reyes-Gibby et al. (2010) [135]	45 %																						
Williams et al. (2010) [136]			34 %																				
Lamino et al. (2011) [140]	46 %																						
Williams et al. (2011) [143]										53 %													
Total number of studies	18	13	10	9	9	8	7	7	5	5	5	4	4	4	2	2	2	2	2	1	1	1	1
Range of %	23–92	17–86	25–91	58–90	13–91	31–85	40–88	20–87	72–100	39–100	14–90	50–90	0–87	39–71	83–89	29–74	5–66	20–100	71–77	–	–	–	–

aStudies reporting prevalence in advanced disease or at the end of life caregivers declines relative to the growing number of patients who need care [3]. Much more work is needed to study the epidemiology of pain in palliative care and community populations, rather than in specialist centres. Standardised assessments and longitudinal studies would allow the changes in pain over time to be better understood. Further work is also needed on meanings and treatment of pain in different cultural populations and among older people, since existing work already suggests that pain has different meaning in different cultural groups [34]. As cancer treatments change, so may the nature and prevalence of pain in cancer, and this will require careful assessment [151–153].

Clinicians often do not recognise how frequently pain remains untreated or inadequately managed [21]. It should not be assumed that if a person has been receiving cancer care or treatment in a health-care setting, their pain is being adequately controlled [26, 148]. Continual assessment of the response of the patient's pain complaint is essential to ensure continuous pain control and to prevent breakthrough pain [145, 152]. As other chapters in this textbook show, there are now approaches to ensure the development of systems to better manage cancer pain. There is also a need for training and education, a key function of the specialist in palliative care. Health-care professionals in all health-care settings need to monitor pain and know how to treat cancer pain effectively.

Acknowledgments This chapter is based upon a chapter published previously elsewhere [60]. Professor Irene J. Higginson is a National Institute of Health Research senior investigator. Dr. Thomas R. Osborne is funded by King's College Hospital NHS Foundation Trust and Myeloma UK.

References

1. Zech D et al. Validation of World Health Organization guidelines for cancer pain relief: a 10-year prospective study. Pain. 1995;63:65–76.
2. Grond S et al. Validation of World Health Organization guidelines for cancer pain relief during the last days and hours of life. J Pain Symptom Manage. 1991;6:411–22.
3. Stjernsward J, Colleau S, Ventafridda V. The World Health Organization Cancer Pain and Palliative Care Program. Past, present, and future. J Pain Symptom Manage. 1996;12:65–72.
4. Allende S, Carvell HC. Mexico: status of cancer pain and palliative care. J Pain Symptom Manage. 1996;12(2):121–3.
5. Cherny N. Israel: status of cancer pain and palliative care. J Pain Symptom Manage. 1996;12(2):116–7.
6. Fernandez A, Acuna G. Chile: status of cancer pain and palliative care. J Pain Symptom Manage. 1996;12(2):102–3.
7. Goh CR. Singapore: status of cancer pain and palliative care. J Pain Symptom Manage. 1993;8(6):431–3.
8. Larue F et al. France: status of cancer pain and palliative care. J Pain Symptom Manage. 1996;12(2):106–8.
9. Lickiss JN. Australia: status of cancer pain and palliative care. J Pain Symptom Manage. 1996;12(2):99–101.
10. Merriman A. Uganda: status of cancer pain and palliative care. J Pain Symptom Manage. 1996;12(2):141–3.
11. Moyano J. Colombia: status of cancer pain and palliative care. J Pain Symptom Manage. 1996;12(2):104–5.
12. Soebadi R, Tejawinata S. Indonesia: status of cancer pain and palliative care. J Pain Symptom Manage. 1996;12(2):112–5.
13. Strumpf M, Zenz M, Donner B. Germany: status of cancer pain and palliative care. J Pain Symptom Manage. 1996;12(2):109–11.
14. Sun W, Hou W, Li J. Republic of China: status of cancer pain and palliative care. J Pain Symptom Manage. 1996;12(2):127–9.
15. Takeda F. Results of field-testing in Japan of the WHO draft interim guideline on relief of cancer pain. Pain Clinic. 1986;1:83–9.
16. Wenk R, Ochoa J. Argentina: status of cancer pain and palliative care. J Pain Symptom Manage. 1996;12(2):97–8.
17. Zylicz Z. The Netherlands: status of cancer pain and palliative care. J Pain Symptom Manage. 1996;12(2):136–8.
18. Erdine S. Turkey: status of cancer pain and palliative care. J Pain Symptom Manage. 1996;12(2):139–40.
19. Laudico A. The Philippines: status of cancer pain and palliative care. J Pain Symptom Manage. 1993;8(6):429–30.
20. Zhang H et al. People's Republic of China: status of cancer pain and palliative care. J Pain Symptom Manage. 1996;12(2):124–6.
21. Bonica JJ. Treatment of cancer pain: current status and future needs. In: Fields HL, editor. Advances in pain research and therapy. New York: Raven Press; 1985. p. 589–616.
22. Foley K. Pain syndromes in patients with cancer. In: Bonica J, Ventafridda V, editors. Advances in pain research and therapy. New York: Raven Press; 1979. p. 59–75.
23. Portenoy RK. Cancer pain. Epidemiology and syndromes. Cancer. 1989;63(11):2298–307.
24. Solano JP, Gomes B, Higginson IJ. A comparison of symptom prevalence in far advanced cancer, AIDS, heart disease, chronic obstructive pulmonary disease and renal disease. J Pain Symptom Manage. 2006;31(1):58–69.
25. Grond S et al. Prevalence and pattern of symptoms in patients with cancer pain: a prospective evaluation of

1635 cancer patients referred to a pain clinic. J Pain Symptom Manage. 1994;9(6):372–82.

26. Higginson IJ, Hearn J. A multicenter evaluation of cancer pain control by palliative care teams. J Pain Symptom Manage. 1997;14(1):29–35.

27. Banning A, Sjogren P, Henriksen H. Pain causes in 200 patients referred to a multidisciplinary cancer pain clinic. Pain. 1991;45(1):45–8.

28. Portenoy RK. Cancer pain: pathophysiology and syndromes. Lancet. 1992;339(8800):1026–31.

29. Welsh Health Planning Forum. Pain, discomfort and palliative care. Cardiff: Welsh Office of NHS Directorate; 1992.

30. Twycross R. Attention to detail. Prog Palliat Care. 1994;2:222–7.

31. Twycross R. Cancer pain classification. Acta Anaesthesiol Scand. 1997;41(1 Pt 2):141–5.

32. International Association for the Study of Pain. Subcommittee on taxonomy of pain terms: a list with definitions and notes on usage. Pain. 1979;6(3):249–52.

33. Foley KM. Pain assessment and cancer pain. In: Doyle D, Hanks G, MacDonald N, editors. Oxford textbook of palliative medicine. Oxford: Oxford University Press; 1993. p. 140–8.

34. Koffman J et al. Cultural meanings of pain: a qualitative study of Black Caribbean and White British patients with advanced cancer. Palliat Med. 2008;22(4):350–9.

35. Coyle N. The last four weeks of life. Am J Nurs. 1990;90(12):75–6.

36. Daut RL, Cleeland CS. The prevalence and severity of pain in cancer. Cancer. 1982;50(9):1913–8.

37. Serlin RC et al. When is cancer pain mild, moderate or severe? Grading pain severity by its interference with function. Pain. 1995;61(2):277–84.

38. Cherny NI, Portenoy RK. Cancer pain management. Current strategy. Cancer. 1993;72(11 Suppl):3393–415.

39. Baines M, Kirkham SR. Cancer pain. In: Wall PD, Melzack R, editors. Textbook of pain. Edinburgh: Churchill Livingstone; 1993.

40. Jensen MP, Karoly P, Braver S. The measurement of clinical pain intensity: a comparison of six methods. Pain. 1986;27(1):117–26.

41. Moinpour CM et al. Quality of life end points in cancer clinical trials: review and recommendations. J Natl Cancer Inst. 1989;81(7):485–95.

42. Cleeland CS et al. Dimensions of the impact of cancer pain in a four country sample: new information from multidimensional scaling. Pain. 1996;67(2–3):267–73.

43. European Palliative Care Research Collaboration. 2008. Available from: www.epcrc.org. Accessed on 25 Mar 2013.

44. Hearn J, Higginson IJ. Outcome measures in palliative care for advanced cancer patients: a review. J Public Health Med. 1997;19(2):193–9.

45. Cleeland C, Ryan K. Pain assessment: global use of the Brief Pain Inventory. Ann Acad Med Singapore. 1994;23(2):129–38.

46. Holen J et al. The Brief Pain Inventory: pain's interference with functions is different in cancer pain compared with noncancer chronic pain. Clin J Pain. 2008;24(3):219–25.

47. Bruera E et al. The Edmonton Symptom Assessment System (ESAS): a simple method for the assessment of palliative care patients. J Palliat Care. 1991;7(2):6–9.

48. Carvajal A et al. A comprehensive study of psychometric properties of the Edmonton Symptom Assessment System (ESAS) in Spanish advanced cancer patients. Eur J Cancer. 2011;47(12):1863–72.

49. Nekolaichuk C, Watanabe S, Beaumont C. The Edmonton Symptom Assessment System: a 15-year retrospective review of validation studies (1991–2006). Palliat Med. 2008;22(2):111–22.

50. Richardson LA, Jones GW. A review of the reliability and validity of the Edmonton Symptom Assessment System. Curr Oncol. 2009;16(1):55.

51. Hearn J, Higginson IJ. Development and validation of a core outcome measure for palliative care: the palliative care outcome scale. Palliative Care Core Audit Project Advisory Group. Qual Health Care. 1999;8(4):219–27.

52. Stevens AM et al. Experience in the use of the palliative care outcome scale. Support Care Cancer. 2005;13(12):1027–34.

53. Higginson IJ, McCarthy M. Validity of the support team assessment schedule: do staffs' ratings reflect those made by patients or their families? Palliat Med. 1993;7(3):219–28.

54. Portenoy RK et al. The Memorial Symptom Assessment Scale: an instrument for the evaluation of symptom prevalence, characteristics and distress. Eur J Cancer. 1994;30A(9):1326–36.

55. Aaronson NK et al. The European Organization for Research and Treatment of Cancer QLQ-C30: a quality-of-life instrument for use in international clinical trials in oncology. J Natl Cancer Inst. 1993;85(5):365–76.

56. Higginson IJ, Wei G. Caregiver assessment of patients with advanced cancer: concordance with patients, effect of burden and positivity. Health Qual Life Outcomes. 2008;6:42.

57. Ventafridda V, Caraceni A. Cancer pain classification: a controversial issue. Pain. 1991;46(1):1–2.

58. Bennett M. The LANSS Pain Scale: the Leeds assessment of neuropathic symptoms and signs. Pain. 2001;92(1–2):147–57.

59. Potter J et al. Identifying neuropathic pain in patients with head and neck cancer: use of the Leeds Assessment of Neuropathic Symptoms and Signs Scale. J R Soc Med. 2003;96(8):379–83.

60. Higginson I, Murtagh FE. Cancer pain epidemiology. In: Bruera E, Portenoy R, editors. Cancer pain assessment and management. Cambridge: Cambridge University Press; 2009. p. 37–52.

61. Bonica JJ. Cancer pain. In: Bonica JJ, editor. The management of cancer pain. Philadelphia: Lea and Febiger; 1990. p. 400–60.

62. Ward AW. Terminal care in malignant disease. Soc Sci Med. 1974;8(7):413–20.

63. Parkes CM. Home or hospital? Terminal care as seen by surviving spouses. J R Coll Gen Pract. 1978;28(186):19–30.

64. Trotter JM et al. Problems of the oncology outpatient: role of the liaison health visitor. Br Med J (Clin Res Ed). 1981;282(6258):122–4.

65. Morris JN et al. The effect of treatment setting and patient characteristics on pain in terminal cancer patients: a report from the National Hospice Study. J Chronic Dis. 1986;39(1):27–35.

66. Greenwald HP, Bonica JJ, Bergner M. The prevalence of pain in four cancers. Cancer. 1987;60(10):2563–9.

67. Dorrepaal KL, Aaronson NK, van Dam FS. Pain experience and pain management among hospitalized cancer patients. A clinical study. Cancer. 1989;63(3):593–8.

68. McIllmurray MB, Warren MR. Evaluation of a new hospice: the relief of symptoms in cancer patients in the first year. Palliat Med. 1989;3:135–40.

69. Ventafridda V et al. Comparison of home and hospital care of advanced cancer patients. Tumori. 1989;75(6):619–25.

70. Higginson I, Wade A, McCarthy M. Palliative care: views of patients and their families. BMJ. 1990;301(6746):277–81.

71. Ventafridda V et al. Symptom prevalence and control during cancer patients' last days of life. J Palliat Care. 1990;6(3):7–11.

72. Cartwright A. Changes in life and care in the year before death 1969–1987. J Public Health Med. 1991;13(2):81–7.

73. Chan A, Woodruff RK. Palliative care in a general teaching hospital. 1. Assessment of needs. Med J Aust. 1991;155(9):597–9.

74. Fainsinger R et al. Symptom control during the last week of life on a palliative care unit. J Palliat Care. 1991;7(1):5–11.

75. Hiraga K, Mizuguchi T, Takeda F. The incidence of cancer pain and improvement of pain management in Japan. Postgrad Med J. 1991;67 Suppl 2:S14–25.

76. Simpson KS. The use of research to facilitate the creation of a hospital palliative care team. Palliat Med. 1991;5:122–9.

77. Stein WM, Miech RP. Cancer pain in the elderly hospice patient. J Pain Symptom Manage. 1993;8(7):474–82.

78. Vuorinen E. Pain as an early symptom in cancer. Clin J Pain. 1993;9(4):272–8.

79. Mercadante S, Armata M, Salvaggio L. Pain characteristics of advanced lung cancer patients referred to a palliative care service. Pain. 1994;59(1):141–5.

80. Portenoy RK et al. Pain in ovarian cancer patients. Prevalence, characteristics, and associated symptoms. Cancer. 1994;74(3):907–15.

81. Portenoy RK et al. Symptom prevalence, characteristics and distress in a cancer population. Qual Life Res. 1994;3(3):183–9.

82. Addington-Hall J, McCarthy M. Dying from cancer: results of a national population-based investigation. Palliat Med. 1995;9(4):295–305.

83. Donnelly S, Walsh D, Rybicki L. The symptoms of advanced cancer: identification of clinical and research priorities by assessment of prevalence and severity. J Palliat Care. 1995;11(1):27–32.

84. Ellershaw JE, Peat SJ, Boys LC. Assessing the effectiveness of a hospital palliative care team. Palliat Med. 1995;9(2):145–52.

85. Glover J et al. Mood states of oncology outpatients: does pain make a difference? J Pain Symptom Manage. 1995;10(2):120–8.

86. Larue F et al. Multicentre study of cancer pain and its treatment in France. BMJ. 1995;310(6986):1034–7.

87. Miaskowski C, Dibble SL. The problem of pain in outpatients with breast cancer. Oncol Nurs Forum. 1995;22(5):791–7.

88. Shannon MM et al. Assessment of pain in advanced cancer patients. J Pain Symptom Manage. 1995;10(4):274–8.

89. Vainio A, Auvinen A. Prevalence of symptoms among patients with advanced cancer: an international collaborative study. Symptom Prevalence Group. J Pain Symptom Manage. 1996;12(1):3–10.

90. Elliott TE et al. Improving cancer pain management in communities: main results from a randomized controlled trial. J Pain Symptom Manage. 1997;13(4):191–203.

91. Bernabei R et al. Management of pain in elderly patients with cancer. SAGE Study Group. Systematic Assessment of Geriatric Drug Use via Epidemiology. JAMA. 1998;279(23):1877–82.

92. Ger LP et al. The prevalence and severity of cancer pain: a study of newly-diagnosed cancer patients in Taiwan. J Pain Symptom Manage. 1998;15(5):285–93.

93. Rummans TA et al. Quality of life and pain in patients with recurrent breast and gynecologic cancer. Psychosomatics. 1998;39(5):437–45.

94. Wells N, Johnson RL, Wujcik D. Development of a short version of the Barriers Questionnaire. J Pain Symptom Manage. 1998;15(5):294–8.

95. Berry DL et al. Cancer pain and common pain: a comparison of patient-reported intensities. Oncol Nurs Forum. 1999;26(4):721–6.

96. Bucher JA, Trostle GB, Moore M. Family reports of cancer pain, pain relief, and prescription access. Cancer Pract. 1999;7(2):71–7.

97. Chaplin JM, Morton RP. A prospective, longitudinal study of pain in head and neck cancer patients. Head Neck. 1999;21(6):531–7.

98. Chung JW, Yang JC, Wong TK. The significance of pain among Chinese patients with cancer in Hong Kong. Acta Anaesthesiol Sin. 1999;37(1):9–14.

99. Mercadante S. Pain treatment and outcomes for patients with advanced cancer who receive follow-up care at home. Cancer. 1999;85(8):1849–58.

100. Nowels D, Lee JT. Cancer pain management in home hospice settings: a comparison of primary care and oncologic physicians. J Palliat Care. 1999;15(3):5–9.

101. Chang VT et al. Symptom and quality of life survey of medical oncology patients at a veterans affairs medical center: a role for symptom assessment. Cancer. 2000;88(5):1175–83.

102. Chiu TY, Hu WY, Chen CY. Prevalence and severity of symptoms in terminal cancer patients: a study in Taiwan. Support Care Cancer. 2000;8(4):311–3.

103. Ripamonti C et al. Pain experienced by patients hospitalized at the National Cancer Institute of Milan: research project "towards a pain-free hospital". Tumori. 2000;86(5):412–8.

104. Beck SL, Falkson G. Prevalence and management of cancer pain in South Africa. Pain. 2001;94(1):75–84.

105. Liu Z et al. National survey on prevalence of cancer pain. Chin Med Sci J. 2001;16(3):175–8.

106. Lidstone V et al. Symptoms and concerns amongst cancer outpatients: identifying the need for specialist palliative care. Palliat Med. 2003;17(7):588–95.

107. Potter J et al. Symptoms in 400 patients referred to palliative care services: prevalence and patterns. Palliat Med. 2003;17(4):310–4.

108. Rustoen T et al. The impact of demographic and disease-specific variables on pain in cancer patients. J Pain Symptom Manage. 2003;26(2):696–704.

109. Tranmer JE et al. Measuring the symptom experience of seriously ill cancer and noncancer hospitalized patients near the end of life with the memorial symptom assessment scale. J Pain Symptom Manage. 2003;25(5):420–9.

110. Yun YH et al. Multicenter study of pain and its management in patients with advanced cancer in Korea. J Pain Symptom Manage. 2003;25(5):430–7.

111. Hsieh RK. Pain control in Taiwanese patients with cancer: a multicenter, patient-oriented survey. J Formos Med Assoc. 2005;104(12):913–9.

112. Chen ML, Tseng HC. Symptom clusters in cancer patients. Support Care Cancer. 2006;14(8):825–30.

113. Monestel Umaña R, Solano JR, Herrera IS. Prevalencia y factores predictivos del dolor en pacientes con cáncer metastásico en Costa Rica [Prevalence and predictive factors of pain in patients with metastatic cancer in Costa Rica]. Medicina Palliativa. 2006;13(2):80–4.

114. Peng WL et al. Multidisciplinary management of cancer pain: a longitudinal retrospective study on a cohort of end-stage cancer patients. J Pain Symptom Manage. 2006;32(5):444–52.

115. Reyes-Gibby CC et al. Status of cancer pain in Hanoi, Vietnam: a hospital-wide survey in a tertiary cancer treatment center. J Pain Symptom Manage. 2006;31(5):431–9.

116. Tsai JS et al. Symptom patterns of advanced cancer patients in a palliative care unit. Palliat Med. 2006;20(6):617–22.

117. Walsh D, Rybicki L. Symptom clustering in advanced cancer. Support Care Cancer. 2006;14(8):831–6.

118. Chow E et al. Symptom clusters in cancer patients with bone metastases. Support Care Cancer. 2007;15(9):1035–43.

119. van den Beuken-van Everdingen MHJ et al. High prevalence of pain in patients with cancer in a large population-based study in The Netherlands. Pain. 2007;132(3):312–20.

120. Chow E et al. Symptom clusters in cancer patients with brain metastases. Clin Oncol. 2008;20(1):76–82.

121. Collins S et al. Presence, communication and treatment of fatigue and pain complaints in incurable cancer patients. Patient Educ Couns. 2008;72(1):102–8.

122. Gerbershagen HJ et al. Prevalence, severity, and chronicity of pain and general health-related quality of life in patients with localized prostate cancer. Eur J Pain. 2008;12(3):339–50.

123. Lövgren M et al. Symptoms and problems with functioning among women and men with inoperable lung cancer – a longitudinal study. Lung Cancer. 2008;60(1):113–24.

124. Mercadante S et al. Prevalence and treatment of cancer pain in Italian oncological wards centres: a cross-sectional survey. Support Care Cancer. 2008;16(11):1203–11.

125. Valeberg BT et al. Self-reported prevalence, etiology, and characteristics of pain in oncology outpatients. Eur J Pain. 2008;12(5):582–90.

126. Wang SP, Ma L, Chung J. Survey on the influence of pain on quality of life in breast cancer patients. Chinese J Evid Based Med. 2008;8(4):233–6.

127. Breivik H et al. Cancer-related pain: a pan-European survey of prevalence, treatment, and patient attitudes. Ann Oncol. 2009;20(8):1420–33.

128. Costantini M et al. Prevalence, distress, management, and relief of pain during the last 3 months of cancer patients' life. Results of an Italian mortality follow-back survey. Ann Oncol. 2009;20(4):729–35.

129. Duncan JG et al. Symptom occurrence and associated clinical factors in nursing home residents with cancer. Res Nurs Health. 2009;32(4):453–64.

130. Wilson KG et al. Prevalence and correlates of pain in the Canadian National Palliative Care Survey. Pain Res Manag. 2009;14(5):365–70.

131. Yamagishi A et al. Symptom prevalence and longitudinal follow-up in cancer outpatients receiving chemotherapy. J Pain Symptom Manage. 2009;37(5):823–30.

132. Carr BI, Pujol L. Pain at presentation and survival in hepatocellular carcinoma. J Pain. 2010;11(10):988–93.

133. Mercadante S et al. Breakthrough pain in oncology: a longitudinal study. J Pain Symptom Manage. 2010;40(2):183–90.

134. Molassiotis A et al. Symptoms experienced by cancer patients during the first year from diagnosis: patient and informal caregiver ratings and agreement. Palliat Support Care. 2010;8(3):313–24.

135. Reyes-Gibby C et al. Neuropathic pain in breast cancer survivors: using the ID pain as a screening tool. J Pain Symptom Manage. 2010;39(5):882–9.

136. Williams JE et al. Prevalence of pain in head and neck cancer out-patients. J Laryngol Otol. 2010;124(7):767–73.

137. Dhingra L et al. Pain in underserved community-dwelling Chinese American cancer patients: demographic and medical correlates. Oncologist. 2011;16(4):523–33.

138. Harding R et al. The prevalence and burden of symptoms amongst cancer patients attending palliative care in two African countries. Eur J Cancer. 2011;47(1):51–6.

139. Kirkova J et al. The relationship between symptom prevalence and severity and cancer primary site in

796 patients with advanced cancer. Am J Hosp Palliat Med. 2011;28(5):350–5.

140. Lamino Dde A, Mota DD, Pimenta CA. Prevalence and comorbidity of pain and fatigue in women with breast cancer. Rev Esc Enferm USP. 2011;45(2):496–502.

141. Manitta V et al. The symptom burden of patients with hematological malignancy: a cross-sectional observational study. J Pain Symptom Manage. 2011;42(3):432–42.

142. Spichiger E et al. Symptom prevalence and changes of symptoms over ten days in hospitalized patients with advanced cancer: a descriptive study. Eur J Oncol Nurs. 2011;15(2):95–102.

143. Kuo PY et al. The prevalence of pain in patients attending sarcoma outpatient clinics. Sarcoma. 2011;1–6.

144. Stjernsward J, Koroltchouk V, Teoh N. National policies for cancer pain relief and palliative care. Palliat Med. 1992;6:273–6.

145. Cassell EJ. The relief of suffering. Arch Intern Med. 1983;143(3):522–3.

146. Foley KM, Portenoy RK. World Health Organization-International Association for the Study of Pain: joint initiatives in cancer pain relief. J Pain Symptom Manage. 1993;8(6):335–9.

147. Jacox A, Carr DB, Payne R. New clinical-practice guidelines for the management of pain in patients with cancer. N Engl J Med. 1994;330(9):651–5.

148. Kaasa S et al. Psychological distress in cancer patients with advanced disease. Radiother Oncol. 1993;27(3):193–7.

149. Max M. American Pain Society quality assurance standards for relief of acute pain and cancer pain. In: Bond MR, Charlton JE, Woolf CJ, editors. Proceedings of the VI world congress on pain. Amsterdam: Elsevier; 1990.

150. Portenoy RK. Report from the International Association for the Study of Pain Task Force on cancer pain. J Pain Symptom Manage. 1996;12(2): 93–6.

151. Bruera E et al. The Edmonton staging system for cancer pain: preliminary report. Pain. 1989;37(2): 203–9.

152. Bruera E et al. A prospective multicenter assessment of the Edmonton staging system for cancer pain. J Pain Symptom Manage. 1995;10(5):348–55.

153. Portenoy RK, Foley KM, Inturrisi CE. The nature of opioid responsiveness and its implications for neuropathic pain: new hypotheses derived from studies of opioid infusions. Pain. 1990;43(3):273–86.

Recent Advances in Cancer Treatment

M.J. Lind

Abstract

Despite the rising incidence of many common cancers, 5-year survival rates for many of them are improving. Screening, earlier detection, and better systemic anticancer treatments are the main factors in achieving such a dramatic improvement. Understanding the mechanisms of cytotoxic chemotherapy has allowed a more scientific rationale for use as well as accentuating the practical use for a combination therapy. New targets for cancer therapy are being identified that include tyrosine kinase inhibitors, monoclonal, antibodies, and targeting angiogenesis are but few that can potentially improve outcome for cancer patients in the future. Though cancer incidence is likely to increase in the future, as the population ages, improved basic molecular research in cellular mechanism of cancer cells will lead to further improvement in survival rates.

Keywords

Cancer • Survival rates • Cytotoxic therapy • Kinase inhibitors • Monoclonal antibody • Targeting angiogenesis

Introduction

In 2008 there were 12.7 million new cases and 7.6 million deaths worldwide due to cancer [1]. It is estimated that between 2003 and 2020 cancer incidence rates will rise by 50 % [1]. Despite the rising incidence of many common cancers, 5 year survival rates for many of them are improving [2]. In

some malignancies, such as breast cancer, this has led to dramatic declines in mortality [3] (Fig. 3.1). Even in the advanced stages of the disease, patients are now living much longer [4] (Fig. 3.2). Therefore, advanced cancer should now be considered a chronic disease, with all the attendant problems for patients and challenges for their doctors.

These advances in survival are probably a reflection of several different processes, e.g., screening, earlier detection, improved mortality following radical surgery, and better systemic anticancer treatments. Cancer is by and large a systemic disease. Even patients with apparently localised disease often have micrometastatic disease [5]. The past 50

M.J. Lind, BSc, MD, FRCP
Academic Department of Oncology,
Hull York Medical School, University of Hull,
Cottingham Rd, Hull, Yorkshire HU6 7RX, UK
e-mail: m.j.lind@hull.ac.uk

M. Hanna, Z. Zylicz (eds.), *Cancer Pain*,
DOI 10.1007/978-0-85729-230-8_3, © Springer-Verlag London 2013

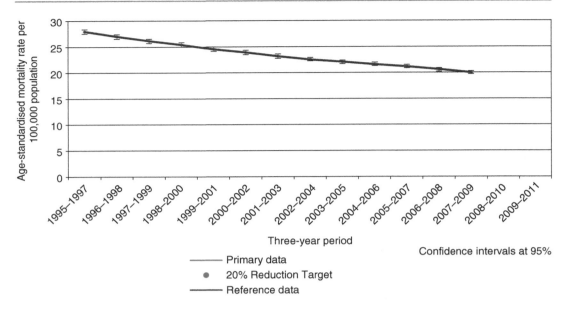

Fig. 3.1 Decline in breast mortality (NCIN)

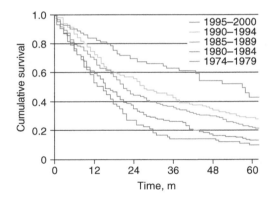

Fig. 3.2 Survival from metastatic breast cancer Giordano et al. [4]

years has seen a huge growth in systemic anticancer therapy, from crude derivatives of chemical warfare (see below) to molecularly targeted anticancer agents which disrupt processes essential to cancer cell survival such as tumour growth, cell cycle progression, apoptosis, and metastases.

Cytotoxic Chemotherapy

Extrapolating from his observation that chemical dyes could interact differentially with tissues and cellular structures, Paul Ehrlich postulated that small molecules could be used to exert a therapeutic effect on microorganisms and cancers [6]; Ehrlich used the word chemotherapy to describe this approach. The release of mustard gas from the bombing of the SS John Harvey in December 1943 while moored in Bari Harbor in Italy resulted in a number of causalities. An American expert in chemical warfare managed to show that the deaths were largely due to mustard gas exposure, which resulted in lymphoid and bone marrow atrophy. Two American pharmacologists at the University of Yale, Goodman and Gilman, injected mustine, a mustard gas derivative, into a patient with non-Hodgkin's lymphoma with good results [5]. In 1948, the observation by Sidney Farber that folic acid when administered to children with acute lymphoblastic leukemia caused proliferation of leukemic cells led to the development of the antifolates aminopterin and methotrexate as therapeutic agents in this disease [7]. The discovery of the structure of DNA by Watson and Crick in 1953 led to further understanding of how these agents work [8]. The serendipitous discovery of cisplatin in 1965 by Barnett Rosenberg et al. [9] led to dramatic new therapies for the treatment of previously fatal tumours such as testicular cancers. The use of combination chemotherapy to cure patients with Hodgkin's disease by DeVita

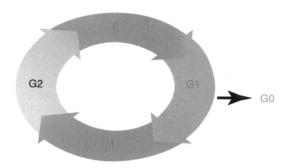

Fig. 3.3 Cell cycle. *M* mitosis, *G1* gap 1, *G2* gap 2, *G0* gap 0, *S* synthesis

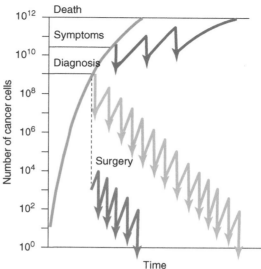

Fig. 3.4 Skipper-Schwabel Proportional cell kill model. The *red line* represents a tumour that is primarily resistant to chemotherapy; the *light blue line* is a curable chemosensitive tumour, the *dark blue* a tumour that is initially sensitive to treatment but then develops secondary resistance, and the *green* the role of adjuvant chemotherapy

ushered in the modern era of cytotoxic chemotherapy [10].

Cytotoxic chemotherapy generally works by interfering with DNA function either by direct binding of small-molecule drugs directly to DNA (alkylating agents, platinum agents, and antitumour antibiotics) or by interference of DNA synthesis (antimetabolites). The resulting DNA damage results in programmed cell death (apoptosis). This mode of action means that such agents only work when cells are in cell cycle (see Fig. 3.3). This results in two problems with cytotoxic chemotherapy. Firstly, not all cancer cells within a tumour are dividing. Indeed many are in a semipermanent resting phase (G0) making them resistant to chemotherapy. Secondly, chemotherapy will damage non-tumour tissues with rapidly dividing cells such as the bone marrow, hair follicles, gut, and mucous membranes resulting in toxicity to these end organs.

A single dose of cytotoxic chemotherapy will kill a certain proportion of cancer cells. This is called the proportional cell kill model [11] (Fig. 3.4). The exact percentage will depend on the sensitivity and dose of chemotherapy used.

Cytotoxic chemotherapy may then be used for four main clinical indications. Firstly in some rare sensitive tumours such as leukemias, lymphomas, and testicular cancers, chemotherapy may be curative. More commonly chemotherapy is used to shrink tumours which will then regrow and become resistant. In these cases, the role of chemotherapy is palliative. Thirdly chemotherapy may be used after surgery to eradicate micrometastatic disease. This is known as adjuvant

chemotherapy and can lead to modest improvements in survival, e.g., breast cancer. Finally chemotherapy may be used to downstage tumours prior to surgery, e.g., rectal cancer.

Mechanisms of Action of Cytotoxic Chemotherapy (Fig. 3.5)

1. Alkylating agents (cyclophosphamide, ifosfamide, melphalan, chlorambucil, etc.) These agents work by forming interstrand cross-linking of opposing DNA strands thus interfering with DNA synthesis and transcription.
2. Heavy metals (cisplatin, carboplatin, and oxaliplatin) are activated intracellularly to form reactive intermediates which form covalent bonds with nucleotides to in turn form inter- and intrastand cross-links.
3. Antimetabolites are small molecules that structurally resemble pyrimidines and purines. They work by inhibiting key enzymes in DNA synthesis and by misincorporation into DNA and RNA strands causing premature strand termination and breakages:

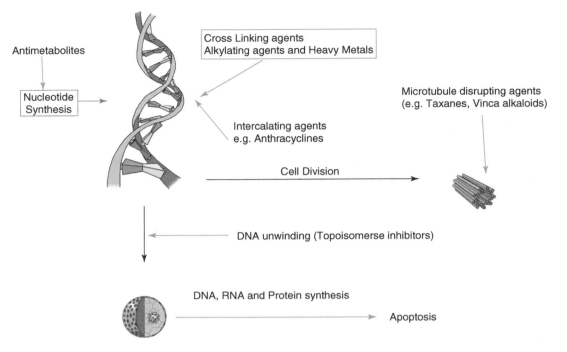

Fig. 3.5 Mechanisms of action of cytotoxic chemotherapy

(a) Antifolates (methotrexate) inhibit the enzyme dihydrofolate reductase (DHFR) which is responsible for the regeneration of oxidised folates following thymidine synthesis following DNA synthesis.

(b) Thymidylate synthase inhibitors (5-fluorouracil, capecitabine, pemetrexed). These small molecules work by inhibiting the enzyme thymidylate synthase, thus preventing the conversion of deoxyuridine monophosphate to deoxythymidine mono, thereby inhibiting DNA synthesis.

(c) Arabinosides (cytosine arabinoside and gemcitabine) are activated intracellularly and inhibit the enzyme DNA polymerase.

(d) Antipurines. Two antipurines are used in clinical practice – 6-mercaptopurine and 6-thioguanine. Both drugs readily enter the cell and are metabolised intracellularly to active forms that inhibit de novo purine synthesis and are misincorporated into DNA.

4. The antitumour antibiotics (doxorubicin, daunorubicin, epirubicin) have multiple modes of action including DNA minor groove binding, generation of cytotoxic free radicals, and inhibition of topoisomerase inhibition.

5. Topoisomerase inhibitors (etoposide, irinotecan, and topotecan). The topoisomerases are a group of enzymes that control the three-dimensional structure of DNA. They allow strand passage of DNA during replication and transcription, by cleavage followed by religation.

6. Tubulin-binding drugs (vinca alkaloids, taxanes, epothilones, and halichondrins).

Tubulin is the basic subunit of microtubules, which have many important, diverse roles in cell function including maintenance of cell shape, mitosis, meiosis, secretion, intracellular transport, and axonal function.

Targeted Agents

The growth of our understanding of the biology of cancer, through modern-day molecular biology techniques such as genomics and proteomics has led to the identification of numerous novel targets for anticancer therapy. The potential

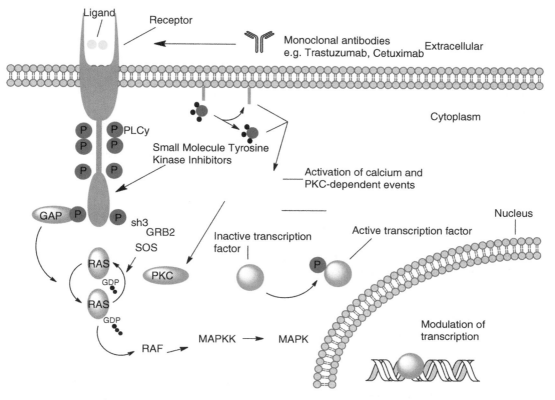

Fig. 3.6   Tyrosine kinase inhibition in cancer

advantages of such an approach may be less toxicity to normal tissues and the ability to personalise anticancer treatment to patients who harbour these molecular abnormalities. These agents have tended to be either small molecules or monoclonal antibodies.

Small-Molecule Tyrosine Kinase Inhibitors

The tyrosine kinase inhibitors are a diverse group of intracellular enzymes that phosphorylate tyrosine residues within a protein. This action generally leads to a conformational change within the target protein resulting in cell-signalling cascades becoming activated (Fig. 3.6). There are two types of tyrosine kinase, receptor and cytoplasmic.

Tyrosine kinase inhibitors have transformed the treatment of many malignancies which were hitherto largely untreated, e.g., chronic myeloid leukaemia (CML), gastrointestinal stromal tumours (GIST), renal cancer, and non-small lung cancer (NSCLC). NSCLC and the use of the two receptor tyrosine kinase inhibitors, Gefitinib and Erlotinib, is particularly interesting. It would appear that some patients with NSCLC harbour an activating mutation in the epidermal growth factor receptor making them extremely sensitive to these two drugs. These patients would appear to respond better to these agents than conventional cytotoxic chemotherapy where those patients who do not have the mutation do better on conventional cytotoxic chemotherapy [12]. Another stunning example of this technology is in the treatment of malignant melanoma. In 50 % of patients with metastatic melanoma, there is a mutation in the BRAF kinase leading to constitutive activation of this pathway. The BRAF kinase inhibitor Vemurafenib has shown considerable activity in those patients with metastatic melanoma harbouring BRAF mutations [13].

Table 3.1 Common tyrosine kinase inhibitors used in the clinic

Agent	Targets	Indication
Imatinib	BcR-Abl, PGDFR, c-Kit	1. Philadelphia-positive CML
		2. CD117-positive GIST
Dasatinib	BcR-Abl, Src family, PDGFRβ	CML resistant to imatinib
Nilotinib	Bcr-abl, c-Kit, PDGFR	CML resistant to imatinib
Gefitinib	EGFR	1. Second-line NSCLC
		2. First-line NSCL with activating EGFR mutation
Erlotinib	EGFR	Second-line NSCLC
Lapatinib	EGFR, HER2	Second line in combination with capecitabine in HER2-positive breast cancer who have received trastuzumab plus a taxane
Sunitinib	VEGFR-1,2,3, c-Kit, PDGR,	1. GIST after failure of imatinib
		2. Advanced renal cancer
Sorafenib	VEGFR-2,3, c-Kit, PDGFR, Raf	Advanced renal cancer
Vemurafenib	BRAF	Metastatic melanoma harbouring the V600E mutation

PGDFR platelet-derived growth factor, *EGFR* epidermal growth factor receptor, *VEGFR* vascular endothelial growth factor, *NSCLC* non-small cell lung cancer, *GIST* gastrointestinal stromal tumour

A list of the commonly used tyrosine kinase inhibitors and their targets is shown in Table 3.1.

Monoclonal Antibody Targeting of Signal Transduction

An alternative approach to targeting growth factor receptors with small molecule tyrosine kinase inhibitors is the use of monoclonal antibodies. A number of such molecules have been used in the clinic. Most notable of these is the anti-HER2 agent trastuzumab (herceptin). HER2 is the second member of the EGFR family. In approximately 20 % of breast cancers, HER2 is overexpressed on the cell surface. This leads to constitutive activation of this pathway. Patients with HER2-positive breast cancer have a more aggressive disease than negative patients and typically have shortened survival, early metastases (particular to the brain), and resistance to endocrine therapy. The use of the anti-HER2 antibody herceptin has largely transformed the outlook for these patients who have traditionally done very badly [14]. Cetuximab is a monoclonal antibody that is directed against the epidermal growth factor that has proved useful in non-small cell lung cancer and head and neck cancer.

Targeting Angiogenesis

A hallmark of malignant behaviour of cancer cells is metastases. For metastasis to occur tumour cells need to invade surrounding blood vessels, be transported by the circulation to the metastasis site, and then establish a new blood supply at that site. Tumours are able to promote such neovascularisation by the secretion of growth factors that stimulate vessel formation. Normally the development of new blood vessels is kept in balance by secretion of pro- and anti-angiogenic growth factors. However, in malignancy tumour, cells are able to cause an "angiogenic switch" by which pro-angiogenic factors predominate leading to vascularisation of the tumour [15] (Fig. 3.7).

Tumours with a high angiogenic drive are known to have a poor prognosis and metastasise early. A number of inhibitors of angiogenesis have now been used in clinical practice. Many of these act on vascular endothelial growth factor or its receptors (VEGF-A, B, C, and D or VEGFR-1, 2, and 3) (Fig. 3.8).

The VEGF system may be targeted by either monoclonal antibodies or small-molecule receptor tyrosine kinase inhibitors. Bevacizumab is a monoclonal that has a great affinity for VEGF-A. It has been used in combination with chemotherapy and has shown a survival advantage over control in lung and colorectal cancers [16, 17].

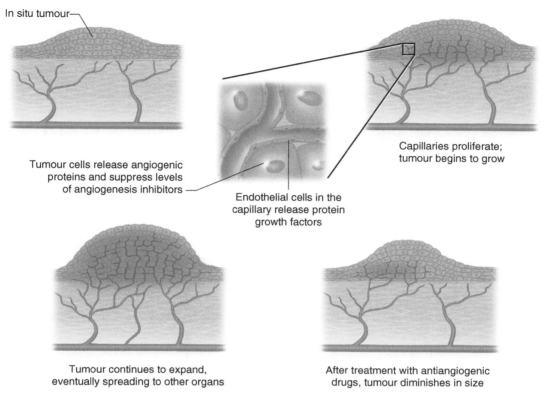

In situ tumour

Tumour cells release angiogenic proteins and suppress levels of angiogenesis inhibitors

Endothelial cells in the capillary release protein growth factors

Capillaries proliferate; tumour begins to grow

Tumour continues to expand, eventually spreading to other organs

After treatment with antiangiogenic drugs, tumour diminishes in size

Fig. 3.7 Tumour angiogenesis

A number of small molecule receptor tyrosine kinase inhibitors such as Sorafenib and Sunitinib are thought to work by a predominantly anti-angiogenic mechanism.

Proteasome Inhibitors

The ubiquitin-proteasome pathways are responsible for the degradation of numerous diverse proteins. As such it is responsible for the control of numerous cellular pathways. The ubiquitin-proteasome cascade works as follows (Fig. 3.9):

1. ATP activation of ubiquitin by ubiquitin-activating ligase enzyme (E1)
2. Transfer of the activated ubiquitin to a cysteine residue of the E2 ubiquitin-conjugating enzyme
3. Transfer of ubiquitin to the target protein

Once the target protein is monoubiquinated, it becomes polyubiquinated. Following this the polyubiquinated is bound to the 26S proteasome and degraded. Key apoptotic proteins are regulated by this system making it an attractive target for anticancer therapy.

The proteasome inhibitor bortezomib has been shown to be incredibly active in multiple myeloma [18].

Modulation of Epigenetic Pathways

Not all aberrations of the cancer cell phenotype are due to changes in DNA; such changes are known as epigenetic changes. Two epigenetic pathways have become targets for anticancer therapy: DNA methylation and histone deacetylase (HDAC). The enzyme DNA methyltransferase methylates the promoter regions of many genes, including many tumour-suppressor genes, leading to gene silencing and loss of function. The DNA methyltransferase inhibitor deoxy-aza-cytidine has been shown to be of great value in treating myelodysplastic patients [18].

Fig. 3.8 The VEGF system

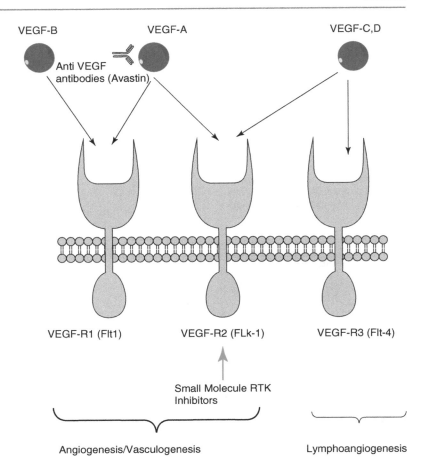

Histones are proteins that surround and interact with DNA. Histones can be acetylated and this leads to activation of gene transcription. They can also be deacetylated by histone deacetylase (HDAC) which leads to silencing of genes. HDAC inhibitors have been used to inhibit this process and thereby reactivate the expression of tumour-suppressor genes. These drugs are in the early stage of development but the oral HDAC inhibitor, vorinostat, has shown great promise in the treatment of mesothelioma and thyroid cancer [19].

Endocrine Treatment of Cancer

Breast Cancer

As far back as 1829, Sir Astley Cooper postulated a relationship between ovarian function and the growth of breast cancer [20]. It was not until 1896 that Beatson demonstrated that surgical oophorectomy resulted in breast cancer regression [21]. In 1944 the Christie Hospital in Manchester performed the world's first phase I trial of stilbestrol in advanced breast cancer-demonstrating activity [22]. In 1971 the Christie Hospital published data on a new ICI synthetic antioestrogen, ICI46474, later known as tamoxifen [23]. Since that time many different antioestrogens have been developed for the treatment and prevention of breast cancer. These act in a variety of different ways (Fig. 3.9).

The modes of action of endocrine manipulation for breast cancer are as follows (Fig. 3.10):
1. Selective oestrogen receptor modulators (SERMS). This group includes tamoxifen. Tamoxifen binds to the intracellular oestrogen receptor in breast cancer cells preventing its transcriptional activities. Tamoxifen has had a huge impact on the treatment of breast

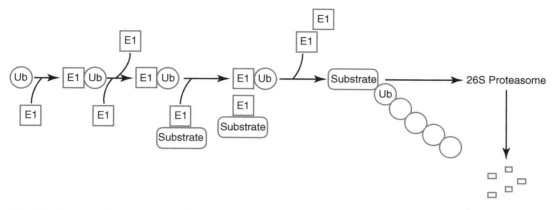

Fig. 3.9 The ubiquitin-proteasome pathway

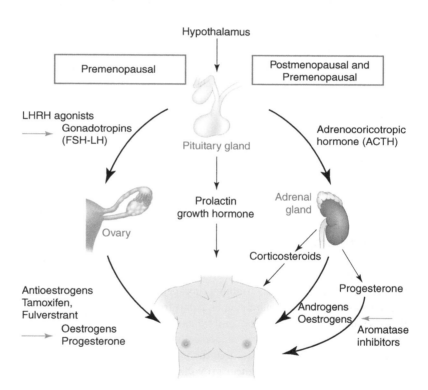

Fig. 3.10 Endocrine treatment of breast cancer

cancer. The use of adjuvant tamoxifen has transformed the prognosis of oestrogen receptor-positive early breast cancer [24]. More recently the use of tamoxifen has been shown to prevent breast cancer developing in women who are at high risk of developing breast cancer [25].

2. Selective oestrogen receptor downregulators. Unlike tamoxifen these agents are pure oestrogen receptor antagonists. The SERD, fulvestrant, is used as a third-line endocrine agent in the treatment of metastatic breast cancer.

3. LHRH agonists (e.g., goserelin) work by downregulating the hypothalamic-pituitary axis. As such they are useful in the treatment of premenopausal women with early or advanced breast cancer.

4. Aromatase inhibitors. In postmenopausal women, the major source of circulating oestrogen comes from the peripheral conversion of androstenedione (derived from the adrenal gland) to estrone which is subsequently converted to estradiol. Three aromatase inhibitors are available: anastrozole, letrozole, and exemestane. In certain circumstance, aromatase inhibitors are superior to tamoxifen [26].

Prostate Cancer

In certain countries prostate cancer is becoming the most common cancer in men. Prostate cancer, even in advanced stages, can be extremely hormone sensitive. The initial treatment of locally advanced prostate cancer is with the LHRH agonists goserelin and leuprolide. A number of antiandrogens (flutamide, bicalutamide, and nilutamide) can also be used for metastatic prostate cancer. More recently, abiraterone, an inhibitor of androgen biosynthesis, has been shown to improve survival in patients whose prostate cancer has become refractory to hormone manipulation [27].

Immunotherapy

It is beyond the scope of this chapter to completely review all the immunotherapeutic approaches to the treatment of cancer. Apart from the obvious use of monoclonal antibodies to target key signalling proteins on cancer cells, it is clear from many clinical studies that the immune system can and does affect cancer growth. Much of the early work on immunotherapy used nonspecific stimulators or modulators of the immune system such as the interferons and interleukins; they have met with little success and considerable toxicity.

Ipilimumab is a monoclonal antibody that blocks cytotoxic T cell lymphocyte A4 (CTLA-4) to promote antitumour immunity. This agent has been shown to improve survival in metastatic melanoma when compared with standard therapy [28].

Conclusions

Cancer remains a major source of morbidity and mortality. This burden is likely to increase over the coming years as populations get older. However, modern treatments have improved the chances of patients surviving their disease. Even in those patients with incurable disease, life expectancy has improved considerably making cancer a chronic disease in many patients. These factors mean that more not less palliative care for cancer patients will be needed in future.

References

1. Globocan, 2008.
2. Verdecchia A et al. Recent cancer survival in Europe: a 2000–02 period analysis of EUROCARE-4 data. Lancet Oncol. 2007;8(9):784–96.
3. Blanks RG et al. Effect of NHS breast screening programme on mortality from breast cancer in England and Wales, 1990–8: comparison of observed with predicted mortality. BMJ. 2000;321(7262):665–9.
4. Giordano SH et al. Is breast cancer survival improving? Cancer. 2004;100(1):44–52.
5. Goodman LS, Wintrobe MM, et al. Nitrogen mustard therapy; use of methyl-bis (beta-chloroethyl) amine hydrochloride and tris (beta-chloroethyl) amine hydrochloride for Hodgkin's disease, lymphosarcoma, leukemia and certain allied and miscellaneous disorders. J Am Med Assoc. 1946;132:126–32.
6. Ehrlich P. Aus Theorie und Praxis der Chemotherapie. Folia Serologica. 1911;7:697–714.
7. Farber S, Diamond LK. Temporary remissions in acute leukemia in children produced by folic acid antagonist, 4-aminopteroyl-glutamic acid. N Engl J Med. 1948;238(23):787–93.
8. Watson JD, Crick FH. Molecular structure of nucleic acids; a structure for deoxyribose nucleic acid. Nature. 1953;171(4356):737–8.
9. Rosenberg B, Vancamp L, Krigas T. Inhibition of cell division in *Escherichia coli* by electrolysis products from a platinum electrode. Nature. 1965;205: 698–9.
10. DeVita VT. Hodgkin's disease. Lancet. 1971;2(7714): 46–7.
11. Skipper HE. The effects of chemotherapy on the kinetics of leukemic cell behavior. Cancer Res. 1965;25(9):1544–50.
12. Mok TS et al. Gefitinib or carboplatin-paclitaxel in pulmonary adenocarcinoma. N Engl J Med. 2009; 361(10):947–57.
13. Chapman PB et al. Improved survival with vemurafenib in melanoma with BRAF V600E mutation. N Engl J Med. 2011;364(26):2507–16.

14. Slamon DJ et al. Use of chemotherapy plus a monoclonal antibody against HER2 for metastatic breast cancer that overexpresses HER2. N Engl J Med. 2001;344(11):783–92.
15. Folkman J. Tumor angiogenesis: therapeutic implications. N Engl J Med. 1971;285(21):1182–6.
16. Hurwitz H et al. Bevacizumab plus irinotecan, fluorouracil, and leucovorin for metastatic colorectal cancer. N Engl J Med. 2004;350(23):2335–42.
17. Sandler A et al. Paclitaxel-carboplatin alone or with bevacizumab for non-small-cell lung cancer. N Engl J Med. 2006;355(24):2542–50.
18. Mateos MV et al. Bortezomib plus melphalan and prednisone compared with melphalan and prednisone in previously untreated multiple myeloma: updated follow-up and impact of subsequent therapy in the phase III VISTA trial. J Clin Oncol. 2010;28(13):2259–66.
19. Schneider BJ et al. Phase I study of vorinostat (suberoylanilide hydroxamic acid, NSC 701852) in combination with docetaxel in patients with advanced and relapsed solid malignancies. Invest New Drugs. 2012;30(1):249–57.
20. Cooper A. Illustration of the diseases of the breast. London; Longman, Rees & Co. 1829.
21. Beatson GT. On the treatment of inoperable cases of carcinoma of the mamma: suggestions for a new method of treatment with illustrative cases. Lancet. 1896;ii:104.
22. Haddow A, Watkinson JM, Patterson E. Influence of synthetic oestrogens upon advanced malignant disease. Br Med J. 1944;2:393–8.
23. Cole MP, Jones CT, Todd ID. A new anti-oestrogenic agent in late breast cancer. An early clinical appraisal of ICI46474. Br J Cancer. 1971;25(2):270–5.
24. Tamoxifen for early breast cancer: an overview of the randomised trials. Early Breast Cancer Trialists' Collaborative Group. Lancet. 1998; 351(9114): 1451–67.
25. Hutchings O et al. Effect of early American results on patients in a tamoxifen prevention trial (IBIS). International Breast Cancer Intervention Study. Lancet. 1998;352(9135):1222.
26. Howell A et al. Results of the ATAC (Arimidex, Tamoxifen, Alone or in Combination) trial after completion of 5 years' adjuvant treatment for breast cancer. Lancet. 2005;365(9453):60–2.
27. de Bono JS et al. Abiraterone and increased survival in metastatic prostate cancer. N Engl J Med. 2011; 364(21):1995–2005.
28. Hodi FS et al. Improved survival with ipilimumab in patients with metastatic melanoma. N Engl J Med. 2010;363(8):711–23.

Pharmacogenetics of Pain in Cancer

4

Pål Klepstad

Abstract

The efficacy of opioids varies between individual cancer pain patients. This relates both to the needed dose and to responses to different opioids. Opioid pharmacology is complex and genes coding several pharmacological elements are proposed to explain some of the variability in opioid response. This includes opioid metabolism, opioid receptors, opioid transport through the blood–brain barrier, inflammation, and mechanisms modifying opioid signalling. Variability in CYP2D6 is established to influence the efficacy from codeine. The two other genes shown in several studies to influence opioids efficacy are the *OPRM1* gene and the *COMT* gene. Variability in other genes are not consistently shown to influence on the efficacy from opioids, and in the only study that included a large patient cohort and a validation sample, no candidate genes were associated with opioid dose. Thus, with the exception of CYP2D6 activity and codeine, there are currently no pharmacogenetic analyses that are able to guide opioid therapy. Still, the biological phenomenon has been established, and it is expected that future research will discover the basis for why individuals vary in terms of opioid response.

Keywords

Opioid • Genetic • Cancer • Pain • Pharmacogenetics

Abbreviations

BBB	Blood–brain barrier
COMT	Catechol-O-methyltransferase
CYP	Cytochrome P
ECF	Extracellular fluid
GWA	Genome-wide association
M6G	Morphine-6-glucuronide
MDR	Multidrug resistance
NKFBIA	Nuclear factor of light polypeptide gene enhancer in B-cell inhibitor alpha
PTGS2	Prostaglandin G/H synthase 2
SNP	Single-nucleotide polymorphism
UGT2B7	UDP-glucuronosyltransferase 2B7
WHO	World Health Organization

P. Klepstad, MD, PhD
Department of Intensive Care Medicine,
St. Olavs University Hospital,
Trondheim 7006, Norway
e-mail: pal.klepstad@ntnu.no

M. Hanna, Z. Zylicz (eds.), *Cancer Pain*,
DOI 10.1007/978-0-85729-230-8_4, © Springer-Verlag London 2013

Introduction

The pain reported by cancer patients and the doses of opioids needed for pain relief vary between individuals. Traditionally, this variation has been explained by variable bioavailability of opioids and differences in intensities of pain stimuli. However, a more complex model that also includes inborn patient characteristics to explain the variability in pain is conceivable.

The patients' disposition for developing cancer pain can be different even before the patient is diagnosed with cancer. Factors that may contribute are demographic variables such as age and gender, chronic nonmalignant pain, psychological distress, addiction, barriers towards the use of analgesics, and cultural factors. After the patients are diagnosed with cancer, both the extent and locations of cancer is important for pain treatment. Antineoplastic treatment can both result in relief from cancer pain and also induce chronic pain as an unwanted adverse effect. Finally, factors related to non-analgesic effects from drug therapy may limit the adequate titration of analgesics to a dose that reduces pain (Fig. 4.1).

Variations in metabolism influence drug efficacy. For opioids with biological inactive metabolites, an increase in metabolism will result in decreased opioid efficacy. For the most used opioid, morphine, a more complicated picture emerges. Because the morphine metabolite morphine-6-glucuronide (M6G) contributes to pain relief, increased metabolism of morphine to M6G may result in a more pronounced opioid effect [1]. However, that serum concentrations of

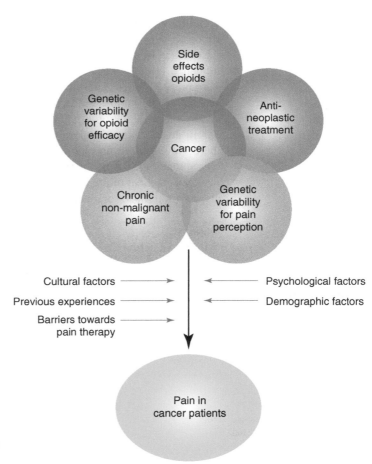

Fig. 4.1 Pain in cancer patients is an end result of several factors

morphine and M6G are not closely associated to clinical outcomes. Therefore, other factors must contribute to the interindividual variability in morphine efficacy. Differences in pharmacodynamics at the mu-opioid receptor, differences in transport of opioids through the blood–brain barrier (BBB), and variability related to non-opioid biological systems that influence opioid pharmacology could all contribute to interindividual variability in opioid efficacy.

The interindividual variability of opioid pharmacology suggests that a patient's genetic disposition influences the response to opioids. This view is strongly supported by observations that ethnicity influences the response to opioids. One example being that Cepeda et al. observed that native Indians had a more pronounced morphine depression of the ventilatory response when compared with Caucasians [2].

Genetic Variability of Cancer Pain

Before reviewing the relationship between genetic dispositions and effects from opioids, it must be recognised that genetic variability also influences pain perception. Animal studies have shown that heritability of nociception ranges from 30 to 76 % in different nociceptive assays [3]. The heritability of pain is believed to be a result of quantitative trait loci; that is, the variability is a result of several genes that – combined – contribute to pain perception [3]. Animal studies have demonstrated numerous genes which may influence nociception. An updated overview of genes observed to be related to pain outcomes in animal transgenic knockout studies is available in the Pain Genes Database [4]. For humans the influence on nociception, both in experimental models and in chronic nonmalignant pain, is, as in animal models, a result from variability in multiple genes. Examples are genes coding transporter proteins, transcription regulators, receptors, cytokines, and ion channels [5]. However, the findings from human pain studies are inconsistent; most studies only assess one or a minor number of gene candidates and many studies are subject to methodological lim-

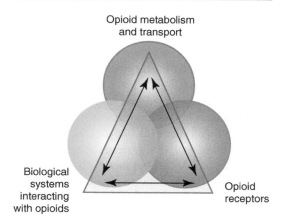

Fig. 4.2 Several mechanisms are involved in opioid pharmacology and may be influenced by genetic variability. Examples of biological mechanisms that interact with opioids are inflammation, nerve transmission, and descending inhibiting pain pathways

itations [6]. A small genome-wide association (GWA) study of postoperative pain did not identify genes that could predict pain intensity [7], and for pain there is a lack of large-scale GWA studies that could potentially identify new pain genes. In cancer pain, a major obstacle in addressing the genetic variability of cancer pain is the influence that genes may have on both pain perception and analgesic efficacy. For obvious reasons a study on untreated cancer pain is not feasible.

For opioids used for moderate or severe cancer pain corresponding to step III on the WHO pain ladder, morphine is the most widely used substance and is the opioid of which genetic links have been the most extensively studied. Therefore, with the exception of data related to genetic variability at the Cytochrome P (CYP) 2D6 gene, the majority of papers address the use of morphine. Given the complexity of morphine pharmacology, variability may be caused by variations in several genes. Candidate genes are genes related to morphine pharmacokinetics, to mu-opioid receptors, and to BBB transport of morphine through multidrug resistance (MDR) transporters. Also genes related to biological systems modifying opioid analgesia or pain perception may alter the efficacy of morphine (Fig. 4.2).

Genetic Variability Related to Analgesics

Metabolism: CYP Enzymes

The influence of genetic variability on the pharmacokinetics of codeine is well recognised. Several variant alleles of the *CYP2D6* gene are nonfunctional and, if they occur as homozygous, will result in codeine poor metabolisers. Because poor metabolisers convert less codeine to the more active metabolite, morphine patients with these variant alleles will experience inferior analgesic treatment with codeine. This is clinically relevant as about 7 % of the Caucasian population are CYP2D6 poor metabolisers [8]. Opposite these observations are poor *CYP2D6* metabolisers, some patients can be fast metabolisers due to variant *CYP2D6* gene alleles. Such variants, which are common in Africans, will increase the opioid efficacy of codeine. Tramadol is metabolised to its active metabolite O-desmethyltramadol by *CYP2D6* and poor metabolisers have decreased analgesic effect from tramadol [9]. However, because tramadol exerts its analgesic effects also through non-opioid mechanism, the efficacy of tramadol is only partly reduced in poor metabolisers. For cancer pain patients the variability in codeine and tramadol represents a minor clinical obstacle because the clinical approach for patients with a lack of pain relief from an opioid for mild pain (WHO pain ladder step II) is to change analgesic treatment to an opioid for moderate and severe pain (WHO pain ladder III). Also many clinicians currently use a two-step pain ladder approach, not using opioids for mild pain at all [51].

Variations in CYP2D6 activity are also shown to influence the metabolism of other opioids than codeine or tramadol. Heiskanen et al. found that inhibition of CYP2D6 alters the metabolism of oxycodone [10] and Andreassen et al. showed that poor metabolisers had different oxycodone-to-metabolites ratios than extensive metabolisers [11]. However, in both studies the altered oxycodone pharmacokinetics did not have any clinical consequences. CYP2D6 genetic variability is also observed to alter the pharmacokinetics of

methadone and suggested by some authors to influence the success of methadone maintenance therapy to addicts [12, 13]. If CYP2D6 genetic variability may also influence the pharmacology for methadone when used for pain is not known.

Other CYP enzymes have also been shown to influence opioid pharmacology. Variability in CYP3A4 and CYP2B6 may be associated with methadone pharmacokinetics and CY3A4 variability may be associated with fentanyl pharmacokinetics, respectively [14, 15]. However, generally most issues are unresolved for the impact of genetic variability in the genes coding CYP enzymes on opioids corresponding to the WHO pain ladder step III.

Metabolism: UGT2B7

The morphine metabolite M6G is found in higher serum concentrations than morphine during chronic oral morphine administration [1]. M6G binds to the mu-opioid receptor, possesses higher analgesic potency in animal models, and contributes to the clinical analgesia produced by morphine [1]. Therefore, differences in the conversion of morphine to M6G could alter the efficacy of morphine treatment. This conversion is catalysed in the liver by the UDP-glucuronosyltransferase 2B7 (UGT2B7) enzyme. In order to assess if genetic variability could explain differences in the activity of this enzyme, a cohort of 239 cancer patients was screened for sequence variation in the coding and regulatory regions of the *UGT2B7* gene. Twelve nucleotide variations (single-nucleotide polymorphisms – SNPs) were identified. This study observed no differences in M6G/morphine ratios between the genotypes, suggesting that genetic variability in the gene coding for the UGT2B7 enzyme is not important for differences in morphine pharmacokinetics [16]. A later study by Sawyer et al. included 99 patients receiving patient-controlled morphine, mostly for postoperative pain [17]. This study observed a significant trend for decreased M6G/morphine ratios in patients homozygous for tyrosine at position 802 at exon 2, patients heterozygous for tyrosine and cytosine at this

Fig. 4.3 The mu-opioid receptor consists of an extracellular, a transmembrane, and an intracellular part. The figure identifies some single-nucleotide polymorphisms (SNP) that result in an altered amino acid sequence in the mu-opioid receptor. SNPs are identified with dbSNP database number or nucleotide position

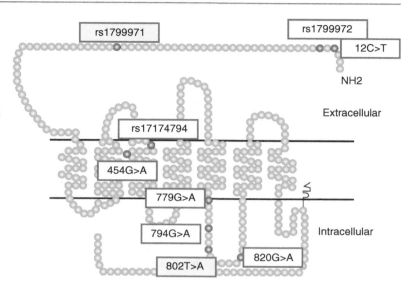

position and patients homozygous for cytosine. The two studies were different in terms of origin of pain (cancer vs. postoperative) and ethnicity (Caucasian only vs. a mixed population of Caucasian and African Americans). Thus, the available data for the genetic influence on clinical pharmacokinetics of morphine is so far uncertain and no firm conclusion can be stated.

Mu-Opioid Receptors

Clinical studies have consistently shown either a lack of, or a low association between, serum concentrations of morphine and M6G and clinical outcomes. These results suggest that pharmacodynamic factors are more important for the interindividual variability in opioid efficacy. Hoehe et al. identified 43 SNPs within the *OPRM1* gene [18]. Most of the SNPs are in the noncoding region of the gene, but as illustrated in Fig. 4.3 several SNPs in the coding regions resulted in an altered amino acid sequence in the mu-opioid receptor (Fig. 4.3). An amino acid substitution at position 268 (SNP 802T>C) strongly impairs receptor signalling after stimulation with opioid agonists including morphine [19]. This observation is of major principal interest since it establishes that genetic variability has the potential to change receptor function. However, because of the low

frequency of this variation, the significance of this SNP for the population variability of opioid efficacy is limited. A more common SNP associated with a change in the amino acid sequence is an A to G substitution in exon 1 (rs1799971), located in the extracellular N-terminal part of the mu-opioid receptor, causing an exchange of asparagine for aspartate at position 40. The frequency of the variant polymorphism is about 10–14 % in Caucasians [18]. Lötsch et al. and Skarke et al. showed in two separate human experimental studies that subjects carrying one or two copies of the variant 118G allele had decreased pupillary constriction after M6G administration [20]. The response to morphine was unaltered in the study by Lötsch et al. and reduced in the volunteers studied by Skarke et al. More evidence for the effect of A118G polymorphisms were supplied by Romberg et al. who in a study on human experimental pain showed that patients with the variant allele needed about threefold M6G serum concentration in order to increase the threshold to painful electric stimulation [21]. Finally, in human volunteers, variability in the rs1799971 influences cortical activation after nociceptive stimuli [22].

Findings in human volunteers must be confirmed in clinical studies in order to establish the clinical significance of biological variability. In a study including 100 cancer patients, the A118G polymorphism resulted in altered function of the mu-opioid receptor as assessed by the level of morphine needed to achieve adequate pain relief from cancer pain. Patients homozygous needed about twice the morphine doses needed by wild-type patients in order to achieve adequate pain relief. This difference was also reflected in serum concentrations of morphine and M6G [23]. The lower efficacy from morphine in patients homozygous for the variant A118G polymorphism supported the results obtained in the human experimental studies. Similar results were observed by Campa et al. who assessed pain relief achieved after the start of morphine to cancer pain patients [24]. Corresponding results supporting the interaction of the rs1799971 polymorphism with morphine analgesia are also reported in studies of opioid efficacy for postoperative pain [25]. These and other studies established a firm belief that this SNP was an important predictor for clinical opioid efficacy. However, a meta-analysis by Walter and Lötsch [26] failed to confirm this finding and, finally, in the first large-scale study assessing genetic variability and opioid doses for cancer pain, Klepstad et al. did not observe any effects from the rs1799971 SNP [27]. Therefore, despite many studies convincingly pointing out an association between genetic variability in the gene coding the mu-opioid receptor and opioid effects, these observations have not been possible to confirm in clinical meta-analyses or large-scale studies.

Genetic variability in the mu-opioid receptor gene can be caused by mechanisms other than SNPs. Animal studies have identified that differences in the selection of exon regions during translation to mRNA give multiple mu-opioid receptor variants (splice variants) that may be responsible for varying analgesic responses and adverse effects from morphine and M6G [28]. Mu-opioid receptor splice variants are also present in the human brain [29, 30]. Despite promising results from the impact of splice variants on some opioid effects in animals, it is still not established if such variants can explain the variable effects from different opioid substances in humans.

MDR Transporters

The effect site, mu-opioid receptors, is primarily located in the extracellular fluid in the central nervous system. Morphine and some other opioids are transported out from the brain through the BBB. Decreased function of the MDR transporters can therefore increase the concentrations of opioids in the extracellular fluid (ECF) of the brain. Human genetic variability within the gene coding MDR transporters is shown to influence the degree of pain relief achieved after the start of morphine in cancer pain [24] and some studies suggest that there is an association with the risk of opioid-induced adverse effects [31, 32]. However, as with gene coding the mu-opioid receptor, a large patient series showed no SNP in the MDR1 gene to interact with opioid efficacy [27]. Therefore, for the MDR1 gene some preclinical and clinical data indicate that genetic variability influences opioid efficacy, but it is still premature for current knowledge to form the basis of any conclusions.

Cellular Response

The binding of morphine to the mu-opioid receptor elicits a response from the cell. Studies of genetic variability in genes coding intracellular processes related to opioid analgesia are scarce. One exception is a study by Ross et al. who in a cohort of 162 patients compared patients successfully treated with morphine with those patients who needed to change to an alternative opioid. In this study it was observed that polymorphisms in the β-arrestin gene, a substance involved at several points in the intracellular sequence of events following opioid agonist stimulation, was associated with the need to switch from morphine [33]. In the large-scale European study by Klepstad et al., genetic variability in the β-arrestin gene was associated with variation in the need for opioid dose in patients receiving opioid treatment for more than 3 months [27]. This finding agrees with the putative role of β-arrestin in the development of opioid tolerance. The study by Ross et al. also observed that polymorphisms in the *stat6* gene were associated with the need for an opioid switch [33]. This observation may be associated with altered stat6 regulation of mu-opioid receptor transcription.

Modifying Systems and Morphine

Opioid analgesia is modified by other biological systems such as descending inhibitory serotinergic and adrenergic neurons. One clinical example illustrating the interaction of non-opioid substances with opioid analgesia is the addition of α_2-agonists in order to enhance the efficacy of opioids. The effects of opioids could be associated with the function of several endogenous substances one example being adrenergic neurotransmitters. Catechol-O-methyltransferase (COMT) metabolises catecholamines such as dopamine, adrenaline, and noradrenaline. A frequent polymorphism (rs4680) in the *COMT* gene results in a valine (Val) to methionine (Met) substitution. The enzyme containing the Met amino has a three- to fourfold reduction in the activity compared to the Val-containing enzyme. Patients with the Met/Met genotype have lower concentrations of enkephalin [34] and might therefore be hypothesised to need more morphine to compensate for a reduction of endogenous enkephalin production. In the same study Zubieta et al. observed an increase of μ-opioid receptors in patients with the Met/Met genotype [34]. This increase in the density of opioid receptors might result in an improved efficacy of morphine, and therefore patients with the Met/Met genotype might need less morphine. The clinical influence from this SNP in the *COMT* gene is supported by several clinical studies. Kim et al. observed that for experimental pain and postoperative pain variations, both the rs4860 and other SNPs within the *COMT* gene influenced pain perception [35, 36]. In 207 cancer patients using morphine, Rakvåg et al. observed that patients with the Val/Val genotype needed more morphine as compared to the Val/Met and the Met/Met genotype groups [37]. Ross et al. observed that other SNPs in the *COMT* gene than the rs4860 influenced the risk for central nervous-associated adverse effects from morphine [31], while

Laugsand et al. observed that both rs4860 and other COMT SNPs were associated with the risk for another adverse effect, nausea [38]. However, none of the SNPs in the *COMT* gene showed a consistent significant association with need for opioid dose in the large-scale studies on cancer pain patients [27].

Multiple other biological systems are reported to have genetic variability associated with opioid effects. These variations share common factors: most findings are reported in only one or two reports and have primarily assessed volunteers or patients with other conditions than cancer pain. Knowing that most genetic associations fail to be replicated in later studies, such findings must be considered with caution. Examples of proposed biological factors to which genetic variability is associated with opioid effects are melanocortin-1 receptors [39], dopamine receptors [40], GTP cyclohydrolase [41], alpha-adrenergic receptors [42], potassium channels (KCNJ6) [43], and nerve transmission [44]. Finally, during recent years new research has developed for the immune system as a biological system that influences opioid analgesia. As reviewed by Hutchinson et al., there is a close link between central immune signalling and opioid analgesia [45, 46]. Some small studies have observed associations between opioid efficacy and genetic variability related to the immune molecules interleukin-1 receptor antagonist [47, 48] and interleukin-6 [49]. Furthermore, genetic variations in immune molecules such as interleukin-6, interleukin-8, tumour necrosis factor, PTGS2, and NKFBIA are reported to influence the intensity of cancer pain [49, 50].

Conclusion

Clinical observations and findings in genetic research strongly argue that opioid efficacy is partly related to inborn properties caused by genetic variability. Such variability may be related to several facets of opioid pharmacology such as opioid metabolism, opioid receptors, opioid signalling, opioid neuroimmunopharmacology, and opioid transporters. Still, several of the hitherto mentioned findings are inconclusive and not supported by the recently published first large-scale study addressing many of the current gene candidates related to opioid efficacy [27]. Also, current studies are only able to predict a minor part of the total interindividual variability in opioid efficacy. Therefore, it is reasonable to believe that other genes are important in order to understand why patients react differently on opioid treatment. New genes must be identified through explorative approaches. One method is GWA studies of which at present have only been done as a pooled DNA analyses for cancer pain [44] and as a small-scale GWA study in postoperative pain [7]. Furthermore, an increased understanding of the interaction between biological systems, in particular the immune system and the pain-signalling system, may elucidate some of the complexity related to cancer pain and analgesia. Future research should be a combination of basic research elucidating genetic variability related to the biological mechanism of opioid signalling and of clinical research that aims to understand the consequences of such variability on patient outcome.

Current guidelines for the treatment of cancer pain are developed with the aim of giving pain treatments to large populations, including those in the undeveloped world. These treatment guidelines have led to improved pain relief for large populations but do, at the same time, fail to result in optimal pain control for all patients. More advanced methods combining clinical observations with genetic technology may predict an individual response to an opioid; the key issue is to evolve from population guidelines to individualised guided treatment.

Key Points
- Cancer pain is an end result of multiple factors related to the patients, the cancer disease, and efficacy of analgesics.
- Genetic variation can influence both pain perception and analgesic efficacy. In studies on cancer pain patients, it is difficult to decipher which of these two pain-related factors are influenced by genetics.
- Genetic variability is reported in genes coding for the metabolism of opioids,

opioid receptors, transport of opioids through the BBB, opioid receptors, and biological systems that interact with opioid pharmacology.
- The hitherto largest study (2,294 cancer pain patients) on the relationship between opioid efficacy and several of the known candidate genes failed to confirm any consistent associations between opioid doses and genetic variability.
- Genetic variability important for opioid efficacy is expected to be identified in new genes.

References

1. Klepstad P, Kaasa S, Borchgrevink PC. Start of oral morphine to cancer patients: effective serum morphine concentrations and contribution from morphine-6-glucuronide to the analgesia produced by morphine. Eur J Clin Pharmacol. 2000;55:713–9.
2. Cepeda MS, Farrar JT, Roa JH, et al. Ethnicity influences morphine pharmacokinetics and pharmacodynamics. Clin Pharmacol Ther. 2001;70:351–61.
3. Mogil JS. Pain genetics: pre- and post-genomic findings. In IASP Newsletter. International Association for the Study of Pain; 2000.
4. Lacroix-Fralish ML, Ledoux JB, Mogil JS. The Pain Genes Database: an interactive web browser of pain-related transgenic knockout studies. Pain. 2007;131(3): e1–4.
5. Diatchenko L, Nackley AG, Tchivileva IE, et al. Genetic architecture of human pain perception. Trends Genet. 2007;23:605–13.
6. Kim H, Clark D, Dionne RA. Genetic contributions to clinical pain and analgesia: avoiding pitfalls in genetic research. J Pain. 2009;10:663–93.
7. Kim H, Ramsay E, Lee H, et al. Genome-wide association study of acute post-surgical pain in humans. Pharmacogenomics. 2009;10:171–9.
8. Sindrup SH, Brøsen K, Bjerring P, et al. Codeine increases pain thresholds to copper vapor laser stimuli in extensive but not poor metabolizers of sparteine. Clin Pharmacol Ther. 1990;48:686–93.
9. Poulsen L, Arendt-Nielsen L, Brøsen K, et al. The hypoalgesic effect of tramadol in relation to CYP2D6. Clin Pharmacol Ther. 1996;60:636–44.
10. Heiskanen T, Olkkola KT, Kalso E. Effects of blocking CYP2D6 on the pharmacokinetics and pharmacodynamics of Oxycodone. Clin Pharmacol Ther. 1998;64:603–11.

11. Andreassen TN, Eftedal I, Klepstad P, et al. Do CYP2D6 genotypes reflect oxycodone requirements for cancer patients treated for cancer pain? A cross-sectional multicentre study. Eur J Clin Pharmacol. 2012;68(1):55–64.

12. Eap CB, Broly F, Mino A, et al. Cytochrome P450 2D6 genotype and methadone steady-state concentrations. J Clin Psychopharmacol. 2001;21:229–34.

13. Crettol S, Deglon JJ, Besson J, Croquette-Krokar M, et al. ABCB1 and cytochrome P450 genotypes and phenotypes: influence on methadone plasma levels and responses to treatment. Clin Pharmacol Ther. 2006;80:668–81.

14. Crettol S, Deglon JJ, Besson J, Croquette-Krokar M, et al. Methadone enantiomer plasma levels, CYP2B6, CYP2C19, and CYP2C9 genotypes, and response to treatment. Clin Pharmacol Ther. 2005;78:593–604.

15. Zhang W, Chang Y-Z, Kan Q-C, et al. CYP3A4*1G genetic polymorphism influences CYP3A activity and response to fentanyl in Chinese gynecologic patients. Eur J Clin Pharmacol. 2010;66:61–6.

16. Holthe M, Rakvåg TN, Klepstad P, et al. Sequence variation in the UDP-glucuronosyltransferase 2B7 (UGT2B7) gene: identification of 10 novel single nucleotide polymorphisms (SNPs) and analysis of their relevance to morphine glucuronidation in cancer patients. Pharmacogenomics J. 2003;3:17–26.

17. Sawyer MB, Innoceti F, Das S, et al. A pharmacogenetic study of uridine diphosphate-glucuronosyltransferase 2B7 in patients receiving morphine. Clin Pharmacol Ther. 2003;73:566–74.

18. Hoehe MR, Köpke K, Wendel B, et al. Sequence variability and candidate gene analysis in complex disease: association of μ opioid receptor gene variation with substance dependence. Hum Mol Genet. 2000;9:2895–908.

19. Befort K, Filliol D, Decalliot FM, et al. A single nucleotide polymorphic mutation in the human mu-opioid receptor severely impairs receptor signaling. J Biol Chem. 2001;276:3130–7.

20. Lotsch J, Geisslinger G. Current evidence for a genetic modulation of the response to analgesics. Pain. 2006;121:1–5.

21. Romberg R, Olufsen E, Bijl H, et al. Polymorphism of μ-opioid receptor gene (OPRM1:c.118A>G) does not protect against opioid-induced respiratory depression despite reduced analgesic response. Anesthesiology. 2005;102:522–30.

22. Lotsch J, Stuck B, Hummel T. The human μ-opioid receptor gene polymorphism 118A>G decreases cortical activation in response to specific nociceptive stimuli. Behav Neurosci. 2006;120:1218–24.

23. Klepstad P, Rakvåg TN, Kaasa S, et al. The 118 A>G polymorphism in the human μ-opioid receptor gene may increase morphine requirements in patients with pain caused by malignant disease. Acta Anaesthesiol Scand. 2004;48:1232–9.

24. Campa D, Gioia A, Tomei A, et al. Association of ABCB1/MDR1 and OPRM1 gene polymorphisms with morphine pain relief. Clin Pharmacol Ther. 2008;83:559–66.

25. Chou WY, Yang LC, Lu HF, et al. Association of mu opioid receptor gene polymorphism (A118G) with variations in morphine consumption for analgesia after total knee arthroplasties. Acta Anaesthesiol Scand. 2006;50:787–92.

26. Walter C, Lötsch J. Meta-analysis of the relevance of the OPRM1 118A>G genetic variant for pain treatment. Pain. 2009;146:270–5.

27. Klepstad P, Fladvad T, Skorpen F, et al. Influence from genetic variability on opioid use for cancer pain: a European genetic association study of 2294 cancer pain patients. Pain. 2011;152:1139–45.

28. Pasternak GW. Incomplete cross tolerance and multiple mu opioid peptide receptors. Trends Pharmacol Sci. 2001;22:67–70.

29. Pan YX, Xu J, Mahurter L, et al. Identification and characterization of two human mu opioid receptor splice variants, hMOR-1O and hMOR-1X. Biochem Biophys Res Commun. 2003;301:1057–61.

30. Kvam TM, Baar C, Rakvåg TT, et al. Genetic analysis of the murine mu opioid receptor: increased complexity of Oprm gene splicing. J Mol Med. 2004;82:250–5.

31. Ross JR, Riley J, Taegtmeyer AB, et al. Genetic variation and response to morphine in cancer patients: catechol-O-methyltransferase (COMT) and multi-drug resistance (MDR-1) gene polymorphism are associated with central side-effects. Cancer. 2007;112:1390–403.

32. Coulbault L, Beaussier M, Verstuyft C, et al. Environmental and genetic factors associated with morphine responses in the postoperative period. Clin Pharmacol Ther. 2006;79:316–24.

33. Ross JR, Ruttler D, Welsh K, et al. Clinical response to morphine in cancer patients and genetic variation in candidate genes. Pharmacogenomics J. 2005;5:324–36.

34. Zubieta JK, Heitzeg MM, Smith YR, et al. COMT val 158 met genotype affects μ-opioid neurotransmitter responses to a pain stressor. Science. 2003;299:1240–3.

35. Kim H, Mittal DP, Iadarola MJ, et al. Genetic predictors for acute experimental cold and heat pain sensitivity in humans. J Med Genet. 2006;43:e40.

36. Kim H, Lee H, Rowan J, et al. Genetic polymorphisms in monoamine neurotransmittor systems show only weak association with acute post-surgical pain in humans. Mol Pain. 2006;2:24.

37. Rakvåg TT, Klepstad P, Baar C, et al. The Val158Met polymorphism of the human catechol-O-methyltransferase (COMT) gene may influence morphine requirements in cancer pain patients. Pain. 2005;116:73–8.

38. Laugsand EA, Fladvad T, Skorpen F, et al. Clinical and genetic factors associated with nausea and vomiting in cancer patients receiving opioids. Eur J Cancer. 2011;47:1682–91.

39. Mogil JS, Ritchie J, Smith SB, et al. Melanonocortin-1 receptor gene variants affect pain and μ-opioid analgesia in mice and humans. J Med Genet. 2005;42:583–7.

40. Crettol S, Besson J, Croquette-Krokar M, et al. Association of dopamine and opioid receptor genetic polymorphisms with response to methadone maintenance treatment. Prog Neuropsychopharmacol Biol Psychiatry. 2008;32:1722–77.

41. Lötsch J, Klepstad P, Doehring A, et al. A GTP cyclo-hydrolase 1 genetic variant delays cancer pain. Pain. 2010;148:103–6.
42. Kohli U, Muszkat M, Sofowora GG, et al. Effects of variation in the human α2A- and α2C-adrenoceptor genes on cognitive tasks and pain perception. Eur J Pain. 2010;14:154–9.
43. Lötsch J, Prüss H, Veh RW, et al. A KCNJ6 (Kir3.2, GIRK2) gene polymorphism modulates opioid effects on analgesia and addiction but not on pupil size. Pharmacogenet Genomics. 2010;20:291–7.
44. Galvan A, Skorpen F, Klepstad P, et al. Multiple loci modulate opioid therapy response for cancer pain. Clin Cancer Res. 2011;17(13):4581–7.
45. Hutchinson MR, Shavit Y, Grace PM, et al. Exploring the neuroimmunopharmacology of opioids: an integrative review of mechanisms of central immune signaling and their implications for opioid analgesia. Pharmacol Rev. 2011;63:772–810.
46. Lewis SS, Hutchinson MR, Rezvani N, et al. Evidence that intrathecal morphine-3-glucuronide may cause pain enhancement via toll-like receptor 4/MD-2 and interleukin-1beta. Neuroscience. 2010;165: 569–83.
47. Bessler H, Shavit Y, Mayburd E, et al. Postoperative pain, morphine consumption, and genetic polymorphism of IL-1beta and IL-1 receptor antagonist. Neurosci Lett. 2006;404:154–8.
48. Candiotti KA, Yang Z, Morris R, et al. Polymorphism in the interleukin-1 receptor antagonist gene is associated with serum interleukin-1 receptor antagonist concentrations and postoperative opioid consumption. Anesthesiology. 2011;114:1162–8.
49. Reyes-Gibby CC, El Osta B, et al. The influence of tumor necrosis factor-alpha −308 G/A and IL-6–174 G/C on pain and analgesia response in lung cancer patients receiving supportive care. Cancer Epidemiol Biomarkers Prev. 2008;17:3262–7.
50. Reyes-Gibby CC, Spitz MR, Yennurajalingam S, et al. Role of inflammation gene polymorphisms on pain severity in lung cancer patients. Cancer Epidemiol Biomarkers Prev. 2009;18:2636–42.
51. Caraceni A, Hanks G, Kaasa S, et al. Use of opioid analgesics in the treatment of cancer pain: evidenced-based recommendation from the EAPC. Lancet Oncol. 2012;13:e58–68.

Mechanisms in Cancer Pain

5

Jerzy Wordliczek and Renata Zajaczkowska

Abstract

Pain in the cancer patient is caused primarily by the development of the disease process (tumours, metastases), which in turn causes, amongst other things, infiltration of soft tissues, bones, nervous system structures, and serous membranes. Cancer may also cause necrosis of solid organs or induce the occlusion of blood vessels.

In addition, pain in the cancer patient may be the consequence of anticancer therapy, which, in the case of radiation therapy, may lead to the development of post-radiation plexopathies or myelopathies. In the case of chemotherapy, related pain syndromes and peripheral neuropathy are the common adverse events of a number of anticancer medications. Surgically treated patients, especially those following thoracotomy, mastectomy, or amputation, may develop persistent postoperative pain (postsurgical neuropathy).

An important kind of pain in cancer patients is acute pain associated with cancer pain treatment, which is due to both diagnostic (i.e., biopsies, blood samples) and therapeutic procedures (acute postoperative pain).

Lastly, the pain in question may be due to mechanisms unrelated to the cancer itself or its treatment, e.g., chronic headache, low-back pain, and pain that the patient may have suffered prior to the diagnosis of cancer.

Keywords

Pain in cancer patients • Somatic pain • Visceral pain • Cancer-related neuropathic pain • Pain caused by anticancer therapy

J. Wordliczek, MD, PhD (✉)
Department of Pain Treatment and Palliative Care, Jagiellonian University Medical College, Sniadeckich Str. 10, 31-531 Krakow, Poland

Department of Anaesthesiology and Intensive Care, University Hospital, Kopernika Str. 50, 31-531 Krakow, Poland
e-mail: j.wordliczek@uj.edu.pl

R. Zajaczkowska, MD, PhD
Department of Anaesthesiology, Intensive Care and Pain Treatment, Province Hospital, Lwowska Str. 60, 35-301 Rzeszow, Poland

Institute of Obstetrics and Emergency Medicine, University of Rzeszow, Pigonia Str. 6, 35-205 Rzeszow, Poland
e-mail: renia356@poczta.onet

M. Hanna, Z. Zylicz (eds.), *Cancer Pain*,
DOI 10.1007/978-0-85729-230-8_5, © Springer-Verlag London 2013

Fig. 5.1 Mechanisms of cancer pain as a direct consequence of tumour

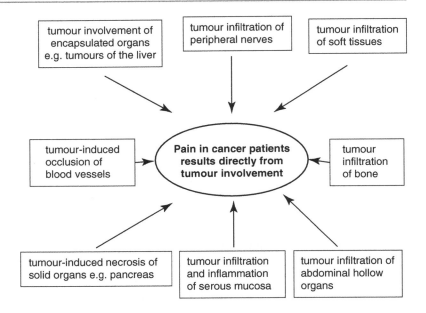

Introduction

The mechanism of cancer pain is a complex pathological process that comprises both cellular, tissue, and systemic changes that occur during the proliferation, invasion, and metastasis of cancer, in addition to mutual interactions between cancer cells, the peripheral and central nervous systems, and the immune system [1].

The intensity of cancer pain is influenced by the histological type of cancer, the location of the primary neoplasm and its metastases, the stage of the cancer, the anticancer therapy received, as well as pain due to coexisting diseases unrelated to cancer and its treatment. Pain felt by the cancer patient is also significantly influenced by psychological and emotional factors (e.g., anxiety, depression).

Pain in the cancer patient is usually due to several causes [2]:

- The presence of a tumour or the appearance and/or growth of a metastasis
- Anticancer therapy (diagnostic procedures, surgical interventions, radiotherapy, chemotherapy)
- Mechanisms indirectly related to cancer and its treatment (infections, metabolic imbalance, myofascial pain)
- Mechanisms unrelated to the cancer itself or its treatment (migraine, painful diabetic neuropathy, low-back pain)

Given the sheer number of factors causing pain in cancer patients, which are not always related to the disease itself or its treatment, this kind of pain should not be called cancer pain, but instead pain in the cancer patient.

Several pain mechanisms that directly accompany tumour growth or its metastases may lead to the appearance of pain or its exacerbation in cancer patients (Fig. 5.1) [2].

In terms of pathophysiological criteria, pain in the cancer patient may be divided into (a) nociceptive (somatic or visceral), (b) neuropathic, and (c) mixed. Nociceptive pain arises as a result of irritation of, or a decreased irritability threshold in, pain receptors, that is, nociceptors located in superficial, skin structures, subcutaneous tissues, muscles, and the osteoarticular system (somatic pain) or in organs located within body cavities, such as the thorax, abdomen, and pelvis (visceral pain). This kind of pain is usually due to the infiltration of tissue by tumour or metastasis or due to tissue injury as a result of anticancer treatment. On the other hand, tumour growth or treatment may lead to lesions in the structures of the central or peripheral nervous system, which causes neuropathic pain. This type of pain is often poorly tolerated and difficult to control. It needs to be stressed, however, that pain in cancer patients is usually of a mixed origin and rarely manifests itself as a purely somatic, visceral, or neuropathic pain syndrome. In most cases, it is a complex phenomenon that is a consequence of various, concurrently occurring factors, including inflammatory, neuropathic, and ischemic elements, that tend to be located in several places simultaneously [3].

The identification of these factors is extremely important due to their therapeutic implications, and, as a consequence, the possibilities of implementing effective therapy.

Pain Due to Tumour Growth and the Appearance or Growth of Metastases

Nociceptive Pain in the Cancer Patient

Somatic Pain in the Cancer Patient

This kind of pain may be caused by neoplastic invasion of the bone, joint, muscle, or connective tissue. The tumour mass produces and/or stimulates local production of inflammatory mediators, which leads to activation of peripheral nociceptors. Other sources of somatic pain in cancer patients include, for example, reactive spasm of muscle in area of tissue damage by cancer, postsurgical incisional pain, or radio-/chemotherapy-induced pain syndromes (e.g., mucositis, proctitis). It may be subdivided into superficial pain (i.e., cutaneous ulceration by malignant involvement) and deep pain (i.e., bone marrow infiltration by malignant cells, osteolytic lesions). Most cutaneous pain is well localised, sharp, or pricking. Deep tissue pain usually appears diffuse and is dull or aching in quality.

In somatic structures, the growing tumour that directly involves tissues triggers the release of potassium ions, ATP, bradykinin, prostanoids, and other inflammatory mediators that activate nociceptors – "pain receptors" – located on the primary endings of afferent sensory neurons (p.e.a.s.n.). The key function of nociceptors is to detect the chemical or physical stimuli and convert them into electrochemical signals transmitted to the central nervous system (CNS) via sensory fibres (unmyelinated C fibres and myelinated Aσ fibres) (Fig. 5.2) [4–6].

Moreover, tissue damage caused by the growing tumour (apart from the orthodromic transmission of nociceptive stimuli to the CNS) induces the release of mediators such as substance P (SP) from primary afferent of Aσ and C fibres along the antidromic pathway. This tissue damage leads to the dilation of the vascular bed (increased capillary permeability) which results in tissue edema and the release of bradykinin (BK) and serotonin (5-HT) from platelets, histamine from mast cells, other tissue mediators such as prostanoids (PG), the nerve growth factor (NGF), and cytokines (TNF-α). These mediators also increase vascular permeability and SP release [6, 7].

NGF, which acts via tyrosine kinase (TrkA) receptors and p74 receptors located on the neuronal membrane, ensures local growth and survival of afferent sensory fibres [8]. However, under pathological conditions this factor can also facilitate cancer invasion (e.g., breast, prostate) and trigger the development of thermal or mechanical hyperalgesia [9, 10]. Moreover, continuous exposure to NGF action increases the expression of ASIC and TRPV1 receptors in afferent sensory fibres, both of which contribute to the development of pain in the cancer patient [11, 12].

The presence of a tumour is accompanied by cytokine production with the tumour necrosis factor-α (TNF-α) that both stimulates the immune cells to produce pronociceptive mediators that act on the nociceptors of primary afferent fibres and itself directly induces hyperalgesia in the cancer microenvironment [13, 14].

Furthermore, the response of inflammatory cells that accompanies neoplastic infiltration of tissue may cause the release of extracellular protons (H^+) that generate local acidosis [15]. This leads to the activation of two acid-sensitive receptors: vanilloid receptors TRPV1 and acid-sensing ion channels ASIC-3, which are expressed by nociceptors and also induce pain stimulation [16].

One of the critical factors in inducing pain in the cancer patient is proteolytic activity. This is because proteases (e.g., trypsin) activate the receptors (protease-activated receptors, PARs) expressed on nociceptors, on the primary afferent fibres within the cancer environment. This, in turn, is caused by the fact that many proteases that activate PARs, either directly or via their peptide products, are synthesised during tissue damage due to the tissue's infiltration by malignant cells.

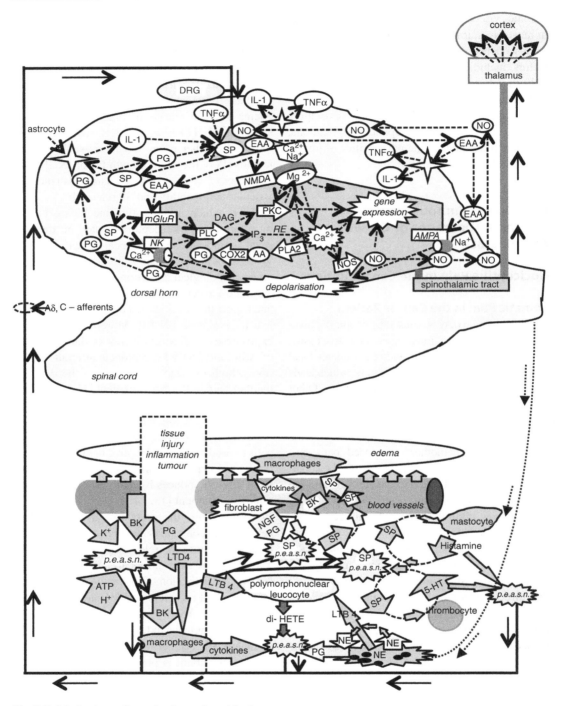

Fig. 5.2 Mechanisms of transduction and sensitisation

For instance cancer-associated trypsin has been identified, among others, in pancreatic cancer, in lung cancer, and in fibrosarcoma [17, 18].

The activation of PARs on nociceptors induces the release of substance P and calcitonin gene-related peptide (CGRP) from C fibres in peripheral tissues, as well as the activation of second messenger pathways, which leads to the sensitisation of vanilloid receptors TRPV1 and to the development of TRPV1-dependent thermal and TRPV4-dependent mechanical hyperalgesia [18–22]. Moreover, in the microenvironment the continuous activation of receptors by proteases released from tumour and nonmalignant cells may lead to the development of mechanical allodynia in cancer patients [1, 23].

Sympathetic postganglionic fibres also release norepinephrine (NE), which stimulates autoreceptors on the same endings, which in turn leads to the release of leukotrienes (LTD4) and prostaglandins (PG) that sensitise nociceptors. Prostaglandins play an important role in the modulation and perception of nociceptive stimuli, since their release at the site of tissue damage and inflammation lowers the excitation threshold for the activation of sensory fibres in response to nociceptive stimulation [24].

As a result of the above mechanisms, neurogenic inflammation develops in damaged tissues. This leads to peripheral sensitisation. It is caused and exacerbated by a direct activation of nociceptors and "extravasation" of algesiogenic and sensitising factors. This sensitisation of nociceptors is responsible for the occurrence of primary hyperalgesia, involves increased sensitivity to noxious stimulation at the injury site, and is mediated by peripheral mechanisms (Fig. 5.2).

The emergence of "pain information" and peripheral sensitisation constitutes a dynamic process that occurs among cancer cells and nociceptors of primary afferent neurons [6, 7].

Nociceptive information, encoded as electrochemical signals, reaches the dorsal root ganglion (DRG) and causes the release of, among others, excitatory amino acids (EAA), substance P (SP), neurokinin A (NKA), and likely other peptides, which are transported from the DRG to the dorsal horn of the spinal cord. Together with other mediators, they act as neurotransmitters or modulators of sensory information [6, 7, 25].

A prolonged and/or powerful surge of nociceptive stimuli to the dorsal horn of the spinal cord, the type of surge that accompanies the development of the disease, causes the release of neurotransmitters EAA and SP from the central endings of nociceptive afferents (Aσ and C fibres) in the dorsal horn. The EAA activate AMPA (α-amino-3-hydroxy-5-methyl-4-isoxazolepropionic acid) receptors and trigger the rapid synaptic potentials and the removal of Mg^{2+} ions that block the ion channel associated with the NMDA (N-methyl-D-aspartate) receptor. As a result of these changes, calcium and sodium ions flow into the cell. Further, SP, by acting on neurokinin receptors (NK), also causes the shift of calcium ions into the cell and, together with EAA, activates metabotropic receptors (mGluR), which, in turn, leads to the activation of phospholipase C (PLC) and the release of inositol triphosphate (IP3) and diacylglycerol (DAG). PLC, IP3, and DAG act as intracellular transmitters of the second signalling system (in molecular biology). IP3 releases calcium ions from the endoplasmic reticulum, which, together with calcium ions coming through the ion channels associated with NMDA and NK receptors, causes the activation of the third signalling system (increased gene expression). DAG stimulates the translocation and activation of protein kinase C (PKC), which itself activates the inflow of calcium ions into the cell via the ion channel associated with the NMDA receptor and, together with calcium ions, increases the gene expression (third signal system). As a result of this process, new protein molecules and new receptors in the cellular membrane may be produced, which alters the activity of the nerve cells for extended periods of time (usually days), but in certain situations the change may be permanent and manifests itself by increasing hypersensitivity of CNS neurons.

Further, the increased concentration of calcium ions activates phospholipase A_2 (PLA2), which, by acting on arachidonic acid (AA), induces prostaglandin synthesis (PG) in the CNS. The elevated level of calcium ions also stimulates nitric oxide synthase (NOS) to produce nitric oxide (NO), which, by free diffusion among the neurons, glial cells, and retroactively the presynaptic endings, induces the windup mechanism, i.e., the activation of NMDA receptors and the release of pronociceptive neurotransmitters. Likewise, prostaglandins may diffuse to the neuroglia and intensify the release of pronociceptive neurotransmitters from the central endings of primary afferents; they may also induce neuroglia cells, i.e., astrocytes, to produce cytokines, a group of proinflammatory mediators in the CNS [6].

The source of cytokines in the CNS is the neuroglia. The activated microglia cells (astroglia, oligodendrocytes, microglia) produce numerous proinflammatory mediators, such as cytokines (TNF-alpha, IL-1a, IL-1b, IL-6), chemokines (fractalkine, Macrophage Inflammatory Protein-1α, Monocyte Chemotactic Protein-1), as well as cytotoxic compounds (free radicals, reactive oxygen and nitrogen), which activate appropriate surface receptors (i.e., the tumour necrosis factor receptor I, CX3C chemokine receptor I) [26, 27]. These mediators are also activated in the case of tumour growth within the CNS [28].

The induction of these mediators and activation of receptors, by acting on adjacent cells in the structures of the spinal cord, cause the spread of the activation process and change the properties of adjacent neurons. Positive feedback occurs between microglia and nerve cells, which brings about changes that manifest themselves clinically as hyperalgesia and allodynia. The above-described process of central sensitisation is a likely cause of (a) secondary hyperalgesia that extends beyond the injury site, (b) referred pain, and (c) the so-called pain memory associated with the hyperexcitability of nociceptive system and WDR cells (Fig. 5.2) [29, 30].

From the dorsal horn of the spinal cord, nociceptive information is transmitted to the higher levels of the CNS, with the final stage of the nociceptive process being the perception that occurs in the brain, which plays a cognitive role and is responsible for the awareness of pain stimulation, its assessment, and affective and emotional response to it. This is where anxiety, aggression, and anger occur and where behaviour models related to the remembered pain are shaped.

Bone Pain in the Cancer Patient

Bone pain is the most common type of pain caused by cancer. It is present in 28–45 % of patients with metastases to the bone [2, 31]. The majority of patients with metastatic bone disease experience moderate to severe pain. The third most common metastatic site is the skeleton (after the lung and the liver) [32, 33]. Metastases may invade bones in 30–69 % of cancer patients, especially in patients with advanced breast, lung, and prostate cancers [34].

In the case of blood cancers, pain syndromes primarily involve bone pain. These syndromes are caused both by osteolytic lesions and the infiltration of bone marrow by malignant cells [35] (Fig. 5.3). These processes induce pain by the activation of sensory and sympathetic nerve fibres which innervate the periosteum, mineralised bone, and bone marrow (especially in patients with multiple myeloma) [33]. In the event of absence of bone lesions, bone pain may be caused by bone marrow edema/ischemia or the stretching of periosteum caused by infiltration of the bone marrow by malignant cells and by mediators released from malignant cells in the bone marrow [33, 36].

Tumour growth in bones results in pain, and it may also be the consequence of skeletal fractures or compression of the spinal cord. Pathological fractures are the most frequent in patients with myeloma and breast cancer and affect primarily vertebral bodies, ribs, and long bones [34]. The most serious complications of vertebral metastases include cord compression caused by vertebral body collapse or spinal cord injury secondary to vascular supply compromised [37]. The collapse of vertebral bodies as a consequence of metastases is frequent in the thoracic spine and may cause compression of thoracic nerve roots and bilateral radicular pain localised to the chest or the upper abdomen [37]. Bone metastases are identified as osteolytic, osteosclerotic, or mixed, according to the appearance of the lesions on radiographs [38]. In patients with multiple myeloma and breast or lung malignancies where bone resorption predominates, the metastases have an osteolytic appearance. In bone metastases characterised by increased osteoblastic activity,

Fig. 5.3 Causes of bone pain in cancer patients

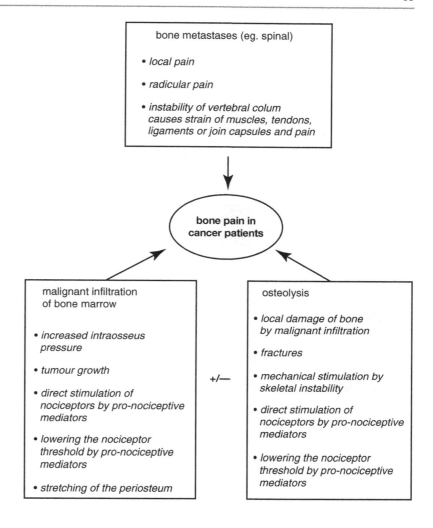

the lesions appear sclerotic and are typical of metastases from the prostate tumour [2]. Both osteolytic and osteosclerotic tumours induce the loss of mechanical strength and stability of the bone affected by the neoplastic process; hence innocuous mechanical stimulation (pressure, movement) may produce a distortion in the mechanosensitive sensory nerve fibres that innervate the bone. Studies on animals and humans have suggested that osteoclasts play a significant role in the mechanism of bone cancer pain development. Both osteolytic and osteoblastic cancers are characterised by osteoclasts proliferation and hypertrophy [39–43].

Osteoclasts are activated both by tumour products and by osteoclast-stimulating substances released by immune cells that are activated by mediators, which are themselves produced by the tumour [2, 44, 45]. Osteoclasts degrade bone minerals by secreting protons through the vacuolar H^+-ATPase, creating acidic microenvironments [46]. Extracellular protons are known to be potent activators of nociceptors; hence osteoclasts cause pain through proton secretion [16, 46].

Two acid-sensing ion channels – the acid-sensitive vanilloid receptor TRPV1 and acid-sensing ion channels-3 ASIC-3 – are expressed by nociceptors on primary afferents of the sensory neurons that innervate the marrow, mineralised bone, and periosteum. It is believed that osteoclasts play a significant part in the induction of bone pain in the cancer patient through the activation

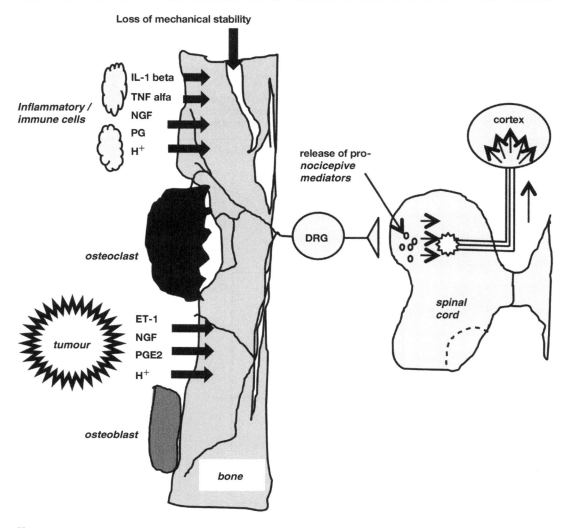

Fig. 5.4 Mechanism of bone pain in cancer patients (With permission from Jimenez-Andrade et al. [34])

of TRPV1 and ASIC-3 [47], because both acid-sensitive vanilloid receptors (TRPV1) and acid-sensing ion channels-3 (ASIC-3) are excited by a decrease in pH in the range of 4.0–5.0 caused by osteoclasts [46]. This is confirmed by the findings of experimental studies, in which the administration of TRPV1 receptor antagonists was found to attenuate nociception in bone pain in mice, in the cancer patient model [47]. Furthermore, immune and inflammatory cells also stimulate tumour cells and tumour stromal cells to release protons that generate local acidosis [16, 47].

It should be stressed that tumour mass is composed of tumour and tumour stromal cells (i.e., macrophages, neutrophils, fibroblasts, endothelial

cells). These cells release various mediators, which sensitise or directly excite nociceptors on primary afferent neurons (Fig. 5.4).

These factors include, among others, prostaglandins, cytokines, endothelins, and nerve growth factor (NGF) [32, 38, 48, 49, 50].

Prostaglandins are mediators which play a complex role in the etiology of bone pain. Prostaglandin concentrations increase at bone metastasis sites. Additionally, they are known to mediate osteolytic and osteoclastic metastatic bone changes. Prostaglandin E_2 is known to sensitise nociceptors and induce hyperalgesia [37, 38].

NGF may directly activate the sensory neurons that express the TrkA receptor and/or modulate

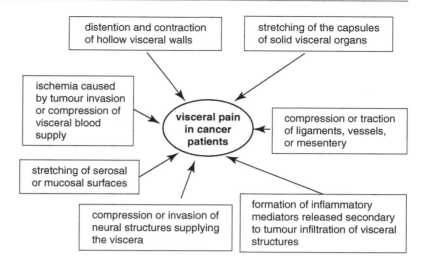

Fig. 5.5 Mechanisms responsible for visceral pain in cancer patients

the expression of proteins of sensory neurons expressing TrkA [8, 51]. NGF also appears to be closely involved in the upregulation, sensitisation, and disinhibition of multiple neurotransmitters, ion channels, and receptors in the primary afferent nerve fibres that synergistically increase nociceptive signals originating from the bone affected by the tumour [34].

Visceral Pain in the Cancer Patient

Visceral pain is caused by pathological processes occurring within the internal organs in the chest, the abdominal cavity, and the pelvis. Pain may result from the distention, impaction, ischemia, inflammation, or traction on the mesentery. Tumour tissue growth within viscera may induce all of the abovementioned mechanisms and, as a consequence, cause the onset of pain. In comparison with somatic pain, visceral pain is poorly localised due to both fewer receptors participating in the process of visceral pain and "scarce representation" within the primary somatosensory cortex [51, 52]. The diffuse nature of visceral pain and its referral to superficial structures are caused by the convergence of visceral and somatic afferents on the same neurons in the dorsal horn of the spinal cord. Convergent receptive fields are generally described as multidermatomal and are significantly larger than the receptive fields of spinal neurons, receiving only somatic input. These observations also explain why visceral pain is difficult to localise

and is often referred to other areas of the body. Viscera are innervated by two distinct classes of nociceptive sensory receptors. High-threshold receptors are activated by stimuli within the noxious range and contribute to the peripheral encoding of noxious events in the viscera. Nevertheless, the low-threshold receptors are activated by a range of stimulation intensity from innocuous to noxious. Visceral afferents are also called polymodal since they generate excitatory responses to inflammation, ischemia, stretching, and distention, in other words excitatory responses to different kinds of stimulation to somatic pain. Inflammation or hypoxia that may occur within the organs affected by the pathology induces the sensitisation and activation of receptors that under normal conditions are not stimulated by innocuous stimuli (e.g., distention) [51]. The main mechanisms responsible for visceral pain in cancer patients are shown in Fig. 5.5.

Obstruction due to neoplastic infiltration or inflammation within the biliary tract or pancreatic duct induced an increase in intralaminar pressure which causes both pain and a release of pronociceptive mediators, which additionally exacerbates the pain [53].

Tumours within certain organs (liver, spleen, kidneys) cause pain due to the stretching of the organ capsule especially in the case of rapidly growing liver tumours, which may lead even to a severalfold increase in the dimensions of this organ. This results in a significant increase in the intraorgan pressure and the ensuing stimulation of intracapsular mechanoreceptors Likewise, distention or traction on the gallbladder leads to deep epigastric pain. On the other hand, tumour growth within the spleen or kidneys does not lead to pain of comparable intensity to tumour growth in the liver. Kidney tumours produce pain only when the kidney has been almost completely destroyed and the tumour has invaded pararenal tissue or when it destroys the renal pelvis. Renal colic is usually secondary to urethral obstruction and the subsequent distention of renal pelvis and the ureter, as is usually the case with tumours located in the lower abdomen.

In pancreatic cancer, pain is caused by the obstruction of the pancreatic ducts; infiltration of pancreatic connective tissue, capillaries, and afferent nerves; and the invasion of adjacent organs by intra- and extrapancreatic perineural invasion by cancer cells. This is observed in 70–97 % of pancreatic cancer patients. It was found that the levels of pronociceptive mediators (NGF and TrKA mRNA) are markedly increased in pancreatic cancer and have been associated with a higher degree of pain. Moreover, overexpression of vanilloid receptors TRPV1 observed in pancreatic cancer patients significantly correlates with the severity of pain [53, 54]. At present, it is also believed that chemokine CX3CL1/fractalkine attracts receptor-positive pancreatic tumour cells to disseminate along peripheral nerves, which may, in part, explain severe pain experienced by patients suffering from pancreatic cancer [55]. The presence of back pain in pancreatic cancer patients may indicate that it has spread into retroperitoneum and para-aortic nodes as well as penetrated into paravertebral muscles [53, 56]. However, it needs to be underscored that an important pain mechanism in cancer patients may involve peritoneal carcinomatosis. In such cases, pain is caused by peritoneal irritation, mesenteric compression/distention, abdominal wall distention with ascites, and bowel obstruction.

Neuropathic Pain

Neuropathic pain is defined as pain arising as a direct consequence of a lesion or disease affecting the somatosensory system. This type of pain develops if the nervous system is damaged, which, in the case of cancer, may occur due to either tumour infiltration of nerves, as a result of tumour-associated or therapy-related toxin activity, or surgical damage [57, 58]. The prevalence of cancer patients with neuropathic pain ranges from a conservative estimate of 19 % to a liberal one of 39 % (if patients with mixed pain were included) [59]. The prevalence of pain with a neuropathic mechanism ranged from 18.7 to 21.4 % of all recorded pain in cancer patients [59]. Findings of the etiology of neuropathic pain in cancer patients indicate that in 63 % of cases it is caused directly by cancer and in 20.3 % by cancer treatment, in 3.5 % it is associated with cancer, in 10.2 % it is unrelated to the cancer, and in 2 % its etiology remains unknown [59]. Neuropathic pain associated with cancer is detailed in Chap. 13 and in the following references [60, 61].

The mechanisms involved are in Fig. 5.6.

Furthermore, nerve damage leads to a pathological interaction between the somatic and autonomous systems. This interaction is caused by the development of pathological points of contact – ephapses – between Aβ afferent fibres that conduct the sensation of touch and nociceptive fibres Aσ and C and efferent sympathetic fibres, both along the nerve and within the neuroma. Additionally, sympathetic fibres sprout and wrap around the DRG in a way that resembles a basket. Thus mutual excitation may occur directly or indirectly by endogenous catecholamines. The abovementioned changes in the proximal part of the damaged nerve cause the sympathetically maintained pain component [62–65].

The mechanism of neuropathic pain may also accompany inflammatory processes. At the nerve damage site, tissues and vessels release substances such as BK, 5-HT, hydrogen ions, prostanoids, NGF, cytokines, and free radicals, which leads to the inflow of immune cells and plasma transudate and the lowering of the excitation threshold in the endings of nerves that innervate the nerve trunks (nervi nervorum). Inflammatory processes may lead to neuropathic pain even without structural nerve damage. In recent years, researchers underlined the role of glia cell excitation and an increased release of proinflammatory cytokines in the development of chronic pain

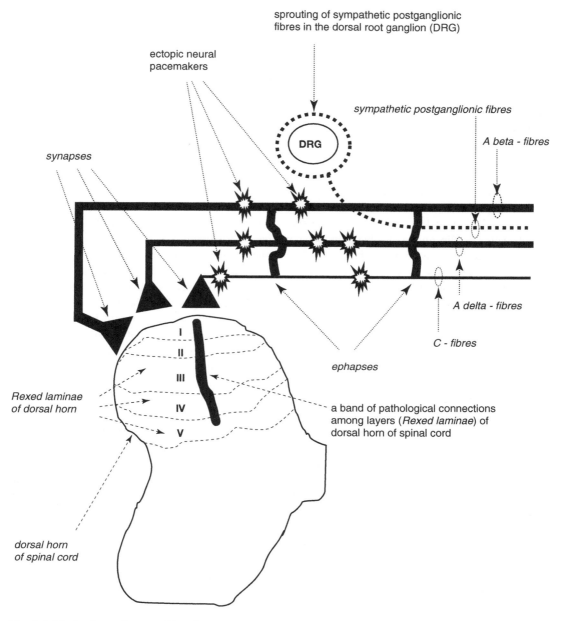

Fig. 5.6 Mechanisms of neuropathic pain

syndromes, both following spinal cord damage and peripheral nerve damage. It is postulated that the excitation of glia cells causes referred pain distant from the damage site as well as mirror-reflection pain syndromes [26, 66–68].

Under normal conditions, pain is transmitted by afferent neuron fibres, whose afferent dendrocytes

reach Rexed laminae I and II in the dorsal horn. On the other hand, Aβ fibres that transmit the sensation of touch reach layer III. However, in the case of peripheral nerve damage, some neurons in the areas of the spinal cord that are not responsible for pain transmission (i.e., Aβ) also sprout into lamina II of the dorsal horn of the spinal cord, which is the area involved in the transmission of nociceptive afferent inputs [69]. As a result of these processes, a band of nerve fibres grow that combine neurons from layer II to layer V. This is followed by increased neuronal activity, expansion of the neuronal receptive field, and hyperexcitability of other regions. This fact enables us to explain the central mechanism behind allodynia or, in other words, why the irritation of neurons Aβ (that transmit the sensation of touch) causes pain [70] (Fig. 5.6). Following nerve damage, central changes not only involve the neurons of the dorsal horns of the spinal cord but also diffuse throughout the entire CNS. Systems of new mutual excitation and feedback loops emerge, which, acting as if in a wave, involve progressively higher CNS levels. In accordance with the principles of cybernetics, feedback loops are bound by certain limits determined by their energy and placement in time. If these limits are exceeded, the mechanism gets "out of control" of other systems and oscillates as if nonsensically beyond the point of return to the normal state [71].

Paraneoplastic Syndrome

Paraneoplastic neurological syndromes (PNS) comprise an infrequent, highly heterogenous group of disorders caused by, or associated with, cancer. These syndromes may affect several areas of the nervous system. The best-known paraneoplastic neurological syndromes include paraneoplastic encephalomyelitis, cerebellar degeneration, sensory neuronopathy, Lambert–Eaton myasthenic syndrome, and paraneoplastic myopathy [72, 73]. Paraneoplastic neurological syndromes (PNS) include clinically distinct nervous system disorders in cancer patients, in whom the malignancy is located outside the nervous system and is unrelated to the presence of metastases or to the local tumour activity. The best-studied pathomechanism of the PNS is immunologic response to an onconeural antigen shared by the tumour and the nervous system. The development of the paraneoplastic syndrome entails prior damage to the blood–brain barrier by cytokines. Immunologic response of the body directed against the cancer cells in which onconeural proteins express themselves also involves the nervous system [72–74]. Some paraneoplastic syndromes are causally

associated with a specific type of cancer, but others appear in the course of various cancers. In as many as 80 % of patients, the cause of the paraneoplastic syndrome is lung cancer, usually microcellular, and rarely lymphoma or gynaecological tumours [75].

The PNS may affect virtually any part of the nervous system, but its most frequent clinical manifestation involves peripheral neuropathy. Most cases represent one of the four types of the condition: sensory, motor, sensorimotor or autonomic. From a clinical point of view, they cannot be distinguished from the more common non-paraneoplastic neuropathy, but they resolve after cancer treatment and are associated with the presence of a paraneoplastic antibody.

Paraneoplastic syndromes constitute an important group of diseases due to the fact that they may be the first signs of an otherwise occult cancer. They may also serve as useful indicators of the efficacy of cancer treatment and supply prognostic information (the paraneoplastic syndrome is usually associated with a poorer prognosis) and often cause symptoms with a significant impact on the patients' quality of life [74, 76–78].

Tumour/Metastasis Compression or Infiltration of the Skull or CNS Structures (Brain)

Central pain syndromes are relatively infrequent in the cancer population. Painful cranial neuralgias may occur secondary to head and neck (especially nasopharynx) cancers and skull and leptomeningeal metastases [79].

In the case of accompanying skull metastases, especially involving the base of the skull, the main symptoms include constant localised aching pain from bone destruction and neurological deficits due to progressive cranial nerve palsies.

Base-of-skull metastases are frequently associated with primary lung tumours and breast and prostate cancers. They produce neuropathic pain syndromes, which coexist with symptoms of dysfunction of one or more cranial nerves. Cranial nerves are often affected at the level of middle or posterior cranial fossae. Clinical symptoms may result from a tumour or a metastasis in the area or from leptomeningeal metastases. The neoplastic process located in the middle cranial fossa induces paresthesias, dysesthesias, and facial numbness involving the innervation of the second and third division of the trigeminal nerve with accompanying episodes of lancinating or throbbing pain. In the case of glossopharyngeal nerve involvement in the area of the jugular foramen, pain is distributed over the ear or mastoid region and may radiate to the neck and shoulder. Concomitant deficits include paresis of the palate, the vocal cords, sternocleidomastoid, or trapezius muscles or Horner syndrome. Sometimes, especially during severe pain attacks, patients may experience syncope [2].

Leptomeningeal Metastases (Carcinomatous Meningitis)

Meningeal carcinomatosis may develop as a result of cancer cells spreading through the cerebrospinal fluid from direct extension of parenchymal brain metastases or from paravertebral lymph node metastases infiltrating along a spinal nerve root into the spinal canal. Cancer cells may also spread haematogenously via the capillaries of the arachnoid villi.

It is estimated that ca. 5–10 % of patients with diffuse cancer develop carcinomatous meningitis [80, 81]. Most patients with meningeal infiltration are those with breast and lung cancer, lymphoma, or melanoma [80].

Patients usually complain of headaches (30–74 %), cranial neuropathies, painful radiculopathies, and confusion. Headaches may be severe and tend to be associated with other symptoms of meningeal irritation such as nausea, vomiting, photophobia, and rigidity. Radicular pain in the buttocks and leg is also frequent and occurs in about one-third of cases [81, 82].

It needs to be noted that about 74 % of patients with carcinomatous meningitis are likely to suffer from brain metastases, which in one-half of them induces severe headaches as a consequence of increased intracranial pressure [83].

Spinal Cord Compression

Epidural spinal cord metastasis is a common complication and occurs in 5–8 % of all cancer patients [84]. It usually accompanies advanced stages of breast, prostate, and lung cancers [85, 86].

In about 69 % of cases, compression occurs in the thoracic region, in 20 % of cases it involves the lumbar spine, and in 10 % of cases it involves the cervical spine. Multiple sites of compression occur in about 20 % of patients [56, 84]. Metastatic pathways involve haematogenous or cerebrospinal fluid spread, or direct invasion from paravertebral tumours [86, 87].

Pain is the first symptom in 89 % of spinal cord compression cases. It results from vertebral metastases, root compression (radicular pain), and/or compression of the long tracts of the spinal cord (funicular pain). Therefore spinal metastases may be accompanied by local pain usually described as aching or gnawing within the segment invaded by the tumour [86] or back pain that exacerbates as the patient moves or during spinal weight-bearing, especially where vertebral bodies have been damaged by the disease. This damage causes instability of the vertebral column, which results in muscle, tendon, ligament, or joint capsule strain and subsequent pain [88].

Radicular pain occurs when metastases compress a nerve root inducing sharp and shooting pain [88].

Tumour/Metastasis Compression or Infiltration of the Peripheral Nervous System

Tumour-Related Mononeuropathy

The most often observed tumour-related painful mononeuropathy is intercostal nerve neuropathy secondary to rib or chest wall metastases. Rib metastases and their pathological fractures are usually observed in the case of breast, prostate, stomach, and colon cancers and multiple myeloma. Their incidence is estimated at 1–5 %. Their main symptom is pain that increases intensity with deep inhalation, body movement, coughing, sneezing, and changing body posture [89].

Tumour-Related Plexopathy

Cervical plexus pathologies usually develop in the case of primary head and neck tumours or metastases to lymph nodes in the neck. Pain in this patient group usually has lancinating or dysesthetic components referred to retroauricular and nuchal areas (lesser and greater auricular nerves), the periauricular area (greater auricular nerve), anterior neck and shoulder (transverse cutaneous), and supraclavicular nerve and jaw. They may be accompanied by other symptoms such as ipsilateral Horner syndrome and diaphragmatic nerve palsy [90].

Brachial plexopathy usually develops as a result of compression or infiltration of the brachial plexus from a tumour originating in the adjacent structures, such as axillary or supraclavicular lymph nodes, or from a tumour in the apex of the lung (Pancoast tumour), metastatic spread of tumours to the plexus, or post-radiation injury causing sensory or motor symptoms [89, 91–93].

In neoplastic brachial plexopathy, pain is the first symptom in 84 % of patients and often precedes neurological deficits [2]. Pain involves the arm, shoulder, and axilla. Its intensity increases substantially during shoulder movement. The pain is neuropathic in nature and is accompanied by numbness, paresthesias, dysesthesias, allodynia, and hyperesthesias [91]. There are several symptoms that make it possible to determine whether brachial plexopathies are secondary to metastatic changes in the plexus or due to radiotherapy. Thus, metastases most commonly involve the lower cords of the brachial plexus causing neurological symptoms in the distribution of C8–T1 nerve roots. In contrast, post-radiation plexopathy most commonly involves upper cords of the plexus, predominantly in the distribution of the C5–C7 roots. Severe pain and Horner syndrome are most commonly associated with metastatic plexopathy rather than with post-radiation plexopathy. Patients with neoplastic plexopathy have symptoms of shorter duration, especially pain prior to the diagnosis of plexopathy [91]. Epidural involvement occurs in a significant number of patients with metastatic plexopathy [37].

Lumbosacral plexopathy is caused by either a direct tumour infiltration from adjacent tissues or lymph nodes, compression from metastases in the bony pelvis, or post-radiation injury [92]. It is estimated that lumbosacral plexopathy due to metastases to retroperitoneal lymph nodes is the most often diagnosed neurological complication in patients with advanced cervical cancer [94].

The lumbosacral plexus is usually locally infiltrated or invaded by metastases of pelvic neoplasms. It may develop as a result of a local extension or nodal metastasis from colorectal cancer and other pelvic tumours (prostate, testicle, cervix, uterus, bladder), sarcomas, and lymphomas. It may also occur with metastases from breast and lung cancer or melanoma [92, 95, 96].

In one-third of cancer patients, neoplastic infiltration may occur involving the upper part of the plexus (L1–L4), and the pain may occur in the back, lower abdomen, iliac crest, or anterolateral thigh. In one-half of cancer patients with infiltration involving the lower plexus (L4–S3), pain occurs in the buttocks and perineum with referral to the posterolateral leg and thigh, and pain is commonly severe burning, cramping, or lancinating [2, 94].

Pain Caused by Anticancer Therapy

Certain pain syndromes diagnosed in cancer patients are due to treatment modalities including surgery, chemotherapy, and radiation therapy. In most cases, pain is the predominant symptom. Its source is in the damaged structures of the peripheral or central (mainly the spinal cord) nervous system. Sometimes, symptoms such as pain and concomitant neurological deficits develop with a delay of several weeks or even months, which may cause difficulties in differential diagnosis between complications of therapy and recurrent disease (Fig. 5.7).

Persistent Postoperative Pain (Postsurgical Neuropathy)

According to Marskey's current definition, persistent postoperative pain is a chronic, pathological pain that develops as a result of a prior surgical procedure, is related to the disruption of tissue continuity, and persists for over 3 months of the surgery despite tissue healing at the site of the surgery [97].

It has some neuropathic pain features resulting from the damage to the peripheral or central

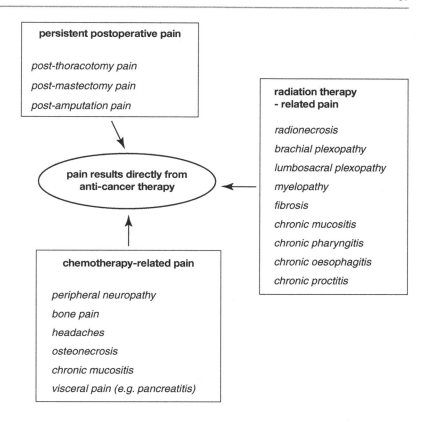

Fig. 5.7 Mechanisms of pain in cancer patients as a direct consequence of anticancer treatment

nervous system. It should be remembered that, especially in cancer patients, psychosocial factors such as anxiety, depression, catastrophizing, illness perception, poor coping strategy, a low sense of control, or poor social support may significantly increase the likelihood of developing persistent postoperative pain [98–100].

Persistent postoperative pain typically occurs in cancer patients following thoracotomy, mastectomy, or amputation [101].

Post-thoracotomy Pain

After thoracotomy, neuropathic pain may develop in the distribution of one or more intercostal nerves close to the thoracotomy scar. The incidence of persistent postoperative pain after thoracotomy varies widely from 5 to 65 % [100].

Traction on the ribs and rib resection are the most common causes of intercostal nerve injury during surgical procedures involving the chest [102]. Pain usually occurs in the area of sensory loss. Pain usually gradually diminishes after

months or years. It should be underlined, however, that whenever pain intensity increases (especially in the thoracotomy area) or occurs more than 3 months after surgery, it is usually due to the recurrence of the cancer [37, 103].

Post-mastectomy Pain

The incidence of persistent postoperative pain after mastectomy varies widely from 20 to 50 % [101, 104]. This pain syndrome most frequently occurs in young women who, apart from the surgery, were subjected to radiotherapy and in those after post-mastectomy breast reconstruction surgery [105–107].

Persistent post-mastectomy pain may present as postaxillary dissection pain which typically develops after several months of the surgery and is usually due to the damage of a section of the intercostobrachial nerve during axillary lymph node dissection [57]. Axillary plexus damage during surgery may also lead to pain and paresthesias in the hand. Persistent post-mastectomy pain may also affect the postoperative scar. This form of pain is characterised by allodynia, which frequently makes it impossible for patients to wear the breast prosthesis. In 7–13 % of patients, chronic pain syndromes present as phantom pain [106, 108, 109]. Persistent post-mastectomy pain more often occurs in female patients with postoperative complications, such as wound infection or local fibrosis [110].

Post-amputation Pain

Phantom pain disables a significant number of patients undergoing amputation of different body parts for malignancy. It is estimated that phantom breast pain occurs in 7–13 % of patients [108, 109], and phantom rectal pain occurs in up to 18 % of patients after surgery for rectal carcinoma [111]. After limb amputation for cancer, the prevalence of phantom limb pain in patients was 46.7 %, phantom sensation 90.7 %, and surgical stump pain 32.0 % [112]. The incidence of post-amputation pain is greater in cases in which pain was present in the body part before the amputation [112, 113]. Phantom sensation may also be related to visceral organs and may be associated with functional sensations, e.g., the urge to urinate or defecate [38].

Post-radiation Therapy Pain

Radiotherapy used in cancer treatment may cause damage to CNS structures, which may manifest as focal radionecrosis. They constitute a response to radiation that primarily affects the white matter of the brain or the spinal cord. It produces necrosis and vascular injuries as well as axonal and oligodendrocyte loss with gliosis and demyelination. Edema, mass effect, increased intracranial pressure, pain, and cognitive dysfunction are also observed [114–116].

Radiotherapy may lead to the damage of peripheral nervous system structures. Typical lesions include brachial and lumbosacral plexopathies or myelopathy [93, 116–118].

Post-radiation plexopathy occurs more often in patients who, apart from radiotherapy, were subjected to chemotherapy [116, 117]. Irradiation of the chest walls and the anatomic structures within the axilla may lead to the development of post-radiation brachial plexopathy [119, 120].

It should be underscored that in patients with a plexopathy caused by tumour growth or a metastasis, pain typically occurs earlier and its intensity is greater than in the case with pain following radiotherapy [93, 121].

Damage to the lumbosacral plexus due to radiotherapy usually develops secondary to intracavitary radium implants for carcinoma of the cervix [122]. Post-radiation plexopathy may also be due to post-radiation fibrosis of the plexus. Less frequently, the damage to the lumbosacral plexus is caused by plexus infiltration by the adjacent neoplasm or its destruction by a metastasis. In this case, pain is the most permanent symptom and is usually characterised by a greater intensity than in the case of post-radiation plexopathy [116, 118, 122].

Pain is an early symptom in about 15 % of patients suffering from post-radiation myelopathy [57]. It may have the form of subacute post-radiation myelopathy most likely secondary to transient demyelination. This kind of myelopathy generally develops one to several months after irradiation and usually involves the cervical spinal cord. It is the consequence of, among other things, irradiation of head and neck cancers. The onset of pain is usually preceded by other neurological symptoms. It involves dermatomes at or below the level of damage [116].

Another pain mechanism associated with local radiotherapy or some forms of chemotherapy is mucositis. It results from the damage of the mucosa by radiation or certain medications used in chemotherapy and the onset of chronic pain syndromes involving the mouth, pharynx, and sometimes the oesophagus [123]. Local radiation may also cause colorectal mucositis, colitis, and proctitis [123, 124].

Chemotherapy-Related Pain Syndromes

The incidence of cancer chemotherapy-induced peripheral neuropathy (CIPN) varies between 3 and 7 % in the case of single-agent use and up to 38 % when using combined medications [125]. Peripheral neuropathy is a common adverse effect of numerous medications used in chemotherapy such as cisplatin, oxaliplatin, vincristine, paclitaxel, and bortezomib [126, 127].

Medications used in cancer chemotherapy have a well-documented direct and indirect neurotoxic action. They affect nerve fibres by altering the amplitude of the action potential and conduction velocity. Medications used in cancer chemotherapy activate the membrane ion channels (sodium, calcium, potassium) or receptors (NMDA) on dorsal root ganglia and dorsal horn neurons to alter the cytosolic ion milieu. A special role in cytotoxic chemotherapy is attributed to the changes in intracellular calcium levels that trigger secondary changes inducing neuropathic pain. Increased intracellular calcium levels, activation of protein kinase C, and the production and release of nitric oxide and free radicals all induce cytotoxicity in axons and neuronal cell bodies [125].

The most frequently observed consequence of neurotoxicity of medications used in cancer chemotherapy is peripheral neuropathy. Chemotherapy-induced peripheral neuropathy may be very painful. It is the source of patients' suffering and also restricts treatment possibilities with potentially useful anticancer drugs [125].

Cisplatin is an anticancer drug widely used for cancer chemotherapy. Its most often observed neurotoxic symptoms include sensory neuropathy that initially manifests itself as pain and paresthesias in the distal parts of extremities [128]. The onset of neuropathy is usually delayed by a few weeks from the start of chemotherapy.

Unlike other drugs containing platinum, oxaliplatin causes an acute painful neuropathy, which becomes apparent within a short time after the administration of the drug [129] Around 90 % of patients experience acute, transient syndromes characterised by cramps, paresthesias, and dysesthesias, which are triggered or exacerbated by exposure to pain [125].

Another medication used in cancer chemotherapy is vincristine, which may cause neuropathy with predominant numbness, tingling and burning of hands and/or feet, numbness around the mouth, and loss of positional sense.

Paclitaxel-induced neurotoxicity usually manifests itself as a sensory neuropathy with symptoms that usually appear in a glove-and-stocking distribution [130]. It is thought that high doses of paclitaxel may also cause axon degeneration of peripheral nerves [131].

Bortezomib, another medication used for cancer chemotherapy, causes peripheral neuropathy that typically occurs during the first course of this drug, reaches a plateau, and usually does not appear to increase [125].

Another group of cancer medications includes the haematopoietic growth factors (HGF). They cause neuropathic pain fairly rarely, but may be the source of other types of pain. Thus, patients receiving granulocyte colony-stimulating factors (G-CSF) in the treatment of neutropenia that accompanies chemotherapy may experience bone pain and headaches secondary to the expansion of the haematopoietic matrix and the sensitisation of nerve endings in the bone marrow [132–134].

Bone marrow edema, ischemia, and the stretching of the periosteum due to bone marrow involvement and the activation of sensory and sympathetic nerve fibres that supply the periosteum, mineralised bone, and bone marrow are the traditionally suspected pain mechanisms in this patient group [34]. It is estimated that pain occurs in approximately 20 % of patients treated with G-CSF [125].

In turn, the therapy with bisphosphonates may cause severe pain and patient suffering secondary to osteonecrosis of the jaw [135]. One of the most painful complications occurring in patients with haematological malignancies under active treatment or in advanced phases of the disease is also oral ulcerative mucositis.

The group of medications that may cause the abovementioned symptoms may include the class of mTOR inhibitors, including sirolimus (rapamycin), temsirolimus, and everolimus [136–138].

Bortezomib and L-asparaginase are well-known agents that cause therapy-related visceral pain due

Fig. 5.8 Mechanisms of acute pain as a direct consequence of cancer management

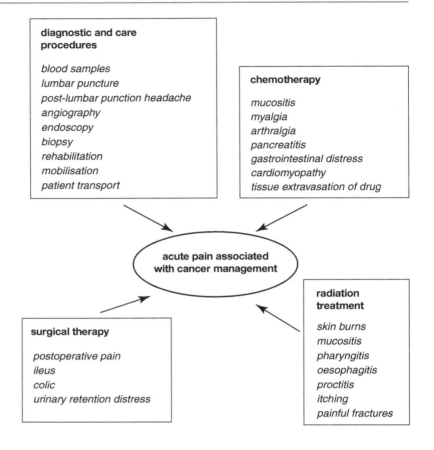

diagnostic and care procedures

blood samples
lumbar puncture
post-lumbar punction headache
angiography
endoscopy
biopsy
rehabilitation
mobilisation
patient transport

chemotherapy

mucositis
myalgia
arthralgia
pancreatitis
gastrointestinal distress
cardiomyopathy
tissue extravasation of drug

acute pain associated with cancer management

radiation treatment

skin burns
mucositis
pharyngitis
oesophagitis
proctitis
itching
painful fractures

surgical therapy

postoperative pain
ileus
colic
urinary retention distress

to acute pancreatitis, intestinal neuropathy, and visceral dysmotility [139].

Acute Pain Associated with Cancer Management

It should be underscored that a significant factor which has a negative impact on the quality of life of cancer patients is acute pain caused both by diagnostic and therapeutic procedures such as chemotherapy, radiotherapy, and surgery (Fig. 5.8) [2]. The acute pain mechanism in this case is associated with the induction of pathophysiological processes described above, but its nature and generally high intensity leads to very intense pain and patient suffering. For this reason, medical staff involved in cancer management must remember to relieve it as a matter of urgency.

Pain Indirectly Related to Cancer or Its Treatment

Infections

Acute herpes zoster is more likely to occur in cancer patients than in the general population because of the higher incidence of immunosuppression in cancer patients. One to two percent of patients have at least one herpes zoster infection during the course of their disease [140]. Approximately 25–50 % of patients develop postherpetic neuralgia following an acute infection [60, 141].

Muscle-Related Pain

The myofascial pain syndrome represents the major cause of muscle-related pain. The mean prevalence of this condition among middle-aged adults (30–60 years) is reported to be 37 % in men and 65 % in women, respectively. In the elderly (>65 years), the prevalence reaches 85 %. This kind of pain frequently occurs in cancer patients [142]. Myofascial pain is a common source of pain in women undergoing surgery for breast cancer. The aetiology of pain includes surgical damage of sensory nerves, axillary dissection, postoperative complications, complications of radiotherapy and chemotherapy, as well as activation of myofascial trigger points [143]. It may develop independent of malignancy or it may be a result of tumour-related tissue changes or treatment-related effects on soft tissues, e.g., surgery, chemotherapy, and radiation therapy [103, 143]. Muscle pain is generally described as aching and cramp-like. It can be difficult to localise and may be referred to other deep somatic structures. Inactivity, which is common in cancer patients in an advanced stage of the disease, predisposes to the development of muscle-related pain [103, 144].

Pain Secondary to Osteoporosis

Osteoporosis may be due to a significant bone mass loss that occurs in the course of glucocorticoid therapy or hypogonadism (i.e., androgen deprivation therapy, bilateral orchiectomy) and may cause pathological fractures of hips or vertebrae with accompanying pain [145].

Pain Related to Wounds/Pressure Ulcers

It is estimated that wounds occur in at least one-third of cancer patients at the end of their lives [146]. Risk factors for tissue breakdown and pressure ulcer development are similar since cancer patients with limited mobility and physical activity are exposed to the highest risk of developing pressure ulcers [146, 147]. Pain that accompanies this pathological process is typically exacerbated by the inflammatory process caused by wound infection.

Pain Caused by Mechanisms Unrelated to the Tumour or Its Treatment

Cancer patients, both during active treatment and in the terminal phase of the disease, may suffer from pain that has a mechanism unrelated to the tumour itself or its treatment. Migraine, tension headaches, osteoarthritis, painful diabetic neuropathy, and low-back pain all may preexist or coexist with cancer. However, consideration should be given that in cachectic patients in the terminal stage of the disease, these pain syndromes may have significantly more influences on the overall quality of life than cancer itself.

Key Points

- The mechanisms involved in the pain of cancer patients are complexed and multifactorial.
- These mechanisms are activated secondary to the disease process, treatment, or both. Due to the complexity of those mechanisms, this pain should not be termed "cancer pain," but pain in a cancer patient.
- Pain in a cancer patient can be classified as nociceptive (somatic, visceral), neuropathic, or mixed.
- A significant negative impact on the quality of life of cancer patients is exerted by acute pain due to both diagnostic (e.g., biopsy, blood sampling) and therapeutic procedures (e.g., acute postoperative pain).

   Understanding the underlying mechanisms of pain in the cancer patient should be the goal for effective management pathways rather than current empirical treatment strategy. Complex pain mechanism, in cancer patients, will require multimodal pharmacological and non-pharmacological treatment.

References

1. Schmidt BL, Hamamoto DT, Simone DA, Wilcox GL. Mechanism of cancer pain. Mol Interv. 2010; 10(3):164–78.

2. Fitzgibbon DR, Chapman CR. Cancer pain: assessment and diagnosis. In: Loeser JD, Butler SH, Chapman CR, Turk DC, editors. Bonica's management of pain. Philadelphia: Lippincott Williams &Wilkins; 2001. p. 623–58.

3. Urch CE. Pathophysiology of cancer pain. In: Walsh D, editor. Palliative medicine. Philadelphia: Saunders Elsevier; 2009. p. 1378–84.

4. Gold MS, Gebhart GF. Peripheral pain mechanisms and nociceptor sensitization. In: Fishman SM, Ballantyne JC, Rathmell JP, editors. Bonica's management of pain. Philadelphia: Wolters Kluwer/ Lippincott Williams & Wilkins; 2010. p. 24–34.

5. Stein C, Clark JD, Uhtaek O, Vasko MR, Wilcox GL, Overland AC, et al. Peripheral mechanisms of pain and analgesia. Brain Res Rev. 2009;60(1):90–113.

6. Basbaum AI, Bautista DM, Scherrer G, Julius D. Cellular and molecular mechanisms of pain. Cell. 2009;139(2):267–84.

7. Meyer RA, Ringkamp M, Campbell JN, Raja SN. Peripheral mechanisms of cutaneous nociception. In: McMahon SB, Koltzenburg M, editors. Wall and Melzack's textbook of pain. Philadelphia: Elsevier; 2008. p. 3–34.

8. Friedman WJ, Greene LA. Neurotrophin signaling via Trks and p75. Exp Cell Res. 1999;253(1):131–42.

9. Descamps S, Toillon RA, Adriaenssens E, Pawlowski V, Cool SM, Nurcombe V, et al. Nerve growth factor stimulates proliferation and survival of human breast cancer cells through two distinct signaling pathways. J Biol Chem. 2001;276(21):17864–70.

10. Geldof AA, Van Haarst EP, Newling DW. Neurotrophic factors in prostate and prostatic cancer. Prostate Cancer Prostatic Dis. 1998;1(5):236–41.

11. Ji RR, Samad TA, Jin SX, Schmoll R, Woolf CJ. p38 MAPK activation by NGF in primary sensory neurons after inflammation increases TRPV1 levels and maintains heat hyperalgesia. Neuron. 2002;36(1):57–68.

12. Mamet J, Baron A, Lazdunski M, Voilley N. Proinflammatory mediators, stimulators of sensory neuron excitability via the expression of acid-sensing ion channels. J Neurosci. 2002;22:10662–70.

13. Woolf CJ, Allchorne A, Safieh-Garabedian B, Poole S. Cytokines, nerve growth factor and inflammatory hyperalgesia: the contribution of tumour necrosis factor α. Br J Pharmacol. 1997;121(3):417–24.

14. Constantin CE, Mair N, Sailer CA, Andratsch M, Xu ZZ, Blumer MJ, et al. Endogenous tumor necrosis factor α (TNFα) requires TNF receptor type 2 to generate heat hyperalgesia in mouse cancer model. J Neurosci. 2008;28:5072–81.

15. Teitelbaum SL. Osteoclasts: what do they do and how do they do it? Am J Pathol. 2007;170(2):427–35.

16. Julius D, Basbaum AI. Molecular mechanisms of nociception. Nature. 2001;413:203–10.

17. DeClerck YA, Mercurio AM, Stack MS, Chapman HA, Zutter MM, Muschel RJ, et al. Proteases, extracellular matrix, and cancer: a workshop of the path B study section. Am J Pathol. 2004;164(4):1131–9.

18. Hoogerwerf WA, Zou L, Shenoy M, Sun D, Micci MA, Lee-Hellmich H, et al. The proteinase-activated receptor 2 is involved in nociception. J Neurosci. 2001;21:9036–42.

19. Alier KA, Endicott JA, Stemkowski PL, Cenac N, Cellars L, Chapman K, et al. Intrathecal administration of proteinase-activated receptor-2 agonists produces hyperalgesia by exciting the cell bodies of primary sensory neurons. J Pharmacol Exp Ther. 2008;324: 224–33.

20. Steinhoff M, Vergnolle N, Young SH, Tognetto M, Amadesi S, Ennes HS, et al. Agonists of proteinase activated receptor 2 induce inflammation by a neurogenic mechanism. Nat Med. 2000;6:151–8.

21. Amadesi S, Cottrell GS, Divino L, Chapman K, Grady EF, Bautista F, et al. Protease-activated receptor2 sensitizes TRPV1 by protein kinase Cε- and A-dependent mechanisms in rats and mice. J Physiol. 2006;575(2): 555–71.

22. Grant AD, Cottrell GS, Amadesi S, Trevisani M, Nicoletti P, Materazzi S, et al. Protease-activated receptor 2 sensitizes the transient receptor potential vanilloid 4 ion channel to cause mechanical hyperalgesia in mice. J Physiol. 2007;578(3):715–33.

23. Lam DK, Schmidt BL. Serine proteases and protease-activated receptor 2-dependent allodynia: a novel cancer pain pathway. Pain. 2010;149(2):263–72.

24. McMahon SB. Mechanisms of sympathetic pain. Br Med Bull. 1991;47(3):584–600.

25. Mercadante S. Pathophysiology of chronic pain. In: Bruera E, Higginson IJ, Ripamonti C, von Gunten C, editors. Textbook of palliative medicine. London: Edward Arnold; 2006. p. 359–66.

26. Erin D, Milligan L, Watkins R. Pathological and protective roles of glia in chronic pain. Nat Rev. 2009;10:23–36.

27. O'Callaghan JP, Miller DB. Spinal glia and chronic pain. Metabolism. 2010;59 Suppl 1:21–6.

28. Khasabov SG, Hamamoto DT, Harding-Rose C, Simone DA. Tumor-evoked hyperalgesia and sensitization of nociceptive dorsal horn neurons in a murine model of cancer pain. Brain Res. 2007;1180:7–19.

29. Watkins LR, Milligan ED, Maier SF. Glial activation: a driving force for pathological pain. Trends Neurosci. 2001;24:450–5.

30. Randich A, Ness T. Modulation of spinal nociceptive processing. In: Fishman SM, Ballantyne JC, Rathmell JP, editors. Bonica's management of pain. Philadelphia: Wolters Kluwer/Lippincott Williams & Wilkins; 2010. p. 48–60.

31. Coleman RE. Clinical features of metastatic bone disease and risk of skeletal morbidity. Clin Cancer Res. 2006;12:6243–9.

32. Middlemiss T, Laird BJA, Fallon MT. Mechanisms of cancer-induced bone pain. Clin Oncol. 2011;23:387–92.

33. Sabino MA, Mantyh PW. Pathophysiology of bone cancer pain. J Support Oncol. 2005;3(1):15–24.

34. Jimenez-Andrade JM, Mantyh WG, Bloom AP, Ferng AS, Geffre CP, Mantyh PW. Bone cancer pain. Ann N Y Acad Sci. 2010;1198:173–81.

35. Niscola P, Arcuri E, Giovannini M, Scaramucci L, Romani C, Palombi F, et al. Pain syndromes in haematological malignancies: an overview. Hematol J. 2004;5:293–303.
36. Niscola P, Tendas A, Scaramucci L, Giovaninni M, Cupelli L, De Sanctis V, et al. Pain in malignant hematology. Expert Rev Hematol. 2011;4(1):81–93.
37. Reddy SK. Causes and mechanisms of pain in palliative care patients. In: Bruera E, Higginson IJ, Ripamonti C, von Gunten C, editors. Textbook of palliative medicine. London: Edward Arnold; 2009. p. 368–79.
38. Theriault RL, Theriault RL. Biology of bone metastases. Cancer Control. 2012;19:92–101.
39. Drake MT, Clarke BL, Khosla S. Bisphosphonates: mechanism of action and role in clinical practice. Mayo Clin Proc. 2008;83(9):1032–45.
40. Chen YC, Sosnoski DM, Mastro AM. Breast cancer metastasis to the bone: mechanisms of bone loss. Breast Cancer Res. 2010;12(6):215. http://breast-cancer-research.com/content/12/6/215,10.1186/bcr2781.
41. Lipton A. Future treatment of bone metastases. Clin Cancer Res. 2006;12:6305–8.
42. Mantyh PW. Cancer pain and its impact on diagnosis, survival and quality of life. Nat Rev Neurosci. 2006;7:797–809.
43. Von Moos R, Strasser F, Gillessen S, Zaugg K. Metastatic bone pain: treatment options with an emphasis on bisphosphonates. Support Care Cancer. 2008;16:1105–15.
44. Yoneda T, Hata K, Nakanishi M, Nagae M, Nagayama T, Wakabayashi H, et al. Involvement of acidic microenvironment in the pathophysiology of cancer-associated bone pain. Bone. 2011;48:100–5.
45. Halvorson KG, Sevcik MA, Ghilardi JR, Rosol TJ, Mantyh PW. Similarities and differences in tumor growth, skeletal remodeling and pain in an osteolytic and osteoblastic model of bone cancer. Clin J Pain. 2006;22:587–600.
46. Nagae M, Hiraga T, Wakabayashi H, Wang L, Iwata K, Yoneda T. Osteoclasts play a part in pain due to the inflammation adjacent to bone. Bone. 2006;39:1107–15.
47. Ghilardi JR, Röhrich H, Lindsay TH, Sevcik MA, Schwei MJ, Kubota K, et al. Selective blockade of the capsaicin receptor TRPV1 attenuates bone cancer pain. J Neurosci. 2005;25:3126–31.
48. Joyce JA, Pollard JW. Microenvironmental regulation of metastasis. Nat Rev Cancer. 2009;9(4):239–52.
49. Schmidt BL, Pickering V, Liu S, Quang P, Dolan J, Connelly ST, et al. Peripheral endothelin A receptor antagonism attenuates carcinoma-induced pain. Eur J Pain. 2007;11:406–14.
50. Pezet S, McMahon SB. Neurotrophins: mediators and modulators of pain. Annu Rev Neurosci. 2006;29:507–38.
51. Abraham J, Ross E, Klickovich RJ. Cancer-related visceral pain. In: Fishman SM, Ballantyne JC, Rathmell JP, editors. Bonica's management of pain. Philadelphia: Wolters Kluwer/Lippincott Williams & Wilkins; 2010. p. 635–44.
52. Larauche M, Mulak A, Taché Y. Stress and visceral pain: from animal models to clinical therapies. Exp Neurol. 2012;233:49–67.
53. Ceyhan GO, Michalski CW, Demir IE, Muller MW, Friess H. Pancreatic pain. Best Pract Res Clin Gastroenterol. 2008;22(1):31–44.
54. Hirai I, Kimura W, Ozawa K, Kudo S, Suto K, Kuzu H, et al. Perineural invasion in pancreatic cancer. Pancreas. 2002;24:15–25.
55. Marchesi F, Piemonti L, Mantovani A, Allavena P. Molecular mechanisms of perineural invasion, a forgotten pathway of dissemination and metastasis. Cytokine Growth Factor Rev. 2010;21:77–82.
56. Twycross R. Cancer pain syndromes. In: Rice ASC, Warfield CA, Justins D, Eccleston C, editors. Cancer pain. London: Arnold; 2003. p. 3–19.
57. Manfredi PI, Gonzales GR, Sady R, Chandler S, Payne R. Neuropathic pain in patients with cancer. J Palliat Care. 2003;19:115–8.
58. Treede RD, Jensen TS, Campbell JN, Cruccu G, Dostrovsky JO, Griffin JW, et al. Neuropathic pain: redefinition and a grading system for clinical and research purposes. Neurology. 2008;70(18):1630–5.
59. Bennett MI, Rayment C, Hjermstad M, Aass N, Caraceni A, Kaasa S. Prevalence and aetiology of neuropathic pain in cancer patients: A systematic review. Pain. 2012;153:359–65.
60. Andrea M, Harriott BS, Gold MS. Contribution of primary afferent channels to neuropathic pain. Curr Pain Headache Rep. 2009;13:197–207.
61. Xua Q, Yaksh TL. A brief comparison of the pathophysiology of inflammatory versus neuropathic pain. Curr Opin Anaesthesiol. 2011;24:400–7.
62. Chung K, Lee BH, Yoon YW, Chung JM. Sympathetic sprouting in the dorsal root ganglia of the injured peripheral nerve in a rat neuropathic pain model. J Comp Neurol. 1996;376:241–51.
63. Lanteri-Minet M. Physiopathology of neuropathic pain syndromes. Therapie. 1999;54(1):117–20.
64. Chien SQ, Li C, Li H, Xie W, Zhang JM. Sympathetic fiber sprouting in chronically compressed dorsal root ganglia without peripheral axotomy. J Neuropathic Pain Symptom Palliation. 2005;1(1):19–23.
65. Dib-Hajj SD, Binshtok AM, Cummins TR, Jarvis MF, Samad T, Zimmermann K. Voltage-gated sodium channels in pain states: role in pathophysiology and targets for treatment. Brain Res Rev. 2009;60(1):65–83.
66. Mika J. Modulation of microglia can attenuate neuropathic pain symptoms and enhance morphine effectiveness. Pharmacol Rep. 2008;60(3):297–307.
67. Leung L, Cahill CM. TNF-α and neuropathic pain – a review. J Neuroinflammation. 2010;7(27):1–11.
68. Gao YJ, Ji RR. Chemokines, neuronal–glial interactions, and central processing of neuropathic pain. Pharmacol Ther. 2010;126(1):56–68.
69. Dickinson BD, Head CA, Gitlow S, Osbahr AJ. Maldynia: pathophysiology and management of neuropathic and maladaptive pain – a report of the AMA

Council on Science and Public Health. Pain Med. 2010;11(11):1635–53.

70. Woolf CJ, Shortland P, Coggeshall RE. Peripheral nerve injury triggers central sprouting of myelinated afferents. Nature. 1992;355:75–8.

71. Baron R, Binder A, Wasner G. Neuropathic pain: diagnosis, pathophysiological mechanisms, and treatment. Lancet Neurol. 2010;9(8):807–19.

72. Law M. Neurological complications. Cancer Imaging. 2009;9(Spec No A):71–4.

73. Blaes F, Tschernatsch M. Paraneoplastic neurological disorders. Expert Rev Neurother. 2010;10(10):1559–68.

74. Storstein A, Vedeler CA. Paraneoplastic neurological syndromes and onconeural antibodies: clinical and immunological aspects. Adv Clin Chem. 2007;44:143–85.

75. Honnorat J, Antoine JC. Paraneoplastic neurological syndromes. Orphanet J Rare Dis. 2007;2:22. http://www.OJRD.com/content/2/1/22.

76. Plantone D, Caliandro P, Iorio R, Frisullo G, Nociti V, Patanella AK, et al. Brainstem and spinal cord involvement in a paraneoplastic syndrome associated with anti-Yo antibody and breast cancer. J Neurol. 2011; 258(5):921–2.

77. Maddison P, Lang B. Paraneoplastic neurological autoimmunity and survival in small-cell lung cancer. J Neuroimmunol. 2008;201–202:159–62.

78. Danko K, Ponyi A, Molnar AP, Andras C, Constantin T. Paraneoplastic myopathy. Curr Opin Rheumatol. 2009;21(6):594–8.

79. Moris G, Perez-Pena M, Miranda E, Lopez Anglada J, Ribacoba R, Gonzalez C. Trigeminal mononeuropathy: first clinical manifestation of breast cancer. Eur Neurol. 2005;54(4):212–3.

80. Van Horn A, Chamberlain MC. Neoplastic meningitis. J Support Oncol. 2012;10(2):45–53.

81. Chamberlain MC. Neoplastic meningitis. Oncologist. 2008;13(9):967–77.

82. Grossman SA, Krabak MJ. Leptomeningeal carcinomatosis. Cancer Treat Rev. 1999;25(2):103–19.

83. Ostgathe C, Voltz R. Brain metastases. In: Walsh D, editor. Palliative medicine. Philadelphia: Saunders-Elsevier; 2009. p. 1240–4.

84. Loblaw DA, Perry J, Chambers A, Laperriere NJ. Systematic review of the diagnosis and management of malignant extradural spinal cord compression: the Cancer Care Ontario Practice Guidelines Initiative's Neuro-Oncology Disease Site Group. J Clin Oncol. 2005;23:2028–37.

85. Maranzano E, Trippa F, Chirico L, Basagni ML, Rossi R. Management of metastatic spinal cord compression. Tumori. 2003;89(5):469–75.

86. Sciubba DM, Gokaslan ZL. Diagnosis and management of metastatic spine disease. Surg Oncol. 2006;15:141–51.

87. Ribas ES, Schiff D. Spinal cord compression. Curr Treat Options Neurol. 2012;14(4):391–401.

88. Janjan N, Lin E, McCutcheon I, Perkins G, Das P, Krishnan S, et al. Vertebral metastases and spinal cord compression. In: Walsh D, editor. Palliative medicine. Philadelphia: Saunders-Elsevier; 2009. p. 1247–60.

89. Griffo Y, Obbens EA. Neurological complications. In: Walsh D, editor. Palliative medicine. Philadelphia: Saunders-Elsevier; 2009. p. 1237–40.

90. Vecht CJ, Hoff AM, Kansen PJ, de Boer MF, Bosch DA. Types and causes of pain in cancer of the head and neck. Cancer. 1992;70(1):178–84.

91. Amato AA, Collins MP. Neuropathies associated with malignancy. Semin Neurol. 1998;18(1):125–44.

92. Jaeckle KA. Neurologic manifestations of neoplastic and radiation-induced plexopathies. Semin Neurol. 2010;30(3):254–62.

93. Iyer VR, Sanghvi DA, Merchant N. Malignant brachial plexopathy: a pictorial essay of MRI findings. Indian J Radiol Imaging. 2010;20(4):274–8.

94. Rigor BM. Pelvic cancer pain. J Surg Oncol. 2000;75(4):280–300.

95. Landha SS, Spinner RJ, Suarez GA, Amrami KK, Dyck PJ. Neoplastic lumbosacral radiculoplexopathy in prostate cancer by direct perineural spread: an unusual entity. Muscle Nerve. 2006;34(5):659–65.

96. Hébert-Blouin MN, Amrami KK, Myers RP, Hanna AS, Spinner RJ. Adenocarcinoma of the prostate involving the lumbosacral plexus: MRI evidence to support direct perineural spread. Acta Neurochir. 2010;152(9):1567–76.

97. Marskey H, Bogduk K. Descriptions of chronic pain syndromes and definitions of pain terms. 2nd ed. Seattle: IASP Press; 1994.

98. Macrae WA. Chronic post-surgical pain: 10 years on. Br J Anaesth. 2008;101(1):77–86.

99. Hinrichs-Rocker A, Schulz K, Jarvinen I, Lefering R, Simanski C, Neugebauer EA. Psychosocial predictors and correlates for chronic post-surgical pain (CPSP) – a systematic review. Eur J Pain. 2009;13(7):719–30.

100. Niraj G, Rowbotham DJ. Persistent postoperative pain: where are we now? Br J Anaesth. 2011;107(1):25–9.

101. Kehlet H, Jensen TS, Woolf CJ. Persistent postsurgical pain: risk factors and prevention. Lancet. 2006; 367(9522):1618–25.

102. Aasvang EK, Gmaehle E, Hansen JB, Gmaehle B, Forman JL, Schwarz J, et al. Predictive risk factors for persistent postherniotomy pain. Anesthesiology. 2010;112(4):957–69.

103. Fitzgibbon DR. Mechanisms, assessment, and diagnosis of pain due to cancer. In: Fishman SM, Ballantyne JC, Rathmell JP, editors. Bonica's management of pain. Philadelphia: Wolters Kluwer/Lippincott Williams & Wilkins; 2010. p. 559–82.

104. Vilholm OJ, Cold S, Rasmussen L, Sindrup SH. The postmastectomy pain syndrome: an epidemiological study on the prevalence of chronic pain after surgery for breast cancer. Br J Cancer. 2008;99(4):604–10.

105. Junga BF, Ahrendt M, Oaklander AL, Dworkin RH. Neuropathic pain following breast cancer surgery: proposed classification and research update. Pain. 2003;104(1–2):1–13.

106. Hansen DM, Kehlet H, Gärtner R. Phantom breast sensations are frequent after mastectomy. Dan Med Bull. 2011;58(4):A4259.

107. Vadivelu N, Schreck M, Lopez J, Kodumudi G, Narayan D. Pain after mastectomy and breast reconstruction. Am Surg. 2008;74(4):285–96.
108. Björkman B, Arnér S, Hydén LC. Phantom breast and other syndromes after mastectomy: eight breast cancer patients describe their experiences over time: a 2-year follow-up study. J Pain. 2008;9(11):1018–25.
109. Dijkstra PU, Rietman JS, Geertzen JH. Phantom breast sensations and phantom breast pain: a 2-year prospective study and a methodological analysis of literature. Eur J Pain. 2007;11(1):99–108.
110. Macdonald L, Bruce J, Scott NW, Smith WC, Chambers WA. Long-term follow-up of breast cancer survivors with post-mastectomy pain syndrome. Br J Cancer. 2005;92(2):225–30.
111. Ovesen P, Krøner K, Ornsholt J, Bach K. Phantom-related phenomena after rectal amputation: prevalence and clinical characteristics. Pain. 1991;44(3):289–91.
112. Probstner D, Thuler LC, Ishikawa NM, Alvarenga RM. Phantom limb phenomena in cancer amputees. Pain Pract. 2010;10(3):249–56.
113. Hanley MA, Jensen MP, Smith DG, Ehde DM, Edwards WT, Robinson LR. Preamputation pain and acute pain predict chronic pain after lower extremity amputation. J Pain. 2007;8(2):102–9.
114. Rinne ML, Lee EQ, Wen PY. Central nervous system complications of cancer therapy. J Support Oncol. 2012;10(4):133–41.
115. Soussain C, Ricard D, Fike JR, Mazeron JJ, Psimaras D, Delattre JY. CNS complications of radiotherapy and chemotherapy. Lancet. 2009;374(9701):1639–51.
116. Chamberlain MC. Neurotoxicity of cancer treatment. Curr Oncol Rep. 2010;12(1):60–7.
117. Dropcho EJ. Neurotoxicity of radiation therapy. Neurol Clin. 2010;28(1):217–34.
118. Westbury CB, Yarnold JR. Radiation fibrosis – current clinical and therapeutic perspectives. Clin Oncol (R Coll Radiol). 2012;24(10):657–72.
119. Schierle C, Winograd JM. Radiation-induced brachial plexopathy: review. Complication without a cure. J Reconstr Microsurg. 2004;20(2):149–52.
120. Chen AM, Hall WH, Li J, Beckett L, Farwell DG, Lau DH, et al. Brachial plexus-associated neuropathy after high-dose radiation therapy for head-and-neck cancer. Int J Radiat Oncol Biol Phys. 2012;84(1):165–9.
121. Gosk J, Rutowski R, Reichert P, Rabczyński J. Radiation-induced brachial plexus neuropathy – aetiopathogenesis, risk factors, differential diagnostics, symptoms and treatment. Folia Neuropathol. 2007;45(1):26–30.
122. Dahele M, Davey P, Reingold S, Shun WC. Radiation-induced lumbo-sacral plexopathy (RILSP): an important enigma. Clin Oncol (R Coll Radiol). 2006;18(5):427–8.
123. Sanguineti G, Sormani MP, Marur S, Gunn GB, Rao N, Cianchetti M, et al. Effect of radiotherapy and chemotherapy on the risk of mucositis during intensity-modulated radiation therapy for oropharyngeal cancer. Int J Radiat Oncol Biol Phys. 2012;83(1):235–42.
124. Rodríguez ML, Martín MM, Padellano LC, Palomo AM, Puebla YI. Gastrointestinal toxicity associated to radiation therapy. Clin Transl Oncol. 2010;12(8):554–61.
125. Jaggi AS, Singh N. Mechanisms in cancer-chemotherapeutic drugs-induced peripheral neuropathy. Toxicology. 2012;291(1–3):1–9.
126. Farquhar-Smith P. Chemotherapy-induced neuropathic pain. Curr Opin Support Palliat Care. 2011;5(1):1–7.
127. Wolf S, Barton D, Kottschade L, Grothey A, Loprinzi C. Chemotherapy induced peripheral neuropathy: prevention and treatment strategies. Eur J Cancer. 2008;44:1507–15.
128. Kelland L. The resurgence of platinum-based cancer chemotherapy. Nat Rev Cancer. 2007;8:573–84.
129. Pasetto LM, D'Andrea MR, Rossi E, Monfardini S. Oxaliplatin-related neurotoxicity: how and why? Crit Rev Oncol Hematol. 2006;59(2):159–68.
130. Dougherty PM, Cata JP, Cordella JV, Burton A, Weng HR. Taxol-induced sensory disturbance is characterized by preferential impairment of myelinated fiber function in cancer patients. Pain. 2004;109(1–2):132–42.
131. Rowinsky EK, Eisenhauer EA, Chaudhry V, Arbuck SG, Donehower RC. Clinical toxicities encountered with paclitaxel (TAXOL). Semin Oncol. 1993;20(4 Suppl 3):1–15.
132. Niscola P, Tendas A, Scaramucci L, Giovannini M, De Sanctis V. Pain in blood cancers. Indian J Palliat Care. 2011;17(3):175–83.
133. Pinto L, Liu Z, Doan Q, Bernal M, Dubois R, Lyman G. Comparison of pegfilgrastim with filgrastim on febrile neutropenia, grade IV neutropenia and bone pain: a meta-analysis of randomized controlled trials. Curr Med Res Opin. 2007;23:2283–95.
134. Niscola P, Romani C, Scaramucci L, Dentamaro T, Cupelli L, Tendas A, et al. Pain syndromes in the setting of haematopoietic stem cell transplantation for haematological malignancies. Bone Marrow Transplant. 2008;41(9):757–64.
135. Hoff AO, Toth B, Hu M, Hortobagyi GN, Gagel RF. Epidemiology and risk factors for osteonecrosis of the jaw in cancer patients. Ann N Y Acad Sci. 2011;1218:47–54.
136. Sweeney MP, Bagg J. The mouth and palliative care. Am J Hosp Palliat Care. 2000;17(2):118–24.
137. Cella D, Pulliam J, Fuchs H, Miller C, Hurd D, Wingard JR, et al. Evaluation of pain associated with oral mucositis during the acute period after administration of high-dose chemotherapy. Cancer. 2003;98(2):406–12.
138. Niscola P. Mucositis in malignant hematology. Expert Rev Hematol. 2010;3(1):57–65.
139. Flores-Calderón J, Exiga-Gonzaléz E, Morán-Villota S, Martín-Trejo J, Yamamoto-Nagano A. Acute pancreatitis in children with acute lymphoblastic leukemia treated with L-asparaginase. J Pediatr Hematol Oncol. 2009;31(10):790–3.
140. Dworkin RH, Johnson RW, Breuer J, et al. Recommendations for the management of herpes zoster. Clin Infect Dis. 2007;44:1–26.

141. Miaskowski C, Cleary J, Burney R, Coyne P, Finley R, Forter R, et al. Guide line for the management of cancer pain in adults and children. Glenview: American Pain Society; 2005.
142. Giamberardino MA, Affaitati G, Fabrizio A, Costantini R. Myofascial pain syndromes and their evaluation. Best Pract Res Clin Rheumatol. 2011; 25(2):185–98.
143. Torres Lacomba M, Mayoral del Moral O, Coperias Zazo JL, Gerwin RD, Goni AZ. Incidence of myofascial pain syndrome in breast cancer surgery: a prospective study. Clin J Pain. 2010;26:320–5.
144. Alvarez P, Ferrari LF, Levine JD. Muscle pain in models of chemotherapy-induced and alcohol-induced peripheral neuropathy. Ann Neurol. 2011;70(1):101–9.
145. Hoff AO, Gagel RF. Osteoporosis in breast and prostate cancer survivors. Oncology (Williston Park). 2005;19(5):651–8.
146. Langemo D. General principles and approaches to wound prevention and care at end of life: an overview. Ostomy Wound Manage. 2012;58:24–34.
147. Stephen-Haynes J. Pressure ulceration and palliative care: prevention, treatment, policy and outcomes. Int J Palliat Nurs. 2012;18:9–16.

Preclinical Cancer Pain Models

6

Joanna Mika, Wioletta Makuch,
and Barbara Przewlocka

Abstract

This chapter describes animal models of cancer pain and the changes observed in these models based on our experience in studying pain and data from the literature. We provide examples of animal models of non-bone cancer pain, including skin, pancreatic, orofacial, and neuroma models. Many of the most common tumours, such as breast, prostate, kidney, thyroid, and lung cancer, undergo bone metastasis in animals; therefore, we also describe models of cancer pain that appear spontaneously and can be induced in bones. Moreover, we discuss models of neuropathic cancer pain, which is the most difficult to treat analgesically treatment in clinical settings and can be induced by both invasion and chemotherapy, and we collected data on immune factors important for cancer pain development in animal models. Furthermore, we also discuss the use of different behavioural methods to measure changes in the nociceptive threshold, which is diminished under cancer pain using electrical, mechanical, and thermal stimulation and the registration of motor disturbances.

Keywords

Animal models of cancer pain • Methods for cancer pain studies • Neuropathic pain • Chemotherapy-induced pain • Preclinical cancer pain models

J. Mika, PhD (✉) • W. Makuch, MSc
B. Przewlocka, PhD
Department of Pain Pharmacology,
Institute of Pharmacology,
Polish Academy of Sciences,
12 Smetna Street,
Kracow 31-343, Poland
e-mail: joamika@if-pan.krakow.pl;
makuch@if-pan.krakow.pl;
przebar@if-pan.krakow.pl

Introduction: Cancer Pain

People with cancer commonly experience pain as a consequence of the disease itself or as a result of the therapy. In 2007, van den Beuken-van Everdingen et al. [1] showed that in patients with advanced cancer, 62–86 % experience significant pain, which is described as moderate to severe in

M. Hanna, Z. Zylicz (eds.), *Cancer Pain*,
DOI 10.1007/978-0-85729-230-8_6, © Springer-Verlag London 2013

approximately 40–50 % and as extremely severe in 25–30 % of patients. Patients with advanced cancer commonly experience pain from bone cancer; two-thirds of humans with metastatic bone disease experience severe pain [2, 3]. It is well known that the skeleton is a preferred site for the metastasis of many of the most common tumours, such as kidney, thyroid, and lung cancer and particularly prostate and breast cancers [4–8]. Pain resulting from tumour growth in the bone remains a significant clinical issue because this condition compromises the patient's survival and quality of life.

Tumours can also cause pain by damage to the nerves. Whether inflammatory or neuropathic pain mechanisms dominate during tumour growth might depend on the interactions between tumour cells and surrounding tissues and nerves [9, 10]. Unfortunately, cancer therapies, such as surgical debridement, radiotherapy, and chemotherapy, can also injure nerves and cause neuropathic pain. The incidence of chemotherapy-induced peripheral neuropathy varies, depending on the conditions, from 3 to 7 % severe neuropathy with a single agent to 38 % with a combination of treatment regimens [11]. Scientists have explored the mechanisms responsible for cancer pathogenesis, and they have also created a variety of useful models to study the mechanisms of chemotherapy-induced peripheral neuropathy and cancer.

Primary and metastatic bone tumours were the first animal models developed to study cancer pain. Subsequently, nonbone cancer pain models were developed. Currently, there are a number of animal models of cancer pain that mimic different types of malignant (pancreatic cancer, breast cancer, sarcoma, melanoma, and prostate cancer) and benign (neuromas) cancers. Moreover, animal models of cancer pain have been developed to study the tumour invasion of peripheral nerves. Some studies have been conducted using naturally (spontaneously) occurring tumours in animals, which are natural models of cancer pain.

Despite numerous experimental and clinical studies, molecular mechanisms involving the onset and persistence of cancer pain are not fully understood. Cancer cells produce many different factors that affect other cells within the cancer microenvironment, such as immune cells. Nociception involves dynamic interactions and cross talk between the cancer and primary afferent nociceptors. Accordingly, it is problematic to study a single cancer cell in isolation; therefore, adequate animal models of cancer pain are needed. Animal models have many desired characteristics that fill the gap between in vitro and in vivo studies, and an investigator must consider the activities of the cancer cell, peripheral and central nervous system, and immune system. The enormous biological complexity of human cancer has stimulated the development of more appropriate experimental models that resemble the physiopathological aspects of cancer pain in a natural and spontaneous manner. Currently, there are a number of different animal models of cancer pain that effectively mirror the clinical conditions observed in humans.

Models of Cancer Pain

Models of Pain from Nonbone Cancer

Skin Cancer Pain Model

In recent years, several laboratories have injected tumour cells into the hindpaws of mice to induce skin cancer [12, 13], and this model provides a useful tool to investigate mechanisms of cancer pain as the measurement of tumour growth and cancer pain is relatively easy in the hindpaws of rats and mice. The changes in the spinal cord after the induction of skin cancer have been previously reported. Animals inoculated with melanoma cells into the plantar of the hindpaw show marked pain hypersensitivity [14, 15]. Given the low incidence of pain in melanoma patients (pain is not a major clinical symptom of melanoma, and only 7 % of patients still experience pain) [16], this model might not be clinically relevant compared with other models, such as bone cancer pain. However, this model is convenient to study mechanisms of cancer pain and tumour growth and to test new treatments.

Pancreatic Cancer Pain Model

Pancreatic cancer is typically detected in humans during its late stages, and pain management becomes a factor in maintaining the quality of life for patients [17]. Recently, a transgenic mouse model of cancer pain was developed in which pancreatic cancer was induced through the expression of the simian virus 40 large T antigen under control of the elastase-1 promoter [18]. This model of spontaneous pancreatic cancer development allowed the quantification of pain-related behaviours at early, intermediate, and late stages of cancer. Precancerous cellular changes were evident at 6 weeks in these mice and included increases in microvascular density, macrophages expressing nerve growth factor, and dense sensory and sympathetic fibres that innervated the pancreas [18, 19]. In this model, changes in pain-related behaviours and loss of opioid effectiveness were observed, which is similar to the effects observed in human patients. Importantly, the administration of the blood–brain-barrier-penetrating opioid antagonist naloxone induced overt pain-related behaviours in mice with pancreatic cancer [18, 19]. Understanding these mechanisms might facilitate the improved treatment and care of patients with pancreatic cancer. Pancreatic cancer cells that infiltrate the perineurium of local intrapancreatic nerves might cause pancreatic neuropathy. The actual mechanisms underlying pancreatic cancer pain are unknown, but the generation and maintenance of pancreatic cancer-related pain might involve neurogenic inflammation [20].

Orofacial Cancer Pain Model

In the rat orofacial cancer model, squamous carcinoma cells are injected into the subperiosteal tissue of the lower gingiva. The inoculation of cancer cells induces marked mechanical allodynia and thermal hyperalgesia in the ipsilateral maxillary and mandibular nerves, and these effects are associated with the increased expression of calcitonin gene-related peptide, substance P, P2X3 receptors, and TRPV1 in the trigeminal ganglia [21]. The clear characterisation of the upregulation of these proteins might lead to the development of novel therapeutics for the treatment of orofacial cancer.

Neuroma Transposition Model

Cancers often cause damage to the nerves, and neuropathic pain can develop as a consequence. The tibial neuroma transposition model is a model for investigating the mechanisms of tumour-induced nerve injury. In the tibial neuroma transposition model, the tibial nerve is ligated superior to the lateral malleolus, which allows a neuroma to form [22, 23]. Mechanical stimulation of the neuroma produces a pain behavioural response in rats. Although this model might be more representative of neuropathic pain than tumour pain, it does provide a useful tool to investigate the various mechanisms underlying the tenderness of the neuroma and mechanical hyperalgesia associated with neuropathic pain [22, 23].

Models of Bone Cancer Pain

The most common cancers, including lung, breast, and prostate cancer, have a remarkable propensity to metastasise to bone [5, 24]; therefore, bone cancer often appears in human patients with advanced cancer. One of the first symptoms of bone cancer is bone pain. When the bone tumour grows, the pain becomes more severe and difficult to treat with standard therapies [24]. Different animal models of bone cancer pain have been developed to better understand the mechanisms contributing to the development of tumour-induced bone pain, and these models share many similarities that occur in human bone cancer conditions, including skeletal remodelling, which accompanies metastatic bone cancer [3].

A frequently used method of inducing bone cancer is the application of different cancer cells directly into various bones—examples of such models are summarised in Table 6.1. Moreover, after the systemic or intracardiac administration of tumour cells, cancer growth can be monitored through an assessment of pain and motor behaviours, bone destruction, and radiographic imaging.

Table 6.1 Bone cancer pain models

Cancer type	Location	Animals	References
Melanoma	Humerus Calcaneus	Mouse (C3H/HeJ, B6C3fe/1)	Wacnik et al. [10]
Breast cancer cells (4T1)	Femur	Mouse (C3H-SCID, C3H/HeJ)	Sabino et al. [175, 176] Erin et al. [177]
Breast cancer cells (MDA-MB 231)	Femoral artery	Rat (nude)	Andersen et al. [178] Bauerle et al. [179]
Mammary gland carcinoma cells (MRMT1)	Tibia	Rat (Sprague–Dawley, Wistar)	Medhurst et al. [34] Urch et al. [180] Fox et al. [35]
Colon adenosarcoma	Femur	Mouse (C3H-SCID, C3H/HeJ)	Sabino et al. [175, 176]
Fibrosarcoma	Humerus Calcaneus	Mouse (C3H/HeJ, B6C3fe/1)	Wacnik et al. [10, 28] Vit at al. [31] Khasabov et al. [33]
Osteosarcoma	Humerus	Mouse (C3H/HeJ, B6C3fe/1)	Kehl et al. [29] Wacnik et al. [28] Vit et al. [31]
Sarcoma	Femur Tibia	Mouse (C3H/He; C3H/HeJ, B6C3-Fe-a/a, C3H/ HeNCrl, nude)	El Mouedden et al. [181] Goblirsch et al. [36] King et al. [32] Luger et al. [27] Menendez et al. [183]
XC Rous sarcoma-virus-transformed rat fibroblasts	Intraplantar	Mouse (Swiss CD1)	Baamonde et al. [182]
Prostate cancer cells (AT3.1, R3327)	Tibia	Rat (Copenhagen)	Zhang et al. [75] Liepe et al. [37]
Prostate cancer (human CWR22)	Intratibial	Rat (nude)	Andersen et al. [178]

Further, the analysis of histopathological, biochemical, and neuroanatomical changes can be performed in the peripheral and central nervous systems. The most common animal models of bone cancer pain have been developed in mice and rats. Mouse models of bone cancer pain are typically developed through the surgical implantation of tumour cells (e.g., sarcoma, fibrosarcoma, melanoma, and osteosarcoma) directly into the femur, calcaneus, or humerus bone [9, 25–33]. The percutaneous injection of cancer cells (e.g., carcinoma, prostate) into the tibia is typically used to generate bone cancer pain in rats [14, 34–39].

The Dunning R-3327 adenocarcinoma is a spontaneously developed prostate tumour in male rats that has a doubling time of 20 days and is androgen sensitive. The continuous subcutane-

ous passage of the R-3327 tumour resulted in the development of a rapidly growing, androgen insensitive, anaplastic tumour cell line with low metastatic potential. At the 60th passage, the R-3327 AT tumour cell line displayed a high metastatic potential and increased growth rate (doubling time about 1.5 days) and was renamed the MAT (metastatic-AT) tumour. The new MAT tumour cell line reproducibly demonstrated the metastatic development of tumours in the lungs and lymph nodes [40]. This tumour cell line was renamed as the MATLyLu, or "metastatic anaplastic tumour capable of spreading to the lymph nodes and lungs," cell line. MATLyLu (MLL) cells have an in vitro doubling time of 19.7 h. In addition, MLL cells have a characteristic spindle or polygonal shape and possess large nuclei [40].

The intra-femoral MLL cell injection results in tumour formation and progressive bone destruction. The induced bone damage leads to the progressive distribution of weight from the ipsilateral to the contralateral hind leg and a reduction in the ipsilateral paw withdrawal threshold. Recently, De Ciantis et al. [41] performed a complete histological and radiographic analysis of rodent femurs and an analysis of rodent behaviour in a model for cancer-induced bone pain in prostate cancer cell lines via measurements of nociceptive scores. This model could be used in the future for therapeutic studies examining the pain associated with cancer-induced bone metastasis.

In 1999, a cancer pain model was developed in B6C3-Fea/a and C3H/HeJ mice through the implantation of fibrosarcoma cells (NCTC 2472) directly into the femur. The important feature of the model is that the tumour cells are confined to the marrow space and do not invade adjacent soft tissues [25]. After injection, both ongoing and movement-evoked pain-related behaviours increased with increasing cancer cell proliferation and tumour development. These behaviours, which mimic those of patients with primary or metastatic bone cancer, are correlated with progressive bone destruction [25, 42, 43]. In 1999, Schwei et al. described the neurochemical changes that occur in the spinal cord and DRG in a mouse model of bone cancer. At 21 days after the intramedullary injection of osteolytic sarcoma cells into the femur, extensive bone destruction and invasion of the tumour into the periosteum was observed, which is similar to observations in patients with osteolytic bone cancer. The normal, non-noxious palpation of bones with cancer induces behaviours indicative of pain, and in this model, changes similar to those observed when neuropathic pain develops are observed in the spinal cord, e.g., an increase in dynorphin (endogenous opioid peptide that acts as a prohyperalgesic in a non-opioid manner) expression in the dorsal horn laminae of the spinal cord [44] and internalisation of substance P (an important neurotransmitter in nociception) receptors on the tumour-injected side of the spinal cord [25, 26]. The alterations in the neurochemistry of the spinal cord and sensitisation of primary afferents

were positively correlated with the extent of bone destruction and tumour growth. The mice showed nocifensive behaviour, such as vocalisation and guarding of the affected limb, and developed mechanical allodynia (a response to non-noxious mechanical stimuli, such as light touch or palpation). Interestingly, this author observed massive astrocyte hypertrophy in the spinal cord dorsal horn in tumour-bearing mice, which is uncommon in inflammatory or neuropathic pain conditions and thus represents a unique signature of cancer pain.

Obtaining measurements from nerves innervating tumours located in the femur or humerus bones was difficult. In 2001, Wacnik et al. developed a new model of tumour-induced bone destruction and pain produced by implantation of fibrosarcoma cells into the mouse calcaneus bone. This model facilitated the assessment of thermal and mechanical hyperalgesia and improved microperfusion access to measure the release of pain mediators and obtain electrophysiological recordings of nerves innervating the tumour. The electrophysiological recordings obtained from primary afferent fibres using this model showed that the spontaneous activity of tumour-induced calcaneus bone destruction was observed in 34 % of pain fibres (C fibres) at 2 weeks after tumour implantation. After fibrosarcoma or osteosarcoma cell implantation into the calcaneus, femur, or humerus bone, similar cancer-related bone destruction developed in mice.

In electrophysiological studies of central sensitisation, a model of bone cancer pain in which rat mammary gland carcinoma cells (MRMT-1; see below) are implanted into the tibia of female rats revealed that superficial (lamina I) dorsal horn neurons had enlarged receptive field areas, exhibiting enhanced responses to innocuous and noxious mechanical and heat stimuli. Central sensitisation has also been shown to follow the implantation of fibrosarcoma cells into the mouse hindpaw. Wide dynamic range (WDR) neurons exhibited an increase in spontaneous activity and enhanced responses to mechanical, heat, and cold stimuli applied to their receptive field [33]. Although the mechanisms that mediate central sensitisation following tumour development are not clear, it has recently been shown that mitogen-activated protein kinases might be involved [45]. There are a number of studies examining the mediators released at the tumour site that have identified a large number of potential algogenic factors (proinflammatory cytokines and neuropeptides) released by the bone or tumour itself and changes in the peripheral and central nervous systems.

In 1976, Harada [46] described the mammary carcinoma model, MRMT-1, which is induced in immunologically impaired rats fed 3-methylcholanthrene. In 2002, Medhurst et al. developed a rat MRMT-1 model of bone cancer using mammary gland carcinoma cells. The rats showed bone destruction at 2 weeks after intratibial injection, accompanied by gradual signs of hyperalgesia in weight-bearing tests and mechanical allodynia using von Frey monofilaments. The number of tartrate-resistant acid phosphatase-positive polykaryocytes, which were activated by prostaglandins, cytokines, and growth factors from tumour cells, was also increased. Astrocyte hypertrophy was observed at 17 days after MRMT-1 injection. Thus, the rat MRMT1 model in which cells are implanted into the tibia is more useful for behavioural studies because, in contrast to the mouse femur model, rats developed both mechanical allodynia and hyperalgesia [34]. Moreover, because of the bone size, the injection of tumour cells into rat bones is easier than in mice. However, mouse models are advantageous because tumour experiments can be performed on knockout or transgenic mice that over- or underexpress various proteins to determine the role of these proteins in cancer-induced pain.

Models of Neuropathic Cancer Pain

Invasion-Induced Neuropathic Pain

Cancer invasion of peripheral nerves often occurs in patients with vertebral metastasis or malignant lymphomas, during tumour progression as the tumour invades surrounding nerve bundles. Each of these conditions can lead to tumour-induced neuropathic pain syndromes [47]. Therefore, animal models that mimic cancer-induced neuropathic pain have been developed and can be broadly classified as cancer invasion pain models

[48]. Inoculation with Meth A sarcoma cells to the immediate proximity of the sciatic nerve in male BALB/c mice produced significant thermal hyperalgesia, mechanical allodynia, and spontaneous pain [48]. The animal behaviour observed in this model is correlated with the increased pain associated with the tumour invasion of nerves in human patients. In addition, the mechanical allodynia present on day 10 of the model changed to mechanical hyposensitivity on day 14. The damage to both myelinated and nonmyelinated fibres was more extensive in this cancer-induced neuropathy model than in sciatic nerve ligation, suggesting that cancer-associated nerve compression differs mechanistically from nerve ligation. Similar to other previous mouse cancer models, animals injected with Meth A cells showed an upregulation of dynorphin, c-Fos, and substance P expression in the spinal cord [49].

Chemotherapy-Induced Neuropathic Pain

Chemotherapeutic agents have been used for many years to treat tumour-induced peripheral neuropathy. Neuropathic pain syndrome occurs in approximately 20 % of patients receiving standard doses and nearly all patients receiving high-dose chemotherapy. Neurotoxicity is the primary reason for the dose reduction and discontinuation of this lifesaving therapy. Unlike the neuropathic pain associated with diabetes, which starts in the feet and spreads to the hands over a time course of months to years, neuropathic pain in chemotherapy-treated patients often begins simultaneously in the hands and feet [50]. Anticancer drugs, such as platinum-based drugs (cisplatin, carboplatin, and oxaliplatin) [51–53], vincristine [54, 55], taxanes (paclitaxel and docetaxel) [52, 56], epothilones [57], and bortezomib [58], have been well reported (Table 6.2) to exert direct and indirect effects on sensory nerves to alter the amplitude of action potential and conduction velocity and induce pain.

Although a variety of neuroprotective approaches have been investigated in both experimental studies and clinical trials, there is no available preventive strategy or effective treatment for chemotherapy-induced neurotoxicity because its aetiology has not been fully elucidated. Therefore,

Table 6.2 Possible mechanisms involved in development of chemotherapeutic agent-induced neuropathic pain

Chemotherapeutic agents	Mechanisms	References
Paclitaxel Vincristine	Loss of epidermal nerve fibres	Siau et al. [162, 184]
Bortezomib Cisplatin Paclitaxel Vincristine	Mitochondrial changes	Flatters and Bennett [61] Melli et al. [163] Broyl et al. [58]
Paclitaxel Suramin Vincristine	Dysregulation of cellular calcium homeostasis (increase in cytosolic calcium from extracellular and intracellular stores from mitochondria)	Sun and Windebank [164] Siau and Bennett [162, 184] Xiao et al. [165] Kaur et al. [145]
Oxaliplatin	Increase in Na+ current in DRG	Ghelardini et al. [146]
Cisplatin Oxaliplatin Paclitaxel	Upregulation of TRPV1, TRPA1, TRPM8, TRPV4 in sensory neurons	Alessandri-Haber et al. [166] Ta et al. [167] Anand et al. [168]
Bortezomib Vincristine Paclitaxel	Increased the level of TNF-alpha, IL-1beta, IL-6, and NO from glial and macrophages cells	Ledeboer et al. [74] Mangiacavalli et al. [169]
Bortezomib	Significant dysfunction of the afferent small fibres (A-beta, A-delta, C)	Mangiacavalli et al. [169]
Oxaliplatin	Activation of p38 and ERK1/2 in DRG neurons along with downregulation of JNK/Sapk	Scuteri et al. [170]
Cisplatin Paclitaxel	Increase the level of neuropeptides (neuropeptide Y, substance P, CGRP, somatostatin) in the spinal cord and/or DRG	Horvath et al. [171] Jamieson et al. [172] Ling et al. [51]
Oxaliplatin Vincristine	Dysfunction of the spinal NO/cGMP pathway	Kamei et al. [173] Mihara et al. [174]
Taxanes Epothilones	Microtubule-stabilising agent	Lee and Swain [57]

defining the mechanisms underlying the pain symptoms of chemotherapy-induced neuropathic pain is critical to develop preventive and treatment strategies and enhance the quality of life and functional status of cancer survivors. Notably, most chemotherapeutic drugs penetrate the blood–brain barrier poorly but readily penetrate the blood–nerve barrier and bind to the dorsal root ganglia (DRG) and peripheral axons [59, 60], which results in patient suffering and limits treatment with potentially useful anticancer drugs. Anticancer agents activate plasma membrane-localised ion channels on DRG and dorsal horn spinal cord neurons, including sodium, calcium, potassium, and glutamate-activated NMDA receptors, to alter ionic milieu in the cytosol, particularly intracellular calcium, which triggers

secondary changes to induce neuropathic pain [60]. These changes might include the opening of the mitochondrial permeability transition pore to induce intracellular calcium release, activation of protein kinase C, phosphorylation of TRPV, and generation of nitric oxide and free radicals to induce cytotoxicity to axons and neuronal cell bodies. Furthermore, the inflammatory process initiated in glial cells and macrophages also induces changes in the sensory neurons to alter nociceptive processing.

It is relatively straightforward to replicate chemotherapy-induced neuropathic pain in animal models. High doses of the drug paclitaxel destroy sensory fibres and motor neurons in rats; however, lower doses (2 mg/kg administered on 4 alternate days for a total of 8 mg/kg) lead to painful peripheral neuropathy in the distal extremities. There is a distinct delay between the last exposure to paclitaxel and onset of hypersensitivity, which mimics the "coasting" phenomenon described in patients [61]. Paclitaxel is used to treat various cancers, including breast cancer, non-small cell lung cancer, ovarian cancer, head and neck cancer, and melanoma [62–65]. Many cancer patients treated with paclitaxel complain of numbness, tingling, and burning pain [52, 62–68]. Paclitaxel is a vinca alkaloid that binds to tubulin, blocking the polymerisation of microtubules and interfering with mitosis; reported side effects include neuropathic pain development [62, 67, 69, 70]. Studies in rats showed that paclitaxel induces neuropathy that appears as mechanical and cold hyperalgesia without motor deficit that lasts for several weeks and is limited to the peripheral nerves [52, 67, 71]. Paclitaxel-treated rats have demonstrated severe axonal degeneration in DRG. This model revealed that paclitaxel produced minimal effects on the general health of the rats, similar to the patterns observed in human patients treated with the drug [72]. Hypersensitivity to heat is common in animal models of traumatic nerve injury pain, such as the CCI model, but heat hypersensitivity is minor or absent in the rat model of paclitaxel-evoked neuropathy. Studies conducted in different mouse strains, such as DBA/2J, CD1, and C57BL/6J, also showed paclitaxel-induced cold allodynia, but neither strain showed evidence of thermal hyperalgesia [73]. In 2007, Ledeboer et al. showed that paclitaxel-induced neuropathic pain is mediated through proinflammatory cytokines (IL-1beta, TNF-alpha) released by activated immune cells in the DRG. In 2012, Zhang et al. suggested that alterations in spinal synaptic transmissions through the downregulation of the glial glutamate transporters GLAST and GLT-1 in spinal astrocytes are involved in the pathogenesis of paclitaxel-induced pain neuropathy. Interestingly, preemptive treatment with minocycline (glial inhibitor) prevented paclitaxel-induced spinal astroglial responses. Thus, spinal astrocytes, immune cells, and/or glutamate transporters could be potential targets for the treatment of paclitaxel-induced neuropathy [74, 75].

Vincristine is also a commonly used chemotherapeutic agent that belongs to the vinca alkaloid family [76]. It is known that vincristine binds to intracellular tubulin and alters microtubular structures, causing a dose-dependent neuropathy that appear as mechanical allodynia but not thermal hyperalgesia in rats [77]. Interestingly, vincristine caused greater mechanical hyperalgesia in female rats [78] and increased electrophysiological responses to suprathreshold stimuli in C-fibre nociceptors; the mean conduction velocities of both C and A fibres were slower, and no histopathological changes were evident [55]. The histopathological examination after vincristine treatment showed dramatically reduced numbers of axonal microtubules of myelinated axons [79]. This mechanical hyperalgesia could be attenuated through morphine or lidocaine administration [80] but not with the mu-opioid agonist DAMGO ([D-Ala2, N-MePhe4, Gly-ol]-enkephalin). Recent work in human patients has shown that chronic vincristine-induced pain is associated with dysfunction in A-beta, A-delta, and C primary afferent fibres [81]. Deficits in A-delta-fibre and C-fibre function were specifically associated with the generation of pain. Recording neural discharge in the fibres of rats treated with paclitaxel and vincristine shows that both A-beta and C fibres have a high incidence of abnormal spontaneous discharge. This spontaneous discharge was rare and did not resemble the pattern observed in trauma models of neuropathic pain [82].

Cisplatin is commonly used for treating ovarian and small cell lung cancers and causes ototoxicity, nephrotoxicity, neurotoxicity, peripheral polyneuropathy, and mechanical allodynia development in rats [83]. These neuropathy symptoms are described as numbness and tingling, which increases in severity with increasing cumulative doses [84]. Cisplatin-induced polyneuropathy in humans can last for more than 10 years, and the severity of the resulting neuropathy depends on the dose and duration used [53]. In an animal model designed to mimic this condition, rats received three different cisplatin injections at a cumulative dose of 15 mg/kg. These animals showed mechanical allodynia that lasted as long as 15 days after injection [83]. Moreover this treatment regimen caused gait disturbance within 8 weeks of administration [85]. Electrophysiological recordings revealed a significant reduction of sensory nerve conduction velocity, but the motor nerve conduction velocity was unaffected [86]. Histologically, cisplatin affects large axons with normal myelin levels but has no effects on nonmyelinated axons. In addition, DRG apoptosis might contribute in part to cisplatin neurotoxicity, which can be blocked through the administration of a high dose of nerve growth factor [87, 88]. Cisplatin-induced neuropathy was also blocked by treatment with neurotrophic factor, the ACTH4-9 Analogue (ORG 2766) [36, 56] and recombinant human glial growth factor [89, 90], and the survival of large-fibre sensory neurons was induced by the administration of neurotrophin 3 [91]. Although cisplatin-induced neuropathy progressed for 6 weeks after discontinuation of the drug and slowly reversed over 3 months, this side effect could be prevented with early decompressive surgery [92].

Oxaliplatin is a chemotherapy agent widely used in the treatment of many malignancies, including colon cancer. Side effects include peripheral neuropathy, gastrointestinal toxicity, neutropenia, grade 1/2 hepatocellular injury, and hepatic vascular lesions [93]. It is known that oxaliplatin is metabolised to oxalate and dichloro (1,2-diaminocyclohexane) platinum. In 2009, Sakurai et al. [94] showed the involvement of oxalate in the oxaliplatin-induced peripheral neuropathy in rats. Oxaliplatin induced cold hyperalgesia in the early phase (as measured by cold plate and acetone tests) and mechanical allodynia in the late phase (as measured by von Frey test). Oxalate induced cold hyperalgesia but not mechanical allodynia. However, the administration of dichloro (1,2-diaminocyclohexane) platinum (DACHPt, the oxaliplatin parent complex) induced mechanical allodynia but not cold hyperalgesia. The pre-administration of calcium or magnesium before oxaliplatin or oxalate treatment prevented the onset of cold hyperalgesia. Sakurai et al. [94] suggest the usefulness of prophylactic treatments with calcium and magnesium for peripheral neuropathy.

Bortezomib is a new proteasome inhibitor with high antitumour activity and potentially severe peripheral neurotoxicity. In 2007, Cavaletti et al. [95] established a preclinical model by administration of bortezomib to Wistar rats at different doses for 4 weeks. They examined changes induced in the peripheral nerves, DRG, and spinal cord. Sciatic nerve examination and morphometric determinations demonstrated mild to moderate pathological changes, involving the Schwann cells and myelin, although axonal degeneration was also observed. Bortezomib-induced changes were also observed in DRG, which were represented by satellite cell intracytoplasmic vacuolisation due to mitochondrial and endoplasmic reticulum damage, closely resembling the changes observed in sciatic nerve Schwann cells. Occasionally, the cytoplasm of the DRG neurons appeared dark and clear vacuoles were observed. The spinal cord was morphologically normal. In 2012, a recent study showed strong evidence that bortezomib induces severe autonomic neuropathy [96].

Immune Factors Important for Cancer Pain Development in Animal Cancer Pain Models

In tumour masses, both cancer and immune cells produced neuroimmune factors that interact with a variety of receptors on peripheral nociceptive nerve terminals to promote abnormal discharge and hyperexcitability. Cancer growth near peripheral nerves can injure the integrity of the nerve and induce neuropathic pain development. The influence of the tumours on the peripheral nerve results in central sensitisation, which can further enhance the efficacy of nociceptive transmission through the spinal cord dorsal horn and the perception of spontaneous and breakthrough pain. Cancer cells produce mediators that affect other cells within the microenvironment, such as immune cells. Therefore, neuroimmune changes are now one of the most important issues studied as a potential mechanism for cancer pain development. Nociception almost certainly involves dynamic interactions and cross talk between the cancer and primary afferent nociceptor.

In most cancers, the tumour mass is composed of tumour and tumour stromal cells, the latter of which includes macrophages, neutrophils, T lymphocytes, fibroblasts, and endothelial cells. Tumour and/or tumour stromal cells have been shown to secrete a variety of factors that sensitise or directly excite primary afferent neurons, such as prostaglandins [97], tumour necrosis factor-alpha [98, 99], endothelins [100, 101], interleukin-1beta and interleukin-6 [99, 102, 103], epidermal growth factor [104], transforming growth factor-beta [105], and platelet-derived growth factor [106, 107]. Receptors for many of these factors are expressed by primary afferent neurons.

However, there is increasing evidence that indicates that leucocyte infiltration can promote tumour phenotypes, such as angiogenesis, growth, and invasion. This might be due to inflammatory cells that potentially influence cancer promotion through secreting cytokines, growth factors, chemokines, and proteases, which stimulate the proliferation and invasiveness of cancer cells. Macrophages, mast cells, and neutrophils can also support tumour development through the upregulation of nonspecific proinflammatory and proalgesic cytokines, such as interferon-γ, tumour necrosis factor (TNF), interleukin (IL)-1beta, IL-2, IL-6, IL-15, and IL-18. Macrophages are often the most abundant immune cell population in the tumour microenvironment. Recruitment of monocyte precursors circulating in the blood results in their differentiation into tumour-associated macrophages. It has been reported that once recruited into tumours, macrophages assume two different phenotypes: M1 or M2, based on the environmental stimuli and specialised functional properties. The M1 phenotype is associated with inflammation and microbial killing activity, whereas the M2 phenotype is associated with activities that are predominant and key in cancer development, including the inhibition of T helper 1 adaptive immunity through immunosuppressive mediators, such as transforming growth factor-beta 1 (TGF-beta 1), IL-10, IL-4, or prostaglandin E2 (PGE2), and the production of growth and survival factors (EGF, IL-6, and

CXCL8); secretion of angiogenic factors (VEGF, TGF-α, or PGE2); and production of matrix metalloproteases (MMPs), which degrade extracellular matrix, and chemokines that recruit more inflammatory cells (CX3CL1 (fractalkine), CCL2, CCL17, CCL18, or CCL22). Glial activation results from bone cancer pain. The activation of glial cells, such as astrocytes, has recently gained significant recognition as contributing to the pathogenesis of chronic pain. Painful osteolytic destruction of the femoral bone as a result of experimental tumour growth results in the ipsilateral hypertrophy of astrocytes in the spinal cord, as measured using the glial fibrillary acidic protein (GFAP) marker. In 1999, Schwei et al. observed the activation of astrocytes (GFAP marker) in the spinal cord of mice with fibrosarcoma-induced cancer pain. This increase in GFAP labelling in the dorsal horn was likely due to the hypertrophy of astrocytes and also correlated with the extent of bone destruction. The activation of glia in the spinal cord, including astrocytes and microglia, might contribute to the development or maintenance of persistent pain through the release of algesic substances that excite or sensitise nociceptive dorsal horn neurons [108]. Behavioural studies have shown that substances such as propentofylline and minocycline (selective for microglia), which block the activation of glial cells, attenuate paclitaxel-/vincristine-induced cancer neuropathic pain [109, 110], supporting a role for activated microglial cells. It has been reported that macrophage accumulation and activation in the DRG of paclitaxel-treated rats contributes to the generation and development of neuropathy. The investigator must consider the activities of the cancer cell, peripheral and central nervous system, and immune system. We discuss below several immune nociceptive mediators secreted in high levels during cancer development in the animal models and known to cause pain development.

Cytokines are immunomodulators released in response to cancer development and by the tumour itself. They might also have proinflammatory and anti-inflammatory characteristics, which modulate the surrounding cellular and chemical response to injury. In the peripheral nervous system, proinflammatory cytokines and chemokines not only contribute to axonal damage through inflammatory activation but also modulate spontaneous nociceptor sensitivity and activity, thus linking the immune and peripheral nervous systems. Using biochemical methods to detect immune factors is possible in a clinical model of cancer pain, and this helps to understand the mechanisms underlying cancer pain development.

TNF and INF in Cancer Pain

Recent studies have indicated an important role for tumour necrosis factor-alpha (TNF-alpha) in tumour growth and bone cancer-associated pain. The mechanisms by which TNF, through its receptor subtypes TNF receptor 1 (TNFR1) and 2 (TNFR2), elicits altered sensation and pain behaviour remain incompletely understood. Under pain conditions, an increase in TNF has also been observed in DRGs, the dorsal horn of the spinal cord, the rostral ventromedial medulla, locus coeruleus, and hippocampus, presumably from activated astrocytes and microglia [111–114]. There are a variety of drugs on the market that target TNF signalling for the treatment of human autoimmune diseases (rheumatoid arthritis, inflammatory bowel disease, and psoriasis), including infliximab or etanercept [115]. Recently, Gu et al. [116] showed that thalidomide, which selectively inhibits TNF-α production, can diminish bone cancer pain in a mice model. Tobinick et al. [117] have shown that etanercept can be clinically useful in selected patients with treatment-refractory pain caused by bone metastases. Clinical trials are needed to define the potential benefit of biologic TNF-alpha antagonists in the treatment and prevention of malignant osteolysis, suggesting the possibility that the TNF-alpha receptor antagonists might be useful in treating bone cancer pain.

IFN-γ is a dimerised soluble cytokine, which is the only member of the type II class of interferons, and has been implicated in many chronic pain states. IFN-γ treatment in cancer patients has long been reported to induce spontaneous pain [118, 119], and the intrathecal administration of IFN-γ in naïve but not IFN-γR−/− mice has been shown to induce pain hypersensitivity [120].

Interleukins in Cancer Pain

Interleukins are important factors for cancer pain development in clinical and animal models. Numerous lines of evidence from preclinical and clinical studies have shown that NF-κB and NF-κB-mediated proinflammatory cytokines play a central role in the progression of cancer-related symptoms [121]. For instance, the administration of selective inhibitors of the NF-κB pathway has been shown to abrogate the expression of cytokines, such as IL-1β and TNF-α, in animal models of chronic inflammation. In patients with myelodysplastic syndrome and acute leukaemia, a correlation was observed between the severity of symptoms and increased levels of cytokines (TNF-α, IL-6, IL-8) [122]. Similarly, patients without cancer have also been shown to display many of the symptoms of cancer patients after receiving cytokine therapy.

It is known that following cancer pain development, immune cells become activated and release proinflammatory cytokines, such as IL-1beta, IL-2, and IL-6, thereby initiating the pain process. Interleukin 1β (IL-1β) is of special interest because it is secreted under conditions associated with pain and hyperalgesia [123] and is elevated in the cerebral spinal fluid of chronic pain patients [124]. In mice, neutralising antibodies for interleukin-1 receptor reduce pain behaviour associated with experimental neuropathy [125]. Moreover, the deletion of IL-1 receptor type 1 or transgenic overexpression of the naturally occurring IL-1 receptor antagonist (IL-1RA) delays the onset and severity of pain associated with peripheral nerve injury [125]. Similar effects are observed in animals lacking the IL-1β gene [126]. In 2008, Zhang et al. [127] showed that in cancer pain, spinal IL-1β enhances NR1 phosphorylation to facilitate bone cancer pain, and IL-1ra attenuates bone cancer pain and inhibits NR1 phosphorylation.

In another study, Tawara et al. [128] suggest that the IL-6 is frequently upregulated and implicated in the ability of cancer cells to metastasise to bone. In addition, IL-6 is able to activate various cell signalling cascades that include the signal transducer and activator of the transcription (STAT) pathway, phosphatidylinositol 3-kinase

(PI3K) pathway, and mitogen-activated protein kinase (MAPK) pathway. Activation of these pathways might explain the ability of IL-6 to mediate various aspects of normal and pathogenic bone remodelling, inflammation, cell survival, proliferation, pain, and pro-tumorigenic effects. The enhancement of tumour growth by IL-17 involves direct effects on tumour cells and tumour-associated stromal cells, which bear IL-17 receptors. IL-17 induces IL-6 production, which in turn activates oncogenic signal transducer and activator of transcription (Stat) 3, upregulating prosurvival and proangiogenic genes [129]. In 2008, Reyes-Gibby suggested that polymorphisms in several cytokine genes are potential markers for genetic susceptibility to both cancer risk and cancer-induced pain symptoms.

Chemokines in Cancer Pain

In recent years, a major role has been assigned to chemokines and their receptors as molecules that affect neoplastic development and progression. Many chemokines and their receptors are expressed in tumours not only by cancer cells but also by cells of the tumour microenvironment, including cells of the stroma (endothelial cells, fibroblasts) and leucocytes, thus contributing to the cross talk between the tumour and its microenvironment to control tumour growth and progression [130]. In the malignancy context, chemokines play diverse roles, which are derived from their ability to induce cell migration [131]. Many solid tumours are highly populated by host leucocytes that have migrated into the tumour from the systemic circulation, suggesting a malignancy-induced immune response. In tumours, leucocyte infiltrates might have either anticancer or cancer-promoting effects, depending on their type, activity, and modes of interaction with the tumour cells. Consistent with their classification as leucocyte chemoattractants, chemokines are released by tumour cells or cells of their microenvironment and are able to induce the recruitment of different hematopoietic cell subtypes to tumours (T lymphocytes, macrophages, natural killer (NK) cells, neutrophils, eosinophils, and B cells). In particular, among the CXC chemokines, CXCL9, CXCL10, and CXCL11 are induced by interferon

and are typical chemoattractants of NK cells [132]. Accordingly, the overexpression of these chemokines through different experimental means leads to limitations in cancer development associated with the elevation in cytotoxic responses and creation of long-term antitumour immunity [133]. Increasing evidence suggests that chemokines at different anatomical locations, including injured nerves, DRG, the spinal cord, and the brain, contribute to chronic pain processing [134–137]. To date, changes in the expression of numerous cytokines have been observed in neuropathic pain, including changes in the expression of CXCL12, CCL3, CCL5, and CCL21 and their receptors; however, the role of these changes has not been well studied. Currently, the role for the chemokines CX3CL1, or fractalkine, and CCL2 in nociception has been well documented. Fractalkine is present in spinal and DRG neurons, and its receptor CX3CR1 is present in microglial cells. CX3CR1 expression increases following neuronal damage, particularly in the dorsal section of the spinal cord. In addition to CCL2 and CX3CL1, other chemokines are involved in pain regulation. Oh et al. [138] demonstrated that the chemokines CXCL12 (SDF-1, stromal cell-derived factor-1), CCL5, and CCL3 produce pain hypersensitivity through directly exciting primary nociceptive neurons. Chemokine receptor antagonists have also shown efficacy in animal models of pain, e.g., AMD3100 inhibits CXCL12-induced GTP binding and attenuates allodynia [139].

These data indicate an important role for interactions between the immune system and cancer. A comprehensive understanding of these relationships and basic mechanisms is essential for the development of improved therapeutic approaches to cancer pain treatment and protocols for the prevention of cancer development and to counteract the effects of chemotherapy.

Clinical Implication of the Use of Cancer Pain Models

Pain secondary to cancer may develop due to the malignant disease itself or subsequent to treatments, such as chemotherapy, surgery, or radiotherapy.

The pathophysiology of pain due to cancer may be complex and include a variety of inflammatory and neuropathic mechanisms. Lately, relevant animal cancer models have facilitated understanding of the pathology and have advanced the pharmacology of cancer pain, with significant translational applicability to clinic. Successful management depends upon understanding of many factors possibly involved in facilitating and sustaining pain in a particular individual, as well as upon familiarity with all established and novel therapeutic approaches. Systemic pharmacologic management aiming at reducing nociceptive input, modulating transmission of pain to the central nervous system, or altering central perception of pain remains as the mainstay of the treatment. All described animal models of cancer pain are now available and effectively mirror the clinical picture observed in humans. The variety of cancer pain models help and make possible to develop novel mechanism-based pharmacotherapies that not only reduce tumour-induced cancer pain but may provide added benefit in synergistically reduced disease progression. The studies in which the cancer pain of different mechanisms is used provide a basic science rationale for analgesic trials and management. Development of new drugs or new drug combination tested in animal cancer pain models can give in the future the opportunity to apply them in clinical use and can have a positive impact on the patient's functional status, quality of life, and survival.

Methods of Cancer Pain Measurement in Animal Models

The development of animal models that exhibit different elements of clinical cancer pain syndromes, coupled with advances in tools for the quantification of pain behaviour, has greatly advanced the understanding of the mechanisms involved in pain. Several methods have been used to assess reflexive pain behaviours, such as tail-flick and paw withdrawal in response to acute painful stimuli, and using these methods, it is possible to examine spinal reflexes [140]. Paw

licking on the hot plate test can be elicited in decerebrate animals [141], indicating spino-bulbo-spinal reflexes. Considerably less effort has been dedicated to measuring integrated supraspinal nocifensive behaviours, which might be more dependent on cortical activity. Scientists have developed fully automated thermal and mechanical pain behaviour assessment tools to evaluate the pain behaviour in response to both thermal innocuous and noxious stimuli. The most commonly used stimulus modalities are electrical, mechanical, and thermal.

To reduce stress, the animals are acclimated to the researcher's hands and conditions inside the apparatus prior to the experiments. In the last few years, more advanced technologically methods for measuring pain-related motor behaviour disturbances in freely moving animals have been developed, e.g., the walking pattern method, which registers traces of the damaged paw, and dynamic weight bearing (DWB), which registers the weight of the paw in animals subjected to paw injury and the development of allodynia and/or hyperalgesia.

In conclusion, there are many adequate behavioural methods for testing pain in various models of cancer, and their use depends on the experiment and working hypothesis. Below is an overview of the most commonly used behavioural methods for testing pain in studies on the mechanisms of tumour growth, consequences of its therapy, and thus the development of pain related to this disease.

Electrical Stimulation

The application of electrical stimuli is measurable, reproducible, and noninvasive: producing synchronised afferent signals. Nevertheless, it also has serious disadvantages because electrical stimuli are not naturally encountered by an animal in its normal environment. Additionally, electrical stimulation of the animal causes high levels of anxiety and stress known to exhibit modulatory effects on nociceptive sensitivity; therefore, electrical stimulation is not the method of choice in cancer pain studies [142, 143].

Mechanical Stimulation

Typical mechanical tests utilise the calculation of paw withdrawal latencies and/or observations of guarding behaviour to certain mechanical stimuli in cancer pain models, such as thresholds of withdrawal to pinpricks or von Frey filaments [144].

Tail-Pinch Test

The cancer pain development in rodents can be measured using a score based on behaviours such as waving or licking a tail pinched with tweezers [145]. The same level of stimulation should be administered to each rodent using an instrument that produces a pinch with constant pressure, such as a clamp or forceps. The tail-pinch test is a simple method that does not require expensive instruments; however, it is difficult to objectively evaluate the level of pain produced.

Paw Pressure Test

The mechanical stimulation can be determined using the paw pressure test in cancer pain models (Fig. 6.1a). This method determines the threshold response to uniformly increasing pressure. Briefly, rats are maintained in a normal/horizontal position in the hand of the researcher. The right hindpaw is placed in an analgesimeter composed of a cone-shaped paw-presser with a rounded tip used to apply linearly increasing force to the test paw. The nociceptive threshold is represented as the weight in grams required to elicit a nociceptive response, such as paw flexion. A maximum pressure force of 250 g is used to prevent damage to the paws [146, 147].

von Frey Filaments

In cancer pain models the mechanical allodynia can be measured using a series of von Frey filaments ranging from 0.6 to 6 g in mice and from 0.6 to 26 g in rats (Fig. 6.1b) [21, 123, 144, 148]. The animals are placed in plastic cages with a wire-mesh floor, allowing them to move freely, and are allowed to acclimate to this environment. In von Frey filaments, the stimulus is terminated when there is no reaction to the bending of the filament, and subsequently, the next filament is applied.

Automatic von Frey Apparatus

The allodynia development in cancer pain models can be also measured by automatic von Frey apparatus. The animals are placed in plastic cages with a wire-net floor, and the operator slides a touch stimulator unit under the animal, using an adjustable angled mirror to position the filament below the target area of the paw. A button press causes a stainless steel filament (0.5 mm diametre) to move up to touch the animal's paw. The filament exerts an increasing force to the plantar surface, starting below the threshold of detection and increasing until the animal removes its paw, so the stimulus is discontinued as soon as the response in grams is saved in an electronic recorder [149].

Pressure Application Measurement

The pressure application measurement device (PAM) is a novel tool for measuring the mechanical pain threshold in experimental cancer pain models in rodents. The PAM device has been designed and validated specifically for the mechanical stimulation and assessment of joint and bone pain. The PAM device applies a quantifiable force for the direct stimulation of the joint and automatic readout of the response. Increasing pressure is applied to the lateral side of the knee joint at the level of the joint space until the animals attempted to escape or vocalised as described previously [150]. The force required to elicit this response is measured in grams.

Thermal Stimulation

Heat is used to selectively stimulate cutaneous receptors. Consequently, specific categories of peripheral axons, including thermosensitive and nociceptive fibres, can be excited. Thermal stimulation as been extensively used to assess cancer pain behaviour in animals [151], and it remains the basis of most pain assessment tools, including the tail-flick [152], hind-limb withdrawal plantar [123, 153], and hot plate [154] tests. The advantage of using heat is the relative constancy of its threshold across body sites, and extensive

Fig. 6.1 Photographs of behavioural tests useful to establish the nociception under cancer pain. (**a**) Paw pressure test, (**b**) von Frey test, (**c**) tail-flick test, (**d**) Hargreaves plantar test, and (**e**) cold/hot plate test

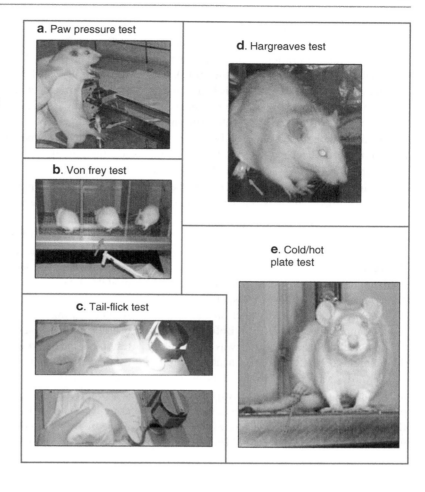

a. Paw pressure test

b. Von frey test

c. Tail-flick test

d. Hargreaves test

e. Cold/hot plate test

research conducted in psychophysical and physiological studies have defined and established the range of temperatures that produce heat nociception and its underlying mechanisms. Thus, responses to painful thermal stimuli remain one of the best behavioural tools for studying cancer pain in animals.

Tail-Flick Test

The nociceptive threshold to a thermal stimulus in naïve animals and those that developed cancer pain can be assessed using tail-flick latency evoked through a noxious hot stimulus, as determined with a tail-flick analgesic meter (Fig. 6.1c). The tail-flick test consists of a beam of light focused on the dorsal tail surface at 1 cm from the tip of the tail. The intensity of the light is adjusted so that the baseline tail-flick latencies

in naïve animals are 3.5–4.5 s, and the cutoff time for the flick of the tail is set to 9 or 10 s [152, 155].

Hargreaves Plantar Test

To assess the pain threshold to thermal stimuli, animals are tested for paw withdrawal latency to noxious thermal stimuli (Fig. 6.1d) using an analgesia meter [153]. Animals are placed into plastic glass-bottomed cages and thermal stimulus in the form of radiant heat emitted from a focused projection bulb, which is placed under the glass floor, is applied to the paw through glass. Noxious thermal stimulus was focused onto the plantar surface of a hindpaw until the animal lifted a paw away from the floor. A cutoff latency of 20 s is used to avoid tissue damage.

Hot/Cold Plate Analgesia Meter

The nociceptive threshold, in cancer pain models, to stimuli of high or low temperatures can be measured using a hot or cold plate (Fig. 6.1e). The high temperature of the cage floor is kept constant at 50–55 °C. The cold temperature is kept at 5 °C for rats and 2 °C for mice [123, 149]. The animal is placed on the hot/cold plate, and reaction time is recorded. The latency period until the animal shows specific responses, such as shaking, licking, lifting hindpaws, or the first escape behaviours, is recorded. The maximal observation time is 30 s to protect the tissues from heat or cold damage due to overstimulation [39, 145].

Acetone Tests

To examine the threshold to cold stimulus (cold allodynia) in cancer pain models, animals underwent behavioural testing to determine sensitivity to low temperatures [145, 156]. Before testing, a 15 min acclimatisation period was allowed for the animal. A small amount of acetone solution (50–100 µL) was applied to the glabrous skin of the ipsilateral paw through polyethylene (PE) ten plastic tubing connected to a 1 mL syringe. During each test session, acetone was applied five times in 5 min intervals. The number of responses was calculated between each application. Responses included hindpaw lifting, licking, and withdrawal of the paw.

Motor Functions

Walking Pattern

The development of motor dysfunction in cancer pain models can be monitored by analysis of the free walking pattern [157], according to De Medinacelli et al. [158] and De Koning et al. [159]. This standardised method yields a reproducible measure of motor deficit of the involved paw. The functional index (FI) of paw motor function is expressed in % as the difference between the ipsi- and contralateral paws. One week before experiments the animals are trained to walk over the strips of paper covering the bottom of a 50 cm long, 6.4 cm wide, upward inclining (10°) corridor ending with a dark box. The rats' hind limbs

are dipped in ink and their footprints are recorded in the corridor on the white paper or the animals walk along a special platform, and the results are automatically analysed using a computer program. The more technically advanced method was presented by Hamers et al. [160]. They described the use of a newly developed automated quantitative gait analysis method that allows for an easy quantitation of a large number of locomotion parameters during walkway crossing, whereas achieving such a number of the parameters with previously used methods was not possible.

Dynamic Weight Bearing (DWB)

Along with the gradual development of mechanical allodynia and thermal hyperalgesia in animal models of cancer pain, behavioural signs of nociception can be also detected using a dynamic weight-bearing apparatus. Hind-limb weight bearing can be assessed using an incapacitance tester that independently measures the weight distributed to each hindpaw. The device consists of a bottomless Plexiglas enclosure and sensor. The sensor is placed on the floor of the enclosure, covering its entire surface. The animal is allowed to move freely within the apparatus, and the weight-bearing information is transmitted live to a laptop computer via an USB interface. The raw data are analysed by a computer. A paw is detected when one sensor recorded a weight of at least 4 g and a minimum of two adjacent sensors recorded a weight of at least 1 g. The paw had to be stable for a minimum of 0.5 s to be included. Using a synchronised video recording of the test and scaled map of the detected zones, each presumed paw is validated by an observer and identified as a left or right and fore- or hindpaw. Other detected zones, representing the tail or another body part, are also included in the analysis. To determine the time course changes of weight-bearing deficit, a baseline weight distribution on each paw is determined prior to cancer pain induction [161].

Presentation of Pain in Animal Models

The presentation of the results in studies of pain requires a special approach due to differences in the individual pain thresholds of each animal. Moreover, nociceptive stimuli are applied only for a specified time to avoid tissue damage. To account for these parameters, the results are presented as percentage of the maximal possible effect %MPE using the following calculation: $\%MPE = [(TL-BL)/(CUTOFF-BL)] \times 100\%$; where BL is the baseline latency; cutoff threshold [e.g. von Frey test is 26 g] and TL is the value obtained after drug injection [123].

The behavioural data-defined response to mechanical allodynia or thermal hyperalgesia can be presented as percentage of maximal possible allodynia ($\%MPA \pm s.e.m.$) using the following equation: $\%MPA = [(BL-TL)/(BL-CUTOFF)] \times 100\%$, where BL is the baseline latency and TL is the respective test latency, or as a percent of maximal possible score ($\%MPS \pm s.e.m.$), where the highest score is assumed to represent 100 % [44].

Conclusion

Our understanding of the basic mechanisms that underlie the development of pain associated with malignancy is important. An understanding of these basic mechanisms is essential for the development of better therapeutic approaches to cancer pain treatment. The efforts of many years of research have resulted in the development of adequate animal tumour models. We provide examples of animal models of nonbone cancer pain, including skin, pancreatic, orofacial, and neuroma models. We also describe models of cancer pain that can be induced in animal bones, like many of the most common tumours, such as breast, prostate, kidney, thyroid, and lung cancer. Moreover, we discuss models of neuropathic cancer pain, which is the most difficult for analgesia treatment in clinical settings and can be induced by both invasion and chemotherapy, and we collected data on immune factors important for cancer pain development in animal models. Furthermore, we also discuss the use of different behavioural methods to measure changes in the nociceptive threshold, which is diminished under cancer pain using electrical, mechanical, and thermal stimulation,

and the registration of motor disturbances. The information generated from these models has provided insight into the mechanisms that initiate and maintain cancer pain to target potential mechanism-based therapies to treat this chronic pain state.

Acknowledgments This study was financed by statutory funds from the Department of Pain Pharmacology.

References

1. van den Beuken-van Everdingen MH, de Rijke JM, Kessels AG, Schouten HC, van Kleef M, Patijn J. High prevalence of pain in patients with cancer in a large population-based study in The Netherlands. Pain. 2007;132:312–20.
2. Coleman RE. Clinical features of metastatic bone disease and risk of skeletal morbidity. Clin Cancer Res. 2006;12(20 Pt 2):6243s–9.
3. Mercadante S, Fulfaro F. Management of painful bone metastases. Curr Opin Oncol. 2007;19:308–14.
4. Fidler IJ. Critical factors in the biology of human cancer metastasis: twenty-eighth G.H.A. Clowes memorial award lecture. Cancer Res. 1990;50:6130–8.
5. Guise TA, Kozlow WM, Heras-Herzig A, Padalecki SS, Yin JJ, Chirgwin JM. Molecular mechanisms of breast cancer metastases to bone. Clin Breast Cancer. 2005;5 Suppl 2:S46–53.
6. Mercadante S. Malignant bone pain: pathophysiology and treatment. Pain. 1997;69:1–18.
7. Miao XR, Gao XF, Wu JX, Lu ZJ, Huang ZX, Li XQ, et al. Bilateral downregulation of Nav1.8 in dorsal root ganglia of rats with bone cancer pain induced by inoculation with Walker 256 breast tumor cells. BMC Cancer. 2010;10:216.
8. Saad F, Lipton A. Bone-marker levels in patients with prostate cancer: potential correlations with outcomes. Curr Opin Support Palliat Care. 2010;4:127–34.
9. Cain DM, Wacnik PW, Eikmeier L, Beitz A, Wilcox GL, Simone DA. Functional interactions between tumor and peripheral nerve in a model of cancer pain in the mouse. Pain Med. 2001;2:15–23.
10. Wacnik PW, Eikmeier LJ, Ruggles TR, Ramnaraine ML, Walcheck BK, Beitz AJ, et al. Functional interactions between tumor and peripheral nerve: morphology, algogen identification, and behavioral characterization of a new murine model of cancer pain. J Neurosci. 2001;21:9355–66.
11. Connelly E, Markman M, Kennedy A, Webster K, Kulp B, Peterson G, et al. Paclitaxel delivered as a 3-hr infusion with cisplatin in patients with gynecologic cancers: unexpected incidence of neurotoxicity. Gynecol Oncol. 1996;62:166–8.
12. Sasamura T, Nakamura S, Iida Y, Fujii H, Murata J, Saiki I, et al. Morphine analgesia suppresses tumor

growth and metastasis in a mouse model of cancer pain produced by orthotopic tumor inoculation. Eur J Pharmacol. 2002;441:185–91.

13. Constantin CE, Mair N, Sailer CA, Andratsch M, Xu ZZ, Blumer MJ, et al. Endogenous tumor necrosis factor alpha (TNFalpha) requires TNF receptor type 2 to generate heat hyperalgesia in a mouse cancer model. J Neurosci. 2008;28:5072–81.

14. Mao-Ying QL, Cui KM, Liu Q, Dong ZQ, Wang W, Wang J, et al. Stage-dependent analgesia of electro-acupuncture in a mouse model of cutaneous cancer pain. Eur J Pain. 2006;10:689–94.

15. Andoh T, Sugiyama K, Fujita M, Iida Y, Nojima H, Saiki I, et al. Pharmacological evaluation of morphine and non-opioid analgesic adjuvants in a mouse model of skin cancer pain. Biol Pharm Bull. 2008;3:520–2.

16. Negin BP, Riedel E, Oliveria SA, Berwick M, Coit DG, Brady MS. Symptoms and signs of primary melanoma: important indicators of Breslow depth. Cancer. 2003;98:344–8.

17. Jemal A, Siegel R, Ward E, Murray T, Xu J, Thun MJ. Cancer statistics. CA Cancer J Clin. 2007;57:43–66.

18. Lindsay TH, Jonas BM, Sevcik MA, Kubota K, Halvorson KG, Ghilardi JR, et al. Pancreatic cancer pain and its correlation with changes in tumor vasculature, macrophage infiltration, neuronal innervation, body weight, and disease progression. Pain. 2005;119:233–46.

19. Sevcik MA, Jonas BM, Lindsay TH, Halvorson KG, Ghilardi JR, Kuskowski MA, et al. Endogenous opioids inhibit early-stage pancreatic pain in a mouse model of pancreatic cancer. Gastroenterology. 2006;131:900–10.

20. di Mola FF, di Sebastiano P. Pain and pain generation in pancreatic cancer. Langenbecks Arch Surg. 2008;393:919–22.

21. Nagamine K, Ozaki N, Shinoda M, Asai H, Nishiguchi H, Mitsudo K, et al. Mechanical allodynia and thermal hyperalgesia induced by experimental squamous cell carcinoma of the lower gingiva in rats. J Pain. 2006;7:659–70.

22. Tyner TR, Parks N, Faria S, Simons M, Stapp B, Curtis B, et al. Effects of collagen nerve guide on neuroma formation and neuropathic pain in a rat model. Am J Surg. 2007;193:e1–6.

23. Dorsi MJ, Chen L, Murinson BB, Pogatzki-Zahn EM, Meyer RA, Belzberg AJ. The tibial neuroma transposition (TNT) model of neuroma pain and hyperalgesia. Pain. 2008;134:320–34.

24. Mercadante S, Arcuri E. Breakthrough pain in cancer patients: pathophysiology and treatment. Cancer Treat Rev. 1998;24:425–32.

25. Schwei MJ, Honore P, Rogers SD, Salak-Johnson JL, Finke MP, Ramnaraine ML, et al. Neurochemical and cellular reorganization of the spinal cord in a murine model of bone cancer pain. J Neurosci. 1999;19: 10886–97.

26. Honore P, Schwei J, Rogers SD, Salak-Johnson JL, Finke MP, Ramnaraine ML, et al. Cellular and

27. Luger NM, Honore P, Sabino MA, Schwei MJ, Rogers SD, Mach DB, et al. Osteoprotegerin diminishes advanced bone cancer pain. Cancer Res. 2001;61: 4038–47.

28. Wacnik PW, Kehl LJ, Trempe TM, Ramnaraine ML, Beitz AJ, Wilcox GL. Tumor implantation in mouse humerus evokes movement-related hyperalgesia exceeding that evoked by intramuscular carrageenan. Pain. 2003;101:175–86.

29. Kehl LJ, Hamamoto DT, Wacnik PW, Croft DL, Norsted BD, Wilcox GL, et al. A cannabinoid agonist differentially attenuates deep tissue hyperalgesia in animal models of cancer and inflammatory muscle pain. Pain. 2003;103:175–86.

30. Goblirsch M, Mathews W, Lynch C, Alaei P, Gerbi BJ, Mantyh PW, et al. Radiation treatment decreases bone cancer pain, osteolysis and tumor size. Radiat Res. 2004;161:228–34.

31. Vit JP, Ohara PT, Tien DA, Fike JR, Eikmeier L, Beitz A, et al. The analgesic effect of low-dose focal irradiation in a mouse model of bone cancer is associated with spinal changes in neuromediators of nociception. Pain. 2006;120:188–201.

32. King T, Vardanyan A, Majuta L, Melemedjian O, Nagle R, Cress AE, et al. Morphine treatment accelerates sarcoma-induced bone pain, bone loss, and spontaneous fracture in a murine model of bone cancer. Pain. 2007;132:154–68.

33. Khasabov SG, Hamamoto DT, Harding-Rose C, Simone DA. Tumor-evoked hyperalgesia and sensitization of nociceptive dorsal horn neurons in a murine model of cancer pain. Brain Res. 2007;1180:7–19.

34. Medhurst SJ, Walker K, Bowes M, Kidd BL, Glatt M, Muller M, et al. A rat model of bone cancer pain. Pain. 2002;96:129–40.

35. Fox A, Medhurst S, Courade JP, Glatt M, Dawson J, Urban L, et al. Antihyperalgesic activity of the COX2 inhibitor lumiracoxib in a model of bone cancer pain in the rat. Pain. 2004;107:33–40.

36. Goblirsch MJ, Zwolak P, Clohisy DR. Advances in understanding bone cancer pain. J Cell Biochem. 2005;96:682–8.

37. Liepe K, Geidel H, Haase M, Hakenberg OW, Runge R, Kotzerke J. New model for the induction of osteoblastic bone metastases in rat. Anticancer Res. 2005;25:1067–73.

38. Zhang RX, Liu B, Wang L, Ren K, Qiao JT, Berman BM, et al. Spinal glial activation in a new rat model of bone cancer pain produced by prostate cancer cell inoculation of the tibia. Pain. 2005;118:125–36.

39. Beyreuther BK, Callizot N, Brot MD, Feldman R, Bain SC, Stohr T. Antinociceptive efficacy of lacosamide in rat models for tumor- and chemotherapy-induced cancer pain. Eur J Pharmacol. 2007;565: 98–104.

40. Wenger AS, Mickey DD, Hall M, Silverman LM, Mickey GH, Fried FA. In vitro characterization of

MAT LyLu: a Dunning rat prostate adenocarcinoma tumor subline. J Urol. 1984;131:1232–6.

41. De Ciantis PD, Yashpal K, Henry J, Singh G. Characterization of a rat model of metastatic prostate cancer bone pain. J Pain Res. 2010;3:213–21.

42. Honore P, Luger NM, Sabino MA, Schwei MJ, Rogers SD, Mach DB, et al. Osteoprotegerin blocks bone cancer-induced skeletal destruction, skeletal pain and pain-related neurochemical reorganization of the spinal cord. Nat Med. 2000;6:521–8.

43. Mantyh PW, Clohisy DR, Koltzenburg M, Hunt SP. Molecular mechanisms of cancer pain. Nat Rev Cancer. 2002;2:201–9.

44. Obara I, Mika J, Schafer MK, Przewlocka B. Antagonists of the kappa-opioid receptor enhance allodynia in rats and mice after sciatic nerve ligation. Br J Pharmacol. 2003;140:538–46.

45. Gao YJ, Cheng JK, Zeng Q, Xu ZZ, Decosterd I, Xu X, et al. Selective inhibition of JNK with a peptide inhibitor attenuates pain hypersensitivity and tumor growth in a mouse skin cancer pain model. Exp Neurol. 2009;219:146–55.

46. Harada Y. Pituitary role in the growth of metastasizing MRMT-1 mammary carcinoma in rats. Cancer Res. 1976;36:18–22.

47. Martin LA, Hagen NA. Neuropathic pain in cancer patients: mechanisms, syndromes, and clinical controversies. J Pain Symptom Manage. 1997;14:99–117.

48. Shimoyama M, Tanaka K, Hasue F, Shimoyama N. A mouse model of neuropathic cancer pain. Pain. 2002;99:167–74.

49. Shimoyama M, Tatsuoka H, Ohtori S, Tanaka K, Shimoyama N. Change of dorsal horn neurochemistry in a mouse model of neuropathic cancer pain. Pain. 2005;114:221–30.

50. Dougherty PM, Cata JP, Cordella JV, Burton A, Weng HR. Taxol-induced sensory disturbance is characterized by preferential impairment of myelinated fiber function in cancer patients. Pain. 2004;109:132–42.

51. Ling B, Authier N, Balayssac D, Eschalier A, Coudore F. Behavioral and pharmacological description of oxaliplatin-induced painful neuropathy in rat. Pain. 2007;128:225–34.

52. Cavaletti G, Bogliun G, Crespi V, Marzorati L, Zincone A, Marzola M, et al. Neurotoxicity and ototoxicity of cisplatin plus paclitaxel in comparison to cisplatin plus cyclophosphamide in patients with epithelial ovarian cancer. J Clin Oncol. 1997;15:199–206.

53. Strumberg D, Brugge S, Korn MW, Koeppen S, Ranft J, Scheiber G, et al. Evaluation of long-term toxicity in patients after cisplatin-based chemotherapy for nonseminomatous testicular cancer. Ann Oncol. 2002;13:229–36.

54. Aley KO, Reichling DB, Levine JD. Vincristine hyperalgesia in the rat: a model of painful vincristine neuropathy in humans. Neuroscience. 1996;73:259–65.

55. Tanner KD, Levine JD, Topp KS. Microtubule disorientation and axonal swelling in unmyelinated sensory axons during vincristine-induced painful neuropathy in rat. J Comp Neurol. 1998;395:481–92.

56. Mimura Y, Kato H, Eguchi K, Ogawa T. Schedule dependency of paclitaxel-induced neuropathy in mice: a morphological study. Neurotoxicology. 2000;21:513–20.

57. Lee JJ, Swain SM. Peripheral neuropathy induced by microtubule-stabilizing agents. J Clin Oncol. 2006;24:1633–42.

58. Broyl A, Corthals SL, Jongen JL, van der Holt B, Kuiper R, de Knegt Y, et al. Mechanisms of peripheral neuropathy associated with bortezomib and vincristine in patients with newly diagnosed multiple myeloma: a prospective analysis of data from the HOVON-65/GMMG-HD4 trial. Lancet Oncol. 2010;11:1057–65.

59. Asai H, Ozaki N, Shinoda M, Nagamine K, Tohnai I, Ueda M, et al. Heat and mechanical hyperalgesia in mice model of cancer pain. Pain. 2005;117:19–29.

60. Wang XM, Lehky TJ, Brell JM, Dorsey SG. Discovering cytokines as targets for chemotherapy-induced painful peripheral neuropathy. Cytokine. 2012;59:3–9.

61. Flatters SJ, Bennett GJ. Ethosuximide reverses paclitaxel- and vincristine-induced painful peripheral neuropathy. Pain. 2004;109:150–61.

62. Kohler DR, Goldspiel BR. Paclitaxel (taxol). Pharmacotherapy. 1994;14:3–34.

63. Rowinsky EK, Chaudhry V, Cornblath DR, Donehower RC. Neurotoxicity of taxol. J Natl Cancer Inst Monogr. 1993;15:107–15.

64. Rowinsky EK, Donehower RC. Paclitaxel (taxol). N Engl J Med. 1995;332:1004–14.

65. Wiernik PH, Schwartz EL, Strauman JJ, Dutcher JP, Lipton RB, Paietta E. Phase I clinical and pharmacokinetic study of taxol. Cancer Res. 1987;47:2486–93.

66. Tamura T, Sasaki Y, Nishiwaki Y, Saijo N. Phase I study of paclitaxel by 3-hour infusion: hypotension just after infusion is one of the major dose-limiting toxicities. Jpn J Cancer Res. 1995;86:1203–9.

67. Polomano RC, Mannes AJ, Clark US, Bennett GJ. A painful peripheral neuropathy in the rat produced by the chemotherapeutic drug paclitaxel. Pain. 2001;94:293–304.

68. Ueda H. Molecular mechanisms of neuropathic pain—phenotypic switch and initiation mechanisms. Pharmacol Ther. 2006;109:57–77.

69. De Brabander M, Geuens G, Nuydens R, Willebrords R, De Mey J. Taxol induces the assembly of free microtubules in living cells and blocks the organizing capacity of the centrosomes and kinetochores. Proc Natl Acad Sci USA. 1981;78:5608–12.

70. Quasthoff S, Hartung HP. Chemotherapy-induced peripheral neuropathy. J Neurol. 2002;249:9–17.

71. Coleman RE. Management of bone metastases. Oncologist. 2000;5:463–70.

72. Cliffer KD, Siuciak JA, Carson SR, Radley HE, Park JS, Lewis DR, et al. Physiological characterization of taxol-induced large-fiber sensory neuropathy in the rat. Ann Neurol. 1998;43:46–55.

73. Smith SB, Crager SE, Mogil JS. Paclitaxel-induced neuropathic hypersensitivity in mice: responses in 10 inbred mouse strains. Life Sci. 2004;74:2593–604.

74. Ledeboer A, Jekich BM, Sloane EM, Mahoney JH, Langer SJ, Milligan ED, et al. Intrathecal interleukin-10 gene therapy attenuates paclitaxel-induced mechanical allodynia and proinflammatory cytokine expression in dorsal root ganglia in rats. Brain Behav Immun. 2007;21:686–98.

75. Zhang H, Yoon SY, Zhang H, Dougherty PM. Evidence that spinal astrocytes but not microglia contribute to the pathogenesis of Paclitaxel-induced painful neuropathy. J Pain. 2012;13:293–303.

76. Higuera ES, Luo ZD. A rat pain model of vincristine-induced neuropathy. Methods Mol Med. 2004;99:91–8.

77. Authier N, Coudore F, Eschalier A, Fialip J. Pain-related behaviour during vincristine-induced neuropathy in rats. Neuroreport. 1999;10:965–8.

78. Joseph EK, Levine JD. Sexual dimorphism for protein kinase C-epsilon signaling in a rat model of vincristine-induced painful peripheral neuropathy. Neuroscience. 2003;119:831–8.

79. Topp KS, Tanner KD, Levine JD. Damage to the cytoskeleton of large diameter sensory neurons and myelinated axons in vincristine-induced painful peripheral neuropathy in the rat. J Comp Neurol. 2000;424:563–76.

80. Nozaki-Taguchi N, Chaplan SR, Higuera ES, Ajakwe RC, Yaksh TL. Vincristine-induced allodynia in the rat. Pain. 2001;93:69–76.

81. Dougherty PM, Cata JP, Burton AW, Vu K, Weng HR. Dysfunction in multiple primary afferent fiber subtypes revealed by quantitative sensory testing in patients with chronic vincristine-induced pain. J Pain Symptom Manage. 2007;33:166–79.

82. Xiao WH, Bennett GJ. Chemotherapy-evoked neuropathic pain: abnormal spontaneous discharge in A-fiber and C-fiber primary afferent neurons and its suppression by acetyl-L-carnitine. Pain. 2008;135: 262–70.

83. Authier N, Fialip J, Eschalier A, Coudore F. Assessment of allodynia and hyperalgesia after cisplatin administration to rats. Neurosci Lett. 2000;291: 73–6.

84. Gispen WH, Hamers FP, Vecht CJ, Jennekens FG, Neyt JP. ACTH/MSH like peptides in the treatment of cisplatin neuropathy. J Steroid Biochem Mol Biol. 1992;43:179–83.

85. Boyle FM, Wheeler HR, Shenfield GM. Amelioration of experimental cisplatin and paclitaxel neuropathy with glutamate. J Neurooncol. 1999;41: 107–16.

86. de Koning P, Neijt JP, Jennekens FG, Gispen WH. ORG2766 protects from cisplatin-induced neurotoxicity in rats. Exp Neurol. 1987;97:746–50.

87. Fischer SJ, Podratz JL, Windebank AJ. Nerve growth factor rescue of cisplatin neurotoxicity is mediated through the high affinity receptor: studies in PC12 cells and p75null mouse dorsal root ganglia. Neurosci Lett. 2001;308:1–4.

88. McDonald ES, Windebank AJ. Cisplatin-induced apoptosis of DRG neurons involves BAX redistribution and cytochrome C release but not FAS receptor signaling. Neurobiol Dis. 2002;9:220–33.

89. Allen JW, Mantyh PW, Horais K, Tozier N, Rogers SD, Ghilardi JR, et al. Safety evaluation of intrathecal substance P-saporin, a targeted neurotoxin, in dogs. Toxicol Sci. 2006;91:286–98.

90. ter Laak MP, Hamers FP, Kirk CJ, Gispen WH. rhGGF2 protects against cisplatin-induced neuropathy in the rat. J Neurosci Res. 2000;60:237–44.

91. Pradat PF, Kennel P, Naimi-Sadaoui S, Finiels F, Scherman D, Orsini C, et al. Viral and nonviral gene therapy partially prevents experimental cisplatin-induced neuropathy. Gene Ther. 2002;9: 1333–7.

92. Tassler P, Dellon AL, Lesser GJ, Grossman S. Utility of decompressive surgery in the prophylaxis and treatment of cisplatin neuropathy in adult rats. J Reconstr Microsurg. 2000;16:457–63.

93. Vietor NO, George BJ. Oxaliplatin-induced hepatocellular injury and ototoxicity: a review of the literature and report of unusual side effects of a commonly used chemotherapeutic agent. J Oncol Pharm Pract. 2012;18:355–9.

94. Sakurai M, Egashira N, Kawashiri T, Yano T, Ikesue H, Oishi R. Oxaliplatin-induced neuropathy in the rat: involvement of oxalate in cold hyperalgesia but not mechanical allodynia. Pain. 2009;147:165–74.

95. Cavaletti G, Gilardini A, Canta A, Rigamonti L, Rodriguez-Menendez V, Ceresa C, et al. Bortezomib-induced peripheral neurotoxicity: a neurophysiological and pathological study in the rat. Exp Neurol. 2007;204:317–25.

96. Stratogianni A, Tosch M, Schlemmer H, Weis J, Katona I, Isenmann S, Haensch CA. Bortezomib-induced severe autonomic neuropathy. Clin Auton Res. 2012;22:199–202.

97. Galasko CS. Diagnosis of skeletal metastases and assessment of response to treatment. Clin Orthop Relat Res. 1995;312:64–75.

98. Watkins LR, Maier SF. Implications of immune-to-brain communication for sickness and pain. Proc Natl Acad Sci USA. 1999;96:7710–3.

99. DeLeo JA, Yezierski RP. The role of neuroinflammation and neuroimmune activation in persistent pain. Pain. 2001;90:1–6.

100. Nelson JB, Carducci MA. The role of endothelin-1 and endothelin receptor antagonists in prostate cancer. BJU Int. 2000;85 Suppl 2:45–8.

101. Davar G. Endothelin-1 and metastatic cancer pain. Pain Med. 2001;2:24–7.

102. Watkins LR, Hansen MK, Nguyen KT, Lee JE, Maier SF. Dynamic regulation of the proinflammatory cytokine, interleukin-1beta: molecular biology for

non-molecular biologists. Life Sci. 1999;65: 449–81.

103. Oprée A, Kress M. Involvement of the proinflammatory cytokines tumor necrosis factor-alpha, IL-1 beta, and IL-6 but not IL-8 in the development of heat hyperalgesia: effects on heat-evoked calcitonin gene-related peptide release from rat skin. J Neurosci. 2000;20:6289–93.

104. Purow BW, Sundaresan TK, Burdick MJ, Kefas BA, Comeau LD, Hawkinson MP, et al. Notch-1 regulates transcription of the epidermal growth factor receptor through p53. Carcinogenesis. 2008;29: 918–25.

105. Roman C, Saha D, Beauchamp R. TGF-beta and colorectal carcinogenesis. Microsc Res Tech. 2001;52: 450–7.

106. Radinsky R. Growth factors and their receptors in metastasis. Semin Cancer Biol. 1991;2:169–77.

107. Lin Z, Sugai JV, Jin Q, Chandler LA, Giannobile WV. Platelet-derived growth factor-B gene delivery sustains gingival fibroblast signal transduction. J Periodontal Res. 2008;43:440–9.

108. Watkins LR, Milligan ED, Maier SF. Glial activation: a driving force for pathological pain. Trends Neurosci. 2001;24:450–5.

109. Cata JP, Weng HR, Chen JH, Dougherty PM. Altered discharges of spinal wide dynamic range neurons and down-regulation of glutamate transporter expression in rats with paclitaxel-induced hyperalgesia. Neuroscience. 2006;138:329–38.

110. Sweitzer SM, Pahl JL, DeLeo JA. Propentofylline attenuates vincristine-induced peripheral neuropathy in the rat. Neurosci Lett. 2006;400:258–61.

111. Ignatowski TA, Covey WC, Knight PR, Severin CM, Nickola TJ, Spengler RN. Brain-derived TNF alpha mediates neuropathic pain. Brain Res. 1999;841: 70–7.

112. Sacerdote P, Franchi S, Trovato AE, Valsecchi AE, Panerai AE, Colleoni M. Transient early expression of TNF-alpha in sciatic nerve and dorsal root ganglia in a mouse model of painful peripheral neuropathy. Neurosci Lett. 2008;436:210–3.

113. Wei F, Guo W, Zou S, Ren K, Dubner R. Supraspinal glial-neuronal interactions contribute to descending pain facilitation. J Neurosci. 2008;28: 10482–95.

114. Jancálek R, Dubový P, Svízenská I, Klusáková I. Bilateral changes of TNF-alpha and IL-10 protein in the lumbar and cervical dorsal root ganglia following a unilateral chronic constriction injury of the sciatic nerve. J Neuroinflammation. 2010;7:11.

115. Sfikakis PP. The first decade of biologic TNF antagonists in clinical practice: lessons learned, unresolved issues and future directions. Curr Dir Autoimmun. 2010;11:180–210.

116. Gu X, Zheng Y, Ren B, Zhang R, Mei F, Zhang J, et al. Intraperitoneal injection of thalidomide attenuates bone cancer pain and decreases spinal tumor necrosis factor-α expression in a mouse model. Mol Pain. 2010;6:64.

117. Tobinick EL. Targeted etanercept for treatment-refractory pain due to bone metastasis: two case reports. Clin Ther. 2003;25:2279–88.

118. Quesada JR, Talpaz M, Rios A, Kurzrock R, Gutterman JU. Clinical toxicity of interferons in cancer patients: a review. J Clin Oncol. 1986;4: 234–43.

119. Mahmoud HH, Pui CH, Kennedy W, Jaffe HS, Crist WM, Murphy SB. Phase I study of recombinant human interferon gamma in children with relapsed acute leukemia. Leukemia. 1992;6:1181–4.

120. Robertson B, Xu XJ, Hao JX, Wiesenfeld-Hallin Z, Mhlanga J, Grant G, et al. Interferon-gamma receptors in nociceptive pathways: role in neuropathic pain-related behaviour. Neuroreport. 1997;8:1311–6.

121. Reyes-Gibby CC, Wu X, Spitz M, Kurzrock R, Fisch M, Bruera E, et al. Molecular epidemiology, cancer-related symptoms, and cytokines pathway. Lancet Oncol. 2008;9:777–85. Review.

122. Meyers CA, Seabrooke LF, Albitar M, Estey EH. Association of cancer-related symptoms with physiological parameters. J Pain Symptom Manage. 2002;24:359–61.

123. Mika J, Korostynski M, Kaminska D, Wawrzczak-Bargiela A, Osikowicz M, Makuch W, et al. Interleukin-1alpha has antiallodynic and antihyperalgesic activities in a rat neuropathic pain model. Pain. 2008;138:587–97.

124. Alexander GM, van Rijn MA, van Hilten JJ, Perreault MJ, Schwartzman RJ. Changes in cerebrospinal fluid levels of pro-inflammatory cytokines in CRPS. Pain. 2005;116:213–9.

125. Sommer C, Petrausch S, Lindenlaub T, Toyka KV. Neutralizing antibodies to interleukin 1-receptor reduce pain associated behavior in mice with experimental neuropathy. Neurosci Lett. 1999;270:25–8.

126. Honore P, Wade CL, Zhong C, Harris RR, Wu C, Ghayur T, et al. Interleukin-1alphabeta gene-deficient mice show reduced nociceptive sensitivity in models of inflammatory and neuropathic pain but not post-operative pain. Behav Brain Res. 2006; 167:355–64.

127. Zhang RX, Liu B, Li A, Wang L, Ren K, Qiao JT, et al. Interleukin 1β facilitates bone cancer pain in rats by enhancing NMDA receptor NR-1 subunit phosphorylation. Neuroscience. 2008;154:1533–8.

128. Tawara K, Oxford JT, Jorcyk CL. Clinical significance of interleukin (IL)-6 in cancer metastasis to bone: potential of anti-IL-6 therapies. Cancer Manag Res. 2011;3:177–89.

129. Wang L, Yi T, Kortylewski M, Pardoll DM, Zeng D, Yu H. IL-17 can promote tumor growth through an IL-6-Stat3 signaling pathway. J Exp Med. 2009;206: 1457–64.

130. Balkwill F. The significance of cancer cell expression of the chemokine receptor CXCR4. Semin Cancer Biol. 2004;14:171–9.

131. Burger JA, Kipps TJ. CXCR4: a key receptor in the crosstalk between tumor cells and their microenvironment. Blood. 2006;107:1761–7.

132. Vandercappellen J, Van Damme J, Struyf S. The role of CXC chemokines and their receptors in cancer. Cancer Lett. 2008;267:226–44.

133. Sheu BC, Chang WC, Cheng CY, Lin HH, Chang DY, Huang SC. Cytokine regulation networks in the cancer microenvironment. Front Biosci. 2008;13:6255–68.

134. Abbadie C, Bhangoo S, De Koninck Y, Malcangio M, Melik-Parsadaniantz S, White FA. Chemokines and pain mechanisms. Brain Res Rev. 2009;60:125–34.

135. Mennicken F, Maki R, de Souza EB, Quirion R. Chemokines and chemokine receptors in the CNS: a possible role in neuroinflammation and patterning. Trends Pharmacol Sci. 1999;20:73–8.

136. Miller RJ, Rostene W, Apartis E, Banisadr G, Biber K, Milligan ED, et al. Chemokine action in the nervous system. J Neurosci. 2008;28:11792–5.

137. White FA, Jung H, Miller RJ. Chemokines and the pathophysiology of neuropathic pain. Proc Natl Acad Sci USA. 2007;104:20151–8.

138. Oh SB, Tran PB, Gillard SE, Hurley RW, Hammond DL, Miller RJ. Chemokines and glycoprotein120 produce pain hypersensitivity by directly exciting primary nociceptive neurons. J Neurosci. 2001;21:5027–35.

139. Bhangoo SK, Ren D, Miller RJ, Chan DM, Ripsch MS, Weiss C, et al. CXCR4 chemokine receptor signaling mediates pain hypersensitivity in association with antiretroviral toxic neuropathy. Brain Behav Immun. 2007;21:581–91.

140. Franklin KBJ, Abbott FV. Techniques for assessing the effects of drugs on nociceptive responses. In: Boultoun M, Baker GB, Greenshaw AJ, editors. Neuromethods, psychopharmacology. Clifton: The Humana Press; 1989. p. 145–215.

141. Woolf CJ. Long term alterations in the excitability of the flexion reflex produced by peripheral tissue injury in the chronic decerebrate rat. Pain. 1984;18:325–43.

142. Basbaum AI, Fields HL. Endogenous pain control systems: brainstem spinal pathways and endorphin circuitry. Annu Rev Neurosci. 1984;7:309–38.

143. Maier SF, Wiertelak EP, Watkins LR. Endogenous pain facilitatory systems: antianalgesia and hyperalgesia. J Pain. 1992;1:191–8.

144. Chaplan SR, Bach FW, Pogrel JW, Chung JM, Yaksh TL. Quantitative assessment of tactile allodynia in the rat paw. J Neurosci Methods. 1994;53:55–63.

145. Kaur G, Jaggi AS, Singh N. Exploring the potential effect of Ocimum sanctum in vincristine-induced neuropathic pain in rats. J Brachial Plex Peripher Nerve Inj. 2010;5:3.

146. Ghelardini C, Desaphy JF, Muraglia M, Corbo F, Matucci R, Dipalma A, et al. Effects of a new potent analog of tocainide on hNav1.7 sodium channels and in vivo neuropathic pain models. Neuroscience. 2010;169:863–73.

147. Machelska H, Schopohl JK, Mousa SA, Labuz D, Schafer M, Stein C. Different mechanisms of intrinsic pain inhibition in early and late inflammation. J Neuroimmunol. 2003;141:30–9.

148. Bennett GJ, Xie YK. A peripheral mononeuropathy in rat that produces disorders of pain sensation like those seen in man. Pain. 1988;33:87–107.

149. Mika J, Osikowicz M, Makuch W, Przewlocka B. Minocycline and pentoxifylline attenuate allodynia and hyperalgesia and potentiate the effects of morphine in rat and mouse models of neuropathic pain. Eur J Pharmacol. 2007;560:142–9.

150. Boettger MK, Hensellek S, Richter F, Gajda M, Stöckigt R, van Banchet GS, et al. Antinociceptive effects of tumor necrosis factor alpha neutralization in a rat model of antigen-induced arthritis: evidence of a neuronal target. Arthritis Rheum. 2008;58:2368–78.

151. Dubner R. Methods of assessing pain in animals. In: Wall PD, Melzack R, editors. Textbook of pain. Edinburgh: Churchville Livingstone; 1989. p. 247–56.

152. Mika J, Wawrzczak-Bargiela A, Osikowicz M, Makuch W, Przewlocka B. Attenuation of morphine tolerance by minocycline and pentoxifylline in naive and neuropathic mice. Brain Behav Immun. 2009;23:75–84.

153. Hargreaves K, Dubner R, Brown F, Flores C, Joris J. A new and sensitive method for measuring thermal nociception in cutaneous hyperalgesia. Pain. 1988;32:77–88.

154. Espejo EF, Mir D. Structure of the rat's behaviour in the hot plate test. Behav Brain Res. 1993;56:171–6.

155. Holtman Jr JR, Crooks PA, Johnson-Hardy J, Wala EP. Antinociceptive effects and toxicity of morphine-6-O-sulfate sodium salt in rat models of pain. Eur J Pharmacol. 2010;648:87–94.

156. Choi Y, Yoon YW, Na HS, Kim SH, Chung JM. Behavioral signs of ongoing pain and cold allodynia in a rat model of neuropathic pain. Pain. 1994;59:369–76.

157. Wang TC, Hsiao IT, Cheng YK, Wey SP, Yen TC, Lin KJ. Noninvasive monitoring of tumor growth in a rat glioma model: comparison between neurological assessment and animal imaging. J Neurooncol. 2011;104:669–78.

158. De Medinacelli L, Freed WJ, Wyatt RJ. An index of the functional condition of rat sciatic nerve based on measurements made from walking tracks. Exp Neurol. 1982;77:634–43.

159. De Koning JH, Brakkee WH, Gispen WH. Methods for producing a reproducible crush in the sciatic and tibial nerve of the rat and rapid and precise testing of return of sensory function. J Neurol Sci. 1986;74:237–56.

160. Hamers FP, Lankhorst AJ, van Laar TJ, Veldhuis WB, Gispen WH. Automated quantitative gait analysis during overground locomotion in the rat: its application to spinal cord contusion and transection injuries. J Neurotrauma. 2001;18:187–201.

161. Doré-Savard L, Otis V, Belleville K, Lemire M, Archambault M, Tremblay L, et al. Behavioral,

medical imaging and histopathological features of a new rat model of bone cancer pain. PLoS One. 2010;5:e13774.

162. Siau C, Bennett GJ. Dysregulation of cellular calcium homeostasis in chemotherapy-evoked painful peripheral neuropathy. Anesth Analg. 2006;102:1485–90.

163. Melli G, Taiana M, Camozzi F, Triolo D, Podini P, Quattrini A, et al. Alpha-lipoic acid prevents mitochondrial damage and neurotoxicity in experimental chemotherapy neuropathy. Exp Neurol. 2008;214:276–84.

164. Sun X, Windebank AJ. Calcium in suramin-induced rat sensory neuron toxicity in vitro. Brain Res. 1996;742:149–56.

165. Xiao W, Boroujerdi A, Bennett GJ, Luo ZD. Chemotherapy-evoked painful peripheral neuropathy: analgesic effects of gabapentin and effects on expression of the alpha-2-delta type-1 calcium channel subunit. Neuroscience. 2007;144:714–20.

166. Alessandri-Haber N, Dina OA, Joseph EK, Reichling DB, Levine JD. Interaction of transient receptor potential vanilloid 4, integrin, and SRC tyrosine kinase in mechanical hyperalgesia. J Neurosci. 2008;28:1046–57.

167. Ta LE, Bieber AJ, Carlton SM, Loprinzi CL, Low PA, Windebank AJ. Transient Receptor Potential Vanilloid 1 is essential for cisplatin-induced heat hyperalgesia in mice. Mol Pain. 2010;6:15.

168. Anand U, Otto WR, Anand P. Sensitization of capsaicin and icilin responses in oxaliplatin treated adult rat DRG neurons. Mol Pain. 2010;6:82.

169. Mangiacavalli S, Corso A, De Amici M, Varettoni M, Alfonsi E, Lozza A, et al. Emergent T-helper 2 profile with high interleukin-6 levels correlates with the appearance of bortezomib-induced neuropathic pain. Br J Haematol. 2010;149:916–8.

170. Scuteri A, Galimberti A, Ravasi M, Pasini S, Donzelli E, Cavaletti G, et al. NGF protects dorsal root ganglion neurons from oxaliplatin by modulating JNK/Sapk and ERK1/2. Neurosci Lett. 2010;486:141–5.

171. Horvath P, Szilvassy J, Nemeth J, Peitl B, Szilasi M, Szilvassy Z. Decreased sensory neuropeptide release in isolated bronchi of rats with cisplatin-induced neuropathy. Eur J Pharmacol. 2005;507:247–52.

172. Jamieson SM, Liu JJ, Connor B, Dragunow M, McKeage MJ. Nucleolar enlargement, nuclear eccentricity and altered cell body immunostaining characteristics of large-sized sensory neurons following treatment of rats with paclitaxel. Neurotoxicology. 2007;28:1092–8.

173. Kamei J, Tamura N, Saitoh A. Possible involvement of the spinal nitric oxide/cGMP pathway in vincris-tine-induced painful neuropathy in mice. Pain. 2005;117:112–20.

174. Mihara Y, Egashira N, Sada H, Kawashiri T, Ushio S, Yano T, et al. Involvement of spinal NR2B-containing NMDA receptors in oxaliplatin-induced mechanical allodynia in rats. Mol Pain. 2011;7:8.

175. Sabino MA, Ghilardi JR, Jongen JL, Keyser CP, Luger NM, Mach DB, et al. Simultaneous reduction in cancer pain, bone destruction, and tumor growth by selective inhibition of cyclooxygenase 2. Cancer Res. 2002;62:7343–9.

176. Sabino MA, Luger NM, Mach DB, Rogers SD, Schwei MJ, Mantyh PW. Different tumors in bone each give rise to a distinct pattern of skeletal destruction, bone cancer-related pain behaviors and neurochemical changes in the central nervous system. Int J Cancer. 2003;104:550–8.

177. Erin N, Boyer PJ, Bonneau RH, Clawson GA, Welch DR. Capsaicin-mediated denervation of sensory neurons promotes mammary tumor metastasis to lung and heart. Anticancer Res. 2004;24:1003–9.

178. Andersen C, Bagi CM, Adams SW. Intratibial injection of human prostate cancer cell line CWR22 elicits osteoblastic response in immunodeficient rats. J Musculoskelet Neuronal Interact. 2003;3:148–55.

179. Bauerle T, Adwan H, Kiessling F, Hilbig H, Armbruster FP, Berger MR. Characterization of a rat model with site-specific bone metastasis induced by MDA-MB231 breast cancer cells and its application to the effects of an antibody against bone sialoprotein. Int J Cancer. 2005;115:177–86.

180. Urch CE, Donovan-Rodriguez T, Dickenson AH. Alterations in dorsal horn neurones in a rat model of cancer-induced bone pain. Pain. 2003;106:347–56.

181. El Mouedden M, Meert TF. Evaluation of pain-related behavior, bone destruction, and effectiveness of fentanyl, sufentanil, and morphine in a murine model of cancer pain. Pharmacol Biochem Behav. 2005;82:109–19.

182. Baamonde A, Lastra A, Fresno MF, Llames S, Meana A, Hidalgo A, et al. Implantation of tumoral XC cells induces chronic, endothelin-dependent, thermal hyperalgesia in mice. Cell Mol Neurobiol. 2004;24:269–81.

183. Menendez L, Lastra A, Fresno MF, Llames S, Meana A, Hidalgo A, et al. Initial thermal heat hypoalgesia and delayed hyperalgesia in a murine model of bone cancer pain. Brain Res. 2003;969:102–9.

184. Siau C, Xiao W, Bennett GJ. Paclitaxel- and vincris-tine-evoked painful peripheral neuropathies: loss of epidermal innervation and activation of Langerhans cells. Exp Neurol. 2006;201:507–14.

Pain Assessment, Recognising Clinical Patterns, and Cancer Pain Syndromes

7

Malgorzata Krajnik and Zbigniew (Ben) Zylicz

Abstract

Pain in cancer is not a single diagnosis or entity. In fact, it is a constellation of many types of pain from which each type needs to be assessed separately in order to choose specific treatment. The pain in cancer can be related to the disease itself, its treatment but also to other, non-cancer-related issues like immobility, atrophy, and degeneration. Here, we present a way to seperate these three large groups from each other and to recognise specific cancer-related pain syndromes. The non-cancer-related syndromes will be discussed in a separate chapter.

Keywords

Cancer Pain • Assessment • Diagnosis • Complex cancer pain • Cancer-related syndromes

Introduction

Pain in patients with cancer cannot be seen as a single disease or entity. It is usually a constellation of many types of pain, non-pain symptoms, and signs. Some of them are related to disease progression and others to immobility and general deterioration. As patients with cancer tend to live longer and the antitumour treatment is now more effective (see Chap. 3), many pains experienced by patients with cancer may be of treatment-related or nonmalignant origin. Patients experiencing pain, however, may still connect it with the progression of disease or a poor prognosis, and this may increase their anxiety, uncertainty, and depression. In extreme situations, aggressive oncology treatment cures some patients at the price of intractable pain, which is the new challenge for pain and palliative medicine [1]. Problems in cancer survivors will be highlighted in Chap. 13.

In this chapter, we shall try to provide some guidance as to how to make sense of multiple signs and symptoms and how to progress to a

M. Krajnik, MD, PhD
Palliative Care Department,
Nicolaus Copernicus University,
Collegium Medium in Bydgoszcz,
Sklodowskiej – Curie 9,
Basel, Bydgoszcz 85-094, Poland
e-mail: malgorzata.krajnik@wp.pl

Z. Zylicz, MD, PhD (✉)
Department of Research and Education,
Hildegard Hospiz, St. Alban Ring 151,
Basel 4020, Switzerland
e-mail: ben.zylicz@hildegard-hospiz.ch

M. Hanna, Z. Zylicz (eds.), *Cancer Pain*,
DOI 10.1007/978-0-85729-230-8_7, © Springer-Verlag London 2013

specific pain diagnosis and treatment. The generic name of "cancer pain" for all kinds of pain affecting patients with cancer is not good enough, as different pains need a different approach and there is no one drug that will ease all of the pains at the same time.

Some symptoms and signs may suggest one mechanism and help to construct a syndrome [2]. In the second half of the chapter, we shall discuss the most important cancer pain syndromes. Even these syndromes, however, may be blurred, complicated, and exacerbated in the course of a disease by pain facilitation, adverse effects of the drugs, effects on the endocrine system, and the influences of psychological and personality factors. For each patient, pain is experienced in a unique way, representing a major challenge for clinicians.

The Strategy for Cancer Pain Assessment

The evaluation of pain should be regarded as a standard of care [3]. It is an essential component of the palliative care approach [4]. Pain, however, is not a simple result of nociception and pain assessment should include psychological, social, and spiritual dimensions. Pain in patients with cancer almost never appears alone and is frequently clustered with other symptoms [5]. Thus, the assessment should also include other symptoms, as the treatment of pain alone may aggravate them, making treatment pointless. The specific diagnosis of pain and its explanation may be reassuring to some patients, as not all pains are related to disease progression and poor prognosis, and may be amenable to simple measures. Therefore, the strategy of pain assessment should address the complex and individual needs of the patient and his or her family.

Taking Pain History

A broad clinical framework of pain assessment includes not only the characterisation of the pain complaint and a formulation of its nature in terms of cause, syndrome, and pathophysiology but also elucidation of the status of the underlying

Table 7.1 Strategy of cancer pain assessment

What should be characterised, clarified, and repeatedly monitored?
Pain dimensions:
Intensity
Temporal features (onset, course, daily fluctuation, and breakthrough pains)
Location and radiation
Quality
Provocative or relieving factors
Response to treatment
Nature of the pain:
Cause
Inferred pathophysiology
Pain syndrome
Effect of the pain on life domains such as:
Physical function and well-being
Mood, coping, and related aspects of psychological well-being
Role functioning and social and familial relationships
Sleep, mood, vitality, and sexual function
Clinical situation and comorbidities:
Extent of neoplastic disease, planned treatment, and prognosis
Nature and quality of previous testing and past treatments
Medical comorbidities
Psychiatric comorbidities (substance-use history, depression and anxiety disorders, personality disorders)
Other needs for palliative care interventions:
Other symptoms
Distress related to psychosocial or spiritual concerns
Caregiver burden and concrete needs
Problems in communication, care coordination, and goal setting
The presence of opioidophobia
Clinician's ability to communicate with the patient and the family

Modified from Portenoy [4] and Ripamonti and Bandieri [6]

disease and comorbidities and an evaluation of the burden and different concerns related to pain and illness [4, 6] (Table 7.1).

Unfortunately, cancer pain is not described particularly accurately in the literature, and the concept of syndromes is used only rarely [7, 8]. The situation is further complicated by the absence of a universally accepted classification system for pain in cancer [9].

To make pain assessment both less time-consuming and more useful, experts and researchers have tried to identify the key variables, which would be important, not only in diagnosing pain but also in defining the treatment plan. A recent multicenter cross-sectional study of cancer patients treated with opioids revealed that breakthrough pain, psychological distress, and sleep and opioid dose were most strongly associated with pain intensity and treatment response and should be included in standard pain assessment [10, 11].

Assessment of Pain Intensity

Taking a history from the patient and from the family members is essential, as pain is a subjective experience. This is why experts have introduced the assessment and reassessment of a clinician's ability to communicate with patients and their families into the guidelines concerning the correct assessment of pain [6]. The evaluation of pain intensity is crucial for taking decisions and the monitoring of treatment dynamics. Optimally, patients should be asked about "pain right now," "pain at its worst," "pain on average," "pain relief," and "pain at its least" (all indicators related to the previous 24 h) [12]. This may be terribly confusing for many patients and is realistic only in a research setting. To keep the number of questions low, some experts suggest limiting them to the first three indicators. "Pain on average" is remarkably valuable in the case of long-term pain treatment, even preferred to "pain right now"; the latter being more adequate for the assessment of acute pain or that felt during parenteral opioid titration [10, 13]. "Pain at its worst" should always be evaluated as the marker of pain fluctuation and interference [14] and as a sensitive indicator of treatment response [15]. Furthermore, "pain on average" and "pain at its worst" correlate well with impaired function [11, 16]. The main value of a pain intensity evaluation is the monitoring of pain management. Not surprisingly, pain evaluation in hospitalised patients in itself reduces pain intensity [17]. In many (out-)

patients, the twice-daily recording of pain in a diary improves pain control and coping skills, as well as communication, and promotes the recording of regular and rescue medication doses [18, 19]. Patients should be taught how to understand and use one of the one-dimensional pain scales, such as the Numerical Rating Scale (NRS), the Verbal Rating Scale (VRS), or the Visual Analogue Scale (VAS) [20]. In the NRS, 0 indicates "no pain at all" and 10 "the worst possible pain" [21]. For the VAS, patients should specify their level of agreement with a statement by indicating a position along a continuous line between two endpoints [21]. Finally, with the VRS, patients rate their pain intensity by choosing from the following descriptors: none, very mild, mild, moderate, severe, and very severe [16].

In clinical practice, the interpretation of the data from pain-rating scales is not as straightforward as it might at first appear. Such scales are often used in pain research. In a systematic review, the NRS showed better compliance than the VAS and VRS in 15 out of the 19 studies reporting this and was the recommended tool in 11 studies on the basis of higher compliance rates, better responsiveness and ease of use, and good applicability relative to the VAS/VRS [22]. Twenty-nine studies gave no preference. However, many studies have shown a wide distribution of NRS scores within each category of the VRS [22]. For example, a patient might describe pain as "severe" (VRS), while indicating "2" or "3" on the NRS. The situation might be even more complicated when a patient has to describe the intensity of two or more coexisting pains or evaluate background and episodic pains. In a multicenter cross-sectional study carried out on a sample of 240 patients with advanced cancer and pain, the NRS revealed a higher discriminatory capability than the VRS in distinguishing between background and peak pain intensity and showed higher reproducibility when measuring pain exacerbation [23]. These results suggest that, in the measurement of cancer pain exacerbation, patients use the NRS more appropriately than the VRS, and as such, the NRS seems to be preferred by patients to the VRS.

Apart from potential errors within the tools used by the same responder, it should be remembered that it is truly erroneous to compare results between different patients. This is also an argument for using a broad clinical framework for pain assessment, such as the Brief Pain Inventory [12] or the McGill Pain Questionnaire [24] and not only pain intensity scales [4, 6]. These two questionnaires have been validated in different languages and appear to be easily completed by those without cognitive deficits [15, 25]. Each pain should be assessed separately and clinicians should pay attention to the details. When a patient indicates a single site of pain, it might be a focal pain experienced in the region of the underlying lesion but could also be pain referred to a site remote from the lesion. For example, visceral pain from the liver due to diaphragmatic irritation is frequently referred to the right shoulder. Neuropathic pain is often referred along the distribution of the affected nerve. Primarily localised pain might change and become more diffuse in the course of disease, for example, due to central sensitisation or as a sign of opioid hyperalgesia [26]. It is useful to determine whether pain exists in a discrete area like a dermatome (as in root compression), in the distribution of a peripheral nerve (as in peripheral nerve compression), or is diffused (as in opioid-induced hyperalgesia). A body diagram helps to document and diagnose the pain sites. There are many more questions the clinician should ask the patient. Is the pain superficial or deep? Is there any radiation? Does it hurt as if burning or is it constant or colic? Which factors evoke or increase the pain (swallowing, constipation, movement, etc.) and which decrease it? Has body position any impact on the pain? Are opioids or any other measures helpful? To what degree? Do drugs have adverse effects? The clinician should also ask about the temporal pattern with regard to pain flares. The time course of pain is also important. Rapidly increasing pain suggests progressive disease or an emergency situation (as with spinal cord compression or bleeding to hepatic tumours). History is also the main (if not only) source of an evaluation of the impact of pain on different dimensions of a patient's life.

Physical Examination

A physical examination focusing on pain includes observation, palpation, percussion, auscultation, movement (active and passive), and neurological assessment [27]. Careful observation allows the noticing of any deformation in the skeleton or joints, muscle wasting, or changes in skin, posture, or gait. Palpation might provoke pain or tenderness or allow an assessment of pathological masses, distended intestines, or enlarged organs. Palpation of the muscles, tendons, and their insertions also reveals trigger and tender points that may be directly associated with the pain experienced [28]. It also tells the investigator if the pain is mechanosensitive, percussion of bone may provoke focal tenderness, auscultation helps to distinguish functional from organic obstruction, and movement may provoke a number of pains, mainly in the musculoskeletal system. To better understand neuropathic pain, a thorough neurological examination is needed, as it may shed light on the localisation of damage in the central nervous system and suggest an appropriate imaging technique to confirm it. Bedside Quantitative Sensory Testing is important in predicting responses to radiotherapy in cancer pain, thus possibly aiding clinical decision making [29].

Additional Investigations

A review of previous laboratory testing and imaging studies might provide useful information on mechanisms of pain and underlying disease. Clinicians should also decide whether there is a need for additional tests and whether these would be appropriate in the light of the patient's condition, prognosis, and goals. Laboratory testing or imaging might be important in defining the cause or pathophysiology of the pain, clarifying the extent of the disease, or assessing comorbidities.

Some laboratory parameters might suggest the cause and mechanisms of pain. For example, an increased level of serum calcium may correlate with bone pain in patients with multiple myeloma [30]. Patients with metastatic prostate cancer and suffering hypercalcemia have significantly higher levels of bone pain than similar patients with normocalcemia [31]. A recent database analysis of patients with prostate cancer showed that a prostate-specific antigen (PSA) response to oncology treatment did not precede pain response and that this serum marker does not anticipate the palliative benefit of chemotherapy [32]. However, a progressive increase in the serum PSA level in a patient after prostatectomy complaining of pain points to the potential recurrence of cancer disease and tumour infiltration as the cause of the painful state [33]. In reverse, severe pain in a patient with prostate cancer without an increase in PSA may point to the possibility of osteoporotic vertebral fractures.

Some other laboratory parameters may help in diagnosing the potential adverse events of an implemented therapy. For example, the measuring of testosterone and its related hormones (estradiol and DHT) in the blood, together with cortisol as an index of adrenal activity, may confirm a diagnosis of hypogonadism as a consequence of opioid treatment [34, 35]. Serum, renal, and liver function test results might be important in the choice of the drugs and doses that may be tolerated by the patient.

Radiological examination may help to diagnose the cause of pain [36]. The diagnostic strategy now should be more and more individually tailored according to the patient's clinical and biological data, such as primary cancer type, markers of aggressiveness, serum levels of the biological markers of bone metabolism, circulating, or disseminating tumour cells, and the availability and diagnostic performance of the imaging modalities [37]. For example, in the case of bone pain in cancer, imaging usually starts from plain bone radiographs, which in many cases will be adequate for identifying skeletal lesions. However, they do not reveal osteolytic lesions until more than 50 % of the bone cortex has been destroyed. The two main anatomical modalities are computed tomography (CT) and magnetic resonance imaging (MRI). The two main functional modalities are scintigraphy and positron emission tomography (PET) [37]. Bone scintigraphy has high sensitivity but low specificity for bone metastases and is useful when identifying the extent of bone lesions throughout the body. Conventional opinion is that nuclear bone scintigraphy is not helpful in the management of pure osteolytic lesions, such as those seen in myeloma bone disease [38]. However, it can sometimes detect bone marrow lesions in myeloma patients which cannot be detected by other imaging methods and is useful, especially in solitary myeloma, for excluding other involved sites [39, 40]. In cases of skeletal metastases, when findings on plain X-rays or bone scans are uncertain, any unexplained region of abnormal uptake should be examined by MRI and/or PET/CT, which has proven more accurate than classical bone scintigraphy, especially when dealing with haematological malignancies [41]. In clinical practice, bone scintigraphy is used also in a different context. When the patient is complaining of pain in a certain part of the skeleton, for example, in left pelvis, and bone scintigraphy discloses presence of a focal accumulation of the isotope, then there is a considerable certainty (the so-called positive match) that the pain is induced by the bone metastases. When the match is negative, the pain is there, but there is lack of isotope accumulation; other causes of pain should be taken into account. In these cases, nerve compression against bony prominence may be apparent (see Chap. 14 on non-cancer-related pain). This differentiation is important, as in the first case, radiotherapy will be the first choice. However, radiotherapy given to a nerve compression pain may only increase the pain intensity.

Cancer Pain Syndromes

According to recent studies, a large majority of cancer patients (>92 %) had one or more pain caused directly by cancer, while more than 20 % of patients had one or more pain caused by the cancer therapies [2, 42]. Almost 25 % of the patients experienced two or more pains [2]. The most common cancerous lesions responsible for pain appear to be those on bones and joints (42 %), visceral organs (28 %), soft tissue infiltration (28 %), and peripheral nerve injury (28 %). Elucidating the cause of pain is important because it might suggest a disease-modifying treatment for analgesic purposes, such as chemotherapy or radiation to a bone secondary.

Clinicians should be aware that defining an inferred pathophysiology is a kind of simplification. Progress in the understanding of the pathogenesis of bone pain has revealed the complexity of the different mechanisms responsible for the so-called bone pain [43, 44]. Cancer pain is often labelled as mixed mechanism pain and is not easily classified as exclusively neuropathic or nociceptive. However, inferring a predominant pathophysiology of pain is very practical and helps to rationalise the treatment. Pain is termed "nociceptive" if it seems to be sustained by ongoing tissue injury, whether somatic or visceral, or neuropathic if sustained through damage to or dysfunction in the nervous system. According to a survey performed by the Task Force on Cancer Pain of the IASP (International Association for the Study of Pain), the predominant type of mechanism was nociceptive somatic pain in 72 % and nociceptive visceral in 35 %, while neuropathic (mostly mixed neuropathic nociceptive) was diagnosed in 40 % of 1,095 patients treated with opioids due to cancer pain [2].

The quality of the pain often suggests its mechanism, although in the large series the results are not specific. Visceral pains originating from solid and hollow organs or tumour masses are diffuse; poorly localised pain described as cramping or gnawing suggests the obstruction of a hollow organ; and sharp, aching, or throbbing pain may indicate the involvement of mesentery or organ capsules. Superficial somatic pains from skin or mucosa are usually well localised and described as sharp, hot, or stinging. Deep somatic pains from muscles, joints, and bones are also well localised but are usually described as throbbing, aching, or dull. Patients with nociceptive pain frequently have a history of progressively worsening localised pain. On physical examination, palpation or percussion often reproduces nociceptive pain. An X-ray, bone scan, or magnetic resonance imaging often helps to identify bone metastases, while CT scans allow the finding of soft tissue masses or abscesses. Neuropathic pain might have nerve or dermatome distribution

and may be experienced by patients as burning, stabbing, shooting, hot, searing, shock like, tingling, or numbness [27]. The presence of comorbidities predisposing to neuropathies such as diabetes should be explored. On physical examination, a sensory assessment should include any gain in function such as allodynia and hyperesthesia or the loss of function which results in a reduction in the sensation caused by mechanical and thermal stimuli and defines an area of abnormal sensation [45]. For routine sensory assessment, such simple tools as a cotton-tipped swab, a toothpick, and a tuning fork should be sufficient.

The third component in understanding the nature of pain is the recognition of the pain syndrome. This is not, however, straightforward, as the same syndromes may have different causative factors and pathophysiologies. The term "cancer pain syndromes" describes rather a constellation of pain features, physical signs, and results of diagnostic testing [46]. Based on a survey of patients with cancer, the Task Force on Cancer Pain of the IASP identified 22 common pain syndromes in cancer-related clusters [46]. For example, patients with prostate cancer were much more likely to experience generalised bone pain and pains from the pelvis and long bones than other patients with different tumour types. Those with lung cancer were more likely to develop chest wall or pleural pain (Table 7.2).

Acute pain syndromes usually accompany diagnostic or therapeutic interventions, whereas chronic pain syndromes are mostly directly related to the neoplasm itself or to an antineoplastic therapy.

Acute Cancer Pain Syndromes
(Table 7.3)

Most acute cancer pain syndromes are iatrogenic, i.e., related to a diagnostic test or treatment [6, 47, 48]. Some of the syndromes are disease related, such as pain due to acute haemorrhage into a tumour, bone pain from a pathological fracture, or visceral pain from the acute obstruction or

Table 7.2 Common disease-related pain syndrome clusters

Lung cancer	Prostate cancer	Colon/rectum cancer	Cancer of upper GI tract
Pleural infiltration (23%) Chest wall syndrome (21%) Vertebral pain Chest and limb infiltration Plexopathy Generalised bone pain	Generalised bone pain (40%) Pelvis and long bones (26%) Vertebral pain (21%) Plexopathy	Suprapubic-perineal pain (40%) Abdominal pain (22%) Pelvis and long bones Liver capsule and biliary distention Plexopathy Vertebral	Rostral retroperitoneal (64%) Liver capsule and biliary distention (22%) Abdominal pain Esophageal mediastinal pain
Breast cancer	Head and neck tumours	Cancer of uterus	Leukaemia, lymphoma
Generalised bone pain (25%) Vertebral pain (21%) Chest and limb infiltration Plexopathy Radiculopathy	Head-neck muscle-fasciae (40%) Oral and skin infiltration (32%) Skull pain (22%) Plexopathy	Suprapubic-perineal pain (45%) Plexopathy (28%) Chest&limb infiltration Abdominal pain	Generalised bone pain Chest and limb infiltration Pelvis and long bones

Extracted from Caraceni and Portenoy [2]

perforation of a hollow organ [48]. Many diagnostic and therapeutic interventions, such as taking a blood sample, cause predictable pain or precipitate incident pain in patients with a preexisting pain syndrome. This happens, for example, during the positioning for radiotherapy of a patient with pathological bone fractures. One of the best-described acute pain syndromes due to a diagnostic procedure is a lumbar puncture headache, which is usually described as a dull occipital discomfort often radiating to the frontal region or to the shoulder. The pain is probably caused by the expansion of intracerebral veins sensitive to pain, as compensation for the reduction in cerebrospinal fluid volume because of leakage through the defect in the dural sheath [49].

Radiotherapy often induces or alters preexisting pain because of the waiting time, treatment manipulations, and transportation, and its prevalence is usually underestimated [50]. Pain syndromes associated with acute radiation toxicity are mostly due to inflammation and ulceration of skin or mucous membranes within the radiation field. As an example, esophagitis may occur after chest irradiation and proctitis following pelvic radiotherapy. Pain due to oral mucositis is the most frequently reported complaint negatively influencing quality of life during cancer therapy. It is related to the rich innervations of the orofacial area and a number of pain-triggering factors, such as oral intake or swallowing. In addition, oral mucosa is susceptible to the toxic effects of chemo- or radiotherapy, and microbial flora may be responsible for secondary infection, which increases the discomfort. Oral mucositis presents initially as erythema of the oral mucosa and frequently progresses to erosion and ulceration, causing severe discomfort. Pain from mucositis following radiotherapy is common (58–75 %) and even more frequent and more severe in cases of combined chemotherapy and radiotherapy [51, 52].

Chemotherapy is very often connected with different acute pain syndromes (see Chap. 13). It might be associated with infusion techniques, such as the intravenous infusion pains due to venous spasm, chemical phlebitis, vesicant extravasation, or anthracycline-associated flare [47]. However, more often clinicians observe acute pains associated with chemotherapy toxicity, such as the paclitaxel acute pain syndrome [53]. A prospective cohort study showed that this chemotherapy-induced peripheral neuropathy peaked 3 days after chemotherapy [53]. Twenty percent of the patients had pain scores of 5–10 out of 10 with the first dose of paclitaxel. Sensory neuropathy symptoms were more prominent than motor or autonomic neuropathy symptoms, and of the sensory neuropathy symptoms, numbness

Table 7.3 Acute cancer pain syndromes

Acute pains due to diagnostic or therapeutic interventions	
Diagnostic interventions and other procedures	Taking blood samples
	Transport and positioning for any procedures which require specific position
	Lumbar puncture headache
	Pain due to biopsies
	Mammography pain
	Radiofrequency tumour ablation
	Cryosurgery
	Pain due to endoscopy
	Pain associated with tumour embolisation techniques
	Pain due to chemical pleurodesis
	Local anaesthetic infiltration pain
	Opioids headache
	Opioid injection pain
	Spinal opioids hyperalgesia syndrome
	Epidural injection pain
Surgery	Postoperative pain
	Ileus, colic pain
	Urinary retention
Chemotherapy	Intravenous infusion pain
	Hepatic artery infusion pain
	Intraperitoneal chemotherapy infusion pain
	Intravesical chemotherapy pain
	Mucositis
	Headache
	Corticosteroid-induced perineal discomfort
	Pain syndrome due to withdrawal of steroids
	Painful peripheral neuropathy
	Diffuse bone pain
	Taxol-induced arthralgia and myalgia
	Ischemic chest pain (5-fluorouracil)
	Hand-foot syndrome
	Post-chemotherapy gynecomastia
	Acute digital ischemia
	Chemotherapy-induced tumour pain
Radiotherapy	Positioning for radiotherapy
	Oropharyngeal mucositis
	Acute radiation enteritis and proctocolitis
	Transient brachial plexopathy
	Subacute radiation myelopathy
	Radiopharmaceutical-induced pain flare
Other antitumour treatments	Luteinising hormone-releasing factor tumour flare in prostate cancer
	Aromatase inhibitor-induced arthralgia
	Hormone-induced pain flare in breast cancer
	Interferon-induced acute pain
	Bisphosphonate-induced bone pain
	Growth factor-induced acute pain

Table 7.3 (continued)

Cancer-induced or cancer-related acute pain syndromes

Acute haemorrhage into a tumour (e.g., in the liver, Wunderlich syndrome)

Spinal cord compression

Pathologic fracture

Acute obstruction or perforation of a hollow structure

Thrombosis (vena cava superior syndrome, acute mesenteric vein thrombosis, deep venous thrombosis, superficial thrombophlebitis, renal vein thrombosis)

Acute pulmonary embolism

Infections (in or around a tumour; acute herpetic neuralgia)

Colic due to constipation

Acute pain not related to cancer or treatment

Trauma

Myocardial infarction

and tingling were more prominent than shooting or burning pain. More than 60 % of breast cancer patients experience this syndrome during treatment with paclitaxel [54]. According to the studies, paclitaxel-induced peripheral neuropathy is a predictor of chronic neuropathic pain, as 27 % of the patients suffering from an acute syndrome were subsequently diagnosed with a chronic one [54]. Patients with higher pain scores after the first dose of paclitaxel appeared later to have more chronic neuropathy [53].

Chronic Cancer Pain Syndromes
(Table 7.4)

Multifocal Bone Pain: Bone Metastases and Bone Marrow Expansion

Bone metastases are the most common cause of chronic pain in cancer patients. As this is often a presenting symptom of bone metastases, focal bone pain in patients with cancer should always be investigated. Bone pain due to metastatic tumours must be differentiated from other causes of pain, such as osteoporotic fracture, osteoarthritis, focal osteonecrosis, or osteomalacia. Patients may experience a deep throbbing punctuated by sharper intense pain, often triggered by movement, coughing, deep breathing, etc. There may be a focal tenderness and swelling. The range of movement might be limited. Pain may be referred in different patterns, for example, a

lesion in the hip causes referred pain to the groin or knee. Bone pain may be focal, multifocal, or generalised, the last possibly a sign of the bone marrow replacement syndrome observed in myeloproliferative malignancies and occasionally in solid tumours [55, 56]. Multifocal pain is commonly experienced by patients with multiple sites of bone metastases. However, even in such cases, patients can complain about pain in one or a few sites. Before the decision of radiotherapy is taken for a painful bone, a positive match should be found between tumour localisation and the patient's complaints of pain. A negative match may suggest musculoskeletal, fascial, or nerve compression pain.

Vertebral Syndromes

Vertebral bodies are the most common site of bone invasion, with more than two-thirds of metastases found in the thoracic spine, 20 % being lumbosacral, and 10 % in the cervical region. Metastases to vertebral bodies often cause midline pain, while those to the vertebral pedicle may present as unilateral nerve root pain.

Occipital pain can indicate the destruction of the atlas or fracture of the odontoid process. It is typically described as severe neck pain radiating over the posterior aspect of the skull to the occiput and vertex which is exacerbated by movement of the neck, particularly flexion [57]. Pathological fracture may lead to subluxation and spinal cord

Table 7.4 Chronic cancer pain syndromes

Pain due to direct tumour involvement

Somatic nociceptive syndromes	Visceral nociceptive syndromes	Neuropathic syndromes
Tumour-related bone pain • Multifocal bone pain: bone metastases, bone marrow expansion (haematological malignancies) • Vertebral syndromes: atlantoaxial destruction and odontoid fracture; C7–T1 syndrome; T12–L1 syndrome; sacral syndrome (back pain secondary to spinal cord compression) • Pain syndromes related to pelvis and hip: pelvic metastases; hip joint syndrome • Base of skull metastases: orbital syndrome; parasellar syndrome; middle cranial fossa syndrome; jugular foramen syndrome; occipital condyle syndrome; clivus syndrome; sphenoid sinus syndrome Tumour-related soft tissue pain • Headache and facial pain • Ear and eye pain syndromes • Pleural pain	• Hepatic distension syndrome • Midline retroperitoneal syndrome • Chronic intestinal obstruction • Peritoneal carcinomatosis • Malignant perineal pain • Adrenal pain syndrome • Ureteric obstruction	• Leptomeningeal metastases • Painful cranial neuralgias • Glossopharyngeal neuralgia • Trigeminal neuralgia • Malignant painful radiculopathy • Plexopathies • Cervical plexopathy • Malignant brachial plexopathy • Malignant lumbosacral plexopathy • Sacral plexopathy • Coccygeal plexopathy • Painful peripheral mononeuropathies

Pain due to cancer therapy

Postoperative pain syndrome	Chronic pain associated with hormonal therapy	Post-chemotherapy pain syndrome	Postradiation pain syndrome
• Postmastectomy pain syndrome • Post-radical neck dissection pain • Post-thoracotomy pain syndrome • Post-thoracotomy frozen shoulder • Postsurgery pelvic floor pain • Stump pain • Phantom pain	Gynecomastia with hormonal therapy for prostate cancer	• Painful peripheral neuropathy • Raynaud's syndrome • Bony complications of long-term steroids • Avascular (aseptic) necrosis of femoral or humeral head • Vertebral compression fractures	• Radiation-induced brachial plexopathy • Chronic radiation myelopathy • Chronic radiation enteritis and proctitis • Lymphedema pain • Burning perineum syndrome • Osteoradionecrosis

Pain due to cancer-related complications

Paraneoplastic sensory neuropathy
Paraneoplastic nociceptive pain syndromes
• Muscle cramps
• Oncogenic osteomalacia
• Hypertrophic pulmonary osteoarthropathy
• Tumour-related gynecomastia
• Paraneoplastic pemphigus
• Paraneoplastic Raynaud's phenomenon
Myofascial pain syndrome
Postherpetic neuralgia
Debility
Constipation
Bed sores
Rectal or bladder spasm
Gastric distention

Pain unrelated to cancer or its treatment or its complications

Osteoarthritis
Myofascial pain
Osteoporosis

Modified from [2, 4, 5, 47, 48]

compression in the cervicomedullary junction. In such a case, the patient may present with progressive sensory, motor, and autonomic dysfunction beginning in the upper limbs.

Bone metastases at the level of the C_7–T_1 vertebral bodies can cause pain to be referred to the infrascapular region in the paraspinal areas radiating to both shoulders. It may also present as unilateral radicular pain radiating to the shoulder and medial aspect of the arm. Physical examination may reveal tenderness on percussion of the spinous processes. It might also be accompanied by paresthesias and numbness in the fourth and fifth fingers and with progressive weakness of the triceps and hand [58]. When T_{12}–L_1 vertebrae are affected, the patient may suffer from aching pain in the mid-back with the referral pattern at the iliac crest or one or both sacroiliac joints. In other cases, it is presented as radicular pain in the groin or thighs. Pain may be exacerbated by sitting or lying and relieved by standing or vice versa. The destruction of the sacrum can lead to severe focal pain radiating to the buttocks, perineum, or posterior tights [59]. Pain is often exacerbated by sitting or lying and may be relieved by standing or walking. If a tumour infiltrates the muscle responsible for the rotation of the hip (the piriformis muscle), it may lead to a "malignant piriformis syndrome" presented as buttock or posterior leg pain exacerbated by internal rotation of the hip [60]. A pain syndrome may be associated with perianal sensory loss, bowel and bladder dysfunction, and/or impotence.

Metastases to the vertebrae can spread posteriorly to the epidural space with eventual epidural spinal cord compression. Back pain is the initial symptom in almost all patients with epidural infiltration and spinal cord compression. As pain usually precedes neurological signs, it should be seen as a red flag and prompt further investigation. The early detection of spinal cord compression improves a patient's prognosis and reduces the chances for para- or even tetraparesis. MRI is the most sensitive test for showing the extension of the disease. The characteristics of the pain depend on the site of compression and the cause of the pain. For example, local pain is not always present but local tenderness is common. Root pain is often unilateral in cervical or lumbar compression

and bilateral in the thoracic spine. Pain may be caused by vertebral metastases, root compression presenting as radicular pain, and/or compression of the long tracts of the spinal cord with the so-called funicular pain. Funicular pain is usually less sharp and more diffuse (like a cuff or garter around the calves, knees, or thighs) and sometimes experienced as an unpleasantly cold sensation. Both funicular and radicular pains are exacerbated by neck flexion or straight-leg raising, recumbence, sneezing, coughing, or straining. If spinal compression is not effectively treated after a period of progressive pain, sometimes of a rapid and crescendo type, it can lead to motor weakness progressing to paraplegia, sensory loss, and loss of bowel and bladder function.

Pain Syndromes Related to the Pelvis and Hip

Metastases may involve the ischiopubic, iliosacral, or periacetabular regions of the pelvis, hip joint, or proximal femur. The pain is often incidental with walking and weight bearing. Localised hip pain due to lesions in the acetabulum or the head of the femur is aggravated by weight bearing and movement of the hip [61]. It may radiate to the knee or to the medial part of the thigh. It may sometimes change its nature when an acetabular tumour extends medially and destroys the lumbosacral plexus.

Base of Skull Metastases

Most commonly, cancer of the breast, lung, or prostate metastasises to this region, or the syndrome may be caused by a tumour spreading directly from the nasopharynx. Usually, the patient complains of a headache and the pain may precede other symptoms by weeks or months. Sometimes, there is only paresthesia or dysesthesia and numbness in the distribution of one or more cranial nerve. Plain radiography is not usually helpful and diagnostic procedures should start with CT, while MRI helps to assess the soft tissue infiltration.

The Most Common Tumour-Related Visceral Nociceptive Syndromes

Hepatic Distension Syndrome

Gross hepatomegaly may produce an aching pain in the right hypochondrium and less commonly in the right mid-back or flank [62]. Referred pain may appear in the right neck or shoulder or in the region of the right scapula. In some patients, the pain is exacerbated by standing, sitting, or prolonged walking, probably because of traction on the hepatic ligaments. Occasionally, patients develop rapidly increasing upper quadrant pain due to a haemorrhage into a metastasis. Physical examination suggests an "acute abdomen." The pain will diminish as the haematoma resolves and/or the capsule adapts. Sometimes, especially in cases of gross hepatomegaly, patients complain about discomfort in the lower rib cage due to outward pressure on the ribs. In other cases, they describe an intermittent sharp pain in the right hypochondrium caused by the enlarged liver pinching the parietal peritoneum against the lower border of the rib cage.

Midline Retroperitoneal Syndrome

This syndrome is the most common cause of pain in the retroperitoneal lymphadenopathy due to pancreatic cancer. The patient usually experiences constant but progressing pain in the upper abdomen, the low thoracic region of the back, or in both locations. It is often diffuse, poorly localised, dull, exacerbated by lying supine, and eased by bending forwards. Some patients cannot lie down at night and keep walking, as this relieves their discomfort. A double dose of morphine nocte sometimes solves this problem.

Chronic Intestinal Obstruction

Patients usually describe abdominal pain both as continuous and colicky, which may be referred to the dermatomes represented by the spinal segments supplying the affected viscera. Usually,

there are also other accompanying symptoms and signs of gastrointestinal obstruction, such as the lack of passage of intestinal contents, nausea, and vomiting. Pain is caused by different factors, such as smooth muscle contractions, mesenteric tension, and mural ischemia. Anticholinergics can be tried. Good results have been reported with the use of octreotide with this syndrome [63].

Malignant Perineal Pain

Perineal pain is most often caused by tumours of the colon or rectum, the female reproductive tract, and the distal genitourinary system. Typically, it is a constant and aching pain, often aggravated by sitting or standing, which may be associated with tenesmus or bladder spasms. Invasion of the muscle of the deep pelvis can result in a syndrome similar to the so-called tension myalgia of the pelvic floor [64]. It presents as a constant ache or heaviness exacerbated by an upright posture.

There are many other cancer-related pain syndromes. This chapter has not exhausted this subject. The authors refer the reader to other sources [46–48, 65]. Knowledge about the syndromes frequently helps in choosing an appropriate diagnostic tool and assists in initiating a specific therapy.

References

1. Levy MH, Chwistek M, Mehta RS. Management of chronic pain in cancer survivors. Cancer J. 2008;14:401–9.
2. Caraceni A, Portenoy RK. An international survey of cancer pain characteristics and syndromes. IASP Task Force on Cancer Pain. International Association for the Study of Pain. Pain. 1999;82:263–74.
3. Dy SM, Asch SM, Naeim A, Sanati H, Walling A, Lorenz KA. Evidence-based standards for cancer pain management. J Clin Oncol. 2008;26:3879–85.
4. Portenoy RK. Treatment of cancer pain. Lancet. 2011;377:2236–47.
5. Kirkova J, Aktas A, Walsh D, Rybicki L, Davis MP. Consistency of symptom clusters in advanced cancer. Am J Hosp Palliat Care. 2010;27:342–6.
6. Ripamonti C, Bandieri E. Pain therapy. Crit Rev Oncol Hematol. 2009;70:145–59.

7. McMillan SC, Tittle M, Hagan S, Laughlin J. Management of pain and pain-related symptoms in hospitalized veterans with cancer. Cancer Nurs. 2000;23:327–36.

8. Dobratz MC. Patterns of advanced cancer pain in home hospice patients. Cancer Nurs. 2001;24:294–9.

9. Hjermstad MJ, Fainsinger R, Kaasa S. Assessment and classification of cancer pain. Curr Opin Support Palliat Care. 2009;3:24–30.

10. Knudsen AK, Brunelli C, Kaasa S, et al. Which variables are associated with pain intensity and treatment response in advanced cancer patients? Implications for a future classification system for cancer pain. Eur J Pain. 2011;15:320–7.

11. Hjermstad MJ, Gibbins J, Haugen DF, Caraceni A, Loge JH, Kaasa S. Pain assessment tools in palliative care: an urgent need for consensus. Palliat Med. 2008;22:895–903.

12. Daut RL, Cleeland CS, Flanery RC. Development of the Wisconsin Brief Pain Questionnaire to assess pain in cancer and other diseases. Pain. 1983;17:197–210.

13. Elsner F, Radbruch L, Loick G, Gartner J, Sabatowski R. Intravenous versus subcutaneous morphine titration in patients with persisting exacerbation of cancer pain. J Palliat Med. 2005;8:743–50.

14. Atkinson TM, Rosenfeld BD, Sit L, et al. Using confirmatory factor analysis to evaluate construct validity of the Brief Pain Inventory (BPI). J Pain Symptom Manage. 2011;41:558–65.

15. Mathias SD, Crosby RD, Qian Y, Jiang Q, Dansey R, Chung K. Estimating minimally important differences for the worst pain rating of the Brief Pain Inventory-Short Form. J Support Oncol. 2011;9:72–8.

16. Caraceni A, Cherny N, Fainsinger R, et al. Pain measurement tools and methods in clinical research in palliative care: recommendations of an Expert Working Group of the European Association of Palliative Care. J Pain Symptom Manage. 2002;23:239–55.

17. Faries JE, Mills DS, Goldsmith KW, Phillips KD, Orr J. Systematic pain records and their impact on pain control. A pilot study. Cancer Nurs. 1991;14:306–13.

18. de Wit R, van Dam F, Hanneman M, et al. Evaluation of the use of a pain diary in chronic cancer pain patients at home. Pain. 1999;79:89–99.

19. Maunsell E, Allard P, Dorval M, Labbe J. A brief pain diary for ambulatory patients with advanced cancer: acceptability and validity. Cancer. 2000;88:2387–97.

20. Williamson A, Hoggart B. Pain: a review of three commonly used pain rating scales. J Clin Nurs. 2005;14:798–804.

21. Dworkin RH, Turk DC, Farrar JT, et al. Core outcome measures for chronic pain clinical trials: IMMPACT recommendations. Pain. 2005;113:9–19.

22. Hjermstad MJ, Fayers PM, Haugen DF, et al. Studies comparing numerical rating scales, verbal rating scales, and visual analogue scales for assessment of pain intensity in adults: a systematic literature review. J Pain Symptom Manage. 2011;41:1073–93.

23. Brunelli C, Zecca E, Martini C, et al. Comparison of numerical and verbal rating scales to measure pain exacerbations in patients with chronic cancer pain. Health Qual Life Outcomes. 2010;8:42.

24. Graham C, Bond SS, Gerkovich MM, Cook MR. Use of the McGill pain questionnaire in the assessment of cancer pain: replicability and consistency. Pain. 1980;8:377–87.

25. Kiss I, Muller H, Abel M. The McGill Pain Questionnaire – German version. A study on cancer pain. Pain. 1987;29:195–207.

26. Zylicz Z, Twycross R. Opioid-induced hyperalgesia may be more frequent than previously thought. J Clin Oncol. 2008;26:1564.

27. Hauser K. Clinical symptom assessment. In: Walsh D, Caraceni A, Fainsinger R, Foley K, Goh C, Lloyd-Williams M, Olarte JN, Radbruch L, editors. Palliative medicine. Philadelphia: Sunders/Elsevier; 2009. p. 325–33.

28. Alvarez DJ, Rockwell PG. Trigger points: diagnosis and management. Am Fam Physician. 2002;65:653–60.

29. Scott AC, McConnell S, Laird B, Colvin L, Fallon M. Quantitative Sensory Testing to assess the sensory characteristics of cancer-induced bone pain after radiotherapy and potential clinical biomarkers of response. Eur J Pain 2012;16:123–33.

30. Wisloff F, Kvam AK, Hjorth M, Lenhoff S. Serum calcium is an independent predictor of quality of life in multiple myeloma. Eur J Haematol. 2007;78:29–34.

31. Tucci M, Mosca A, Lamanna G, et al. Prognostic significance of disordered calcium metabolism in hormone-refractory prostate cancer patients with metastatic bone disease. Prostate Cancer Prostatic Dis. 2009;12:94–9.

32. Berthold DR, Pond GR, Roessner M, de Wit R, Eisenberger M, Tannock AI. Treatment of hormone-refractory prostate cancer with docetaxel or mitoxantrone: relationships between prostate-specific antigen, pain, and quality of life response and survival in the TAX-327 study. Clin Cancer Res. 2008;14:2763–7.

33. Comperat E, Azzouzi AR, Chartier-Kastler E, et al. Late recurrence of a prostatic adenocarcinoma as a solitary splenic metastasis. Urol Int. 2007;78:86–8.

34. Daniell HW. Hypogonadism in men consuming sustained-action oral opioids. J Pain. 2002;3:377–84.

35. Aloisi AM, Ceccarelli I, Carlucci M, et al. Hormone replacement therapy in morphine-induced hypogonadic male chronic pain patients. Reprod Biol Endocrinol. 2011;9:26.

36. Advances in diagnostic radiology and RFA aid cancer detection and treatment. Recent innovations enable earlier treatment with shorter hospital stays and less post-procedure pain. Duke Med Health News. 2007;13:3–4.

37. Talbot J, Paycha F, Balogova S. Diagnosis of bone metastasis: recent comparative studies of imaging modalities. Q J Nucl Med Mol Imaging. 2011;55:374–410.

38. Wang K, Allen L, Fung E, Chan CC, Chan JC, Griffith JF. Bone scintigraphy in common tumors with osteolytic components. Clin Nucl Med. 2005;30:655–71.

39. Alexandrakis MG, Kyriakou DS, Passam F, Koukouraki S, Karkavitsas N. Value of Tc-99 m

sestamibi scintigraphy in the detection of bone lesions in multiple myeloma: comparison with Tc-99 m methylene diphosphonate. Ann Hematol. 2001;80:349–53.

40. McKiernan FE. Technetium-99m-methyl diphosphonate bone scintigraphy may be helpful in preoperative planning for vertebroplasty in multiple myeloma: two cases. J Vasc Interv Radiol. 2010;21:1462–4.

41. Cecchin D, Motta R, Zucchetta P, Bui F, Basso SM, Lumachi F. Imaging studies in hypercalcemia. Curr Med Chem. 2011;18:3485–93.

42. Zech DF, Grond S, Lynch J, Hertel D, Lehmann KA. Validation of World Health Organization Guidelines for cancer pain relief: a 10-year prospective study. Pain. 1995;63:65–76.

43. Mantyh PW, Hunt SP. Mechanisms that generate and maintain bone cancer pain. Novartis Found Symp. 2004;260:221–38; discussion 38–40, 77–9.

44. Urch C. The pathophysiology of cancer-induced bone pain: current understanding. Palliat Med. 2004;18:267–74.

45. Jensen TS, Baron R. Translation of symptoms and signs into mechanisms in neuropathic pain. Pain. 2003;102:1–8.

46. Chang VT, Janjan N, Jain S, Chau C. Update in cancer pain syndromes. J Palliat Med. 2006;9:1414–34.

47. Cherny NI. Pain assessment and cancer pain syndromes. In: Hanks G, Cherny NI, Christiakis NA, Fallon M, Kaasa S, Portenoy RK, editors. Oxford textbook of palliative medicine. Oxford: Oxford University Press; 2010. p. 599–626.

48. Twycross R. Cancer pain syndromes. In: Sykes N, Fallon MT, Patt RB, editors. Cancer pain. 1st ed. London: Arnold; 2003. p. 3–20.

49. Bakshi R, Mechtler LL, Kamran S, et al. MRI findings in lumbar puncture headache syndrome: abnormal dural-meningeal and dural venous sinus enhancement. Clin Imaging. 1999;23:73–6.

50. Pignon T, Fernandez L, Ayasso S, Durand MA, Badinand D, Cowen D. Impact of radiation oncology practice on pain: a cross-sectional survey. Int J Radiat Oncol Biol Phys. 2004;60:1204–10.

51. Trotti A, Bellm LA, Epstein JB, et al. Mucositis incidence, severity and associated outcomes in patients with head and neck cancer receiving radiotherapy with or without chemotherapy: a systematic literature review. Radiother Oncol. 2003;66:253–62.

52. Epstein JB, Wilkie DJ, Fischer DJ, Kim YO, Villines D. Neuropathic and nociceptive pain in head and neck cancer patients receiving radiation therapy. Head Neck Oncol. 2009;1:26.

53. Loprinzi CL, Reeves BN, Dakhil SR, et al. Natural history of paclitaxel-associated acute pain syndrome: prospective cohort study NCCTG N08C1. J Clin Oncol. 2011;29:1472–8.

54. Reyes-Gibby CC, Morrow PK, Buzdar A, Shete S. Chemotherapy-induced peripheral neuropathy as a predictor of neuropathic pain in breast cancer patients previously treated with paclitaxel. J Pain. 2009;10:1146–50.

55. Jamal CY, Islam MM, Rahman SA. Acute lymphoblastic leukaemia presenting with severe hypercalcaemia. Mymensingh Med J. 2011;20:134–7.

56. Hwang JE, Cho SH, Kim OK, et al. Newly developed multiple myeloma in a patient with primary T-cell lymphoma of bone. J Korean Med Sci. 2008;23:544–7.

57. Walid MS, Sanoufa M. Pathologic fracture of the odontoid as the presenting sign of metastatic cancer. Indian J Cancer. 2010;47:475.

58. O'Toole O, O'Hare A, Grogan L, Bolger C, Brett FM. 20 year old lady with a paraspinal mass. Brain Pathol. 2010;20:683–4.

59. Kakutani K, Doita M, Nishida K, Miyamoto H, Kurosaka M. Radiculopathy due to malignant melanoma in the sacrum with unknown primary site. Eur Spine J. 2008;17 Suppl 2:S271–4.

60. Papadopoulos EC, Khan SN. Piriformis syndrome and low back pain: a new classification and review of the literature. Orthop Clin North Am. 2004;35:65–71.

61. Shigemitsu A, Furukawa N, Koike N, Kobayashi H. Endometrial cancer diagnosed by the presence of bone metastasis and treated with zoledronic Acid: a case report and review of the literature. Case Rep Oncol. 2010;3:471–6.

62. Singh V, Sinha SK, Nain CK, et al. Budd-Chiari syndrome: our experience of 71 patients. J Gastroenterol Hepatol. 2000;15:550–4.

63. Mercadante S. Scopolamine butylbromide plus octreotide in unresponsive bowel obstruction. J Pain Symptom Manage. 1998;16:278–80.

64. Sinaki M, Merritt JL, Stillwell GK. Tension myalgia of the pelvic floor. Mayo Clin Proc. 1977;52:717–22.

65. Shaiova L. Difficult pain syndromes: bone pain, visceral pain, and neuropathic pain. Cancer J. 2006;12:330–40.

Opioids, Their Receptors, and Pharmacology

8

R.A.F.J. D'Costa and Magdi Hanna

Abstract

Opioids have a pivotal role in the management of moderate to severe Pain in cancer patients. Appreciating their individual pharmacodynamics, as well as their pharmacokinetic profiles, which create subtle, differences in the way each opioid function. This will enhance the rational rather than the empirical use of opioids and minimise their potential adverse effects.

The management of cancer has changed in recent decades resulting in many patients having a prolonged period in remission. During this time opioids should be adjusted and follow regular assessment of the character and nature of pain to avoid the unnecessary prolong use of opioids and reduce their side effects.

The WHO analgesic ladder, first published over a quarter of a century ago, laid out simple basic guidance for the management of Cancer pain. Although effective for the majority of patients, there is still significant percentage of the world's population that have no access to opioids. This is due to a lack of knowledge and to regulatory controls that form barriers to effective pain control in cancer.

Keywords

Opioids • Analgesics • Opiates • Agonist • Antagonist • Receptors • Pharmacokinetics • Pharmacodynamics • Tolerance • Addiction

R.A.F.J. D'Costa, FFARCSI
Department of Anaesthetics,
King's College Hospital,
Denmark Hill, London SE5 9RS, UK
e-mail: d1costa@yahoo.co.uk

M. Hanna, MBBCH, FCA (✉)
Analgesics and Pain Research Unit (APR LTD),
62 Park Road, Beckenham,
Kent BR3 1QH, UK
e-mail: magdihanna6262@aol.com

Opioids have had a role in the management of pain since antiquity. The earliest record of its use probably dates back to 1500 BC, in the Ebers papyrus [1], which describes the use of an extract of opium to stop excessive crying in children. In more recent times, an understanding of the pharmacokinetics of opioids has allowed for a safer and more effective management of patients, in particular those with impaired renal and liver function. The possibility of drug interactions and

M. Hanna, Z. Zylicz (eds.), *Cancer Pain*,
DOI 10.1007/978-0-85729-230-8_8, © Springer-Verlag London 2013

Table 8.1 Subtypes of opioid receptors

Receptor type	Location	Agonist	Effect
Mu1	Brain stem and medial thalamus	Endorphins	Supraspinal analgesia
Mu2	Brain stem and medial thalamus		Analgesia, respiratory depression, pruritis, prolactin release, dependence, anorexia, and sedation
Kappa	The limbic and diencephalic areas, brain stem, and spinal cord	Dynorphin Ketocyclazocine	Spinal analgesia, sedation, dyspnea, dependence, dysphoria
Delta	Widely expressed in the central nervous system	Delta-alanine-delta-leucine enkephalin	Psychotomimetic, dysopioid, pharmacology phoric effects ? Regulate mu receptors
ORL-1	Widely expressed in the central nervous system	Nociceptine	? Analgesia ? Hyperalgesia

impaired immunity is also of importance when choosing a regime for cancer patients. The variability in the efficacy and tolerability of patients to these drugs is primarily due to the pharmacokinetic, pharmacodynamic, and pharmacogenomic effects of the drug.

The discovery of opioid receptors has underpinned our understanding of their mechanism of action. Recent evidence has suggested the presence of several subtypes, which in part may explain the individual variation in side effect profile to mu agonist opioids. Thus, the presence of multiple opioid receptors opens new perspectives in the actions of analgesics and in the development of new, highly selective analgesics with potentially fewer side effects [2].

Opioid receptors are present not only in the CNS but also in peripheral tissues. These receptors are normally stimulated by endogenous peptides (endorphins, enkephalins, and dynorphins) produced in response to noxious stimulation. Greek letters name the opioid receptors based on their prototype agonists (Table 8.1).

Different genes control each of the three major opioid receptors. Each receptor consists of an extracellular N-terminus, seven transmembrane helical twists, three extracellular and intracellular loops, and an intracellular C-terminus (Fig. 8.1). Once the receptor is activated, it releases a portion of the G protein, which diffuses within the membrane until it reaches its target (either an enzyme or an ion channel). These targets alter protein phosphorylation via inhibition of cyclic AMP (cAMP) which

acts as a second messenger within the cell, resulting in the activation of protein kinases (short-term effects) and gene transcription proteins and/or gene transcription (long-term effects).

Opioid receptors located on the presynaptic terminals of the nociceptive C-fibres and A delta fibres, when activated by an opioid agonist, will indirectly inhibit these voltage-dependent calcium channels, decreasing cAMP levels and blocking the release of pain neurotransmitters such as glutamate, substance P, and calcitonin gene-related peptide from the nociceptive fibres, resulting in analgesia.

Opioids and endogenous opioids activate presynaptic receptors on GABA neurons, which inhibit the release of GABA in the ventral tegmental area. This inhibition of GABA allows dopaminergic neurons to fire more vigorously, resulting in extra dopamine in the nucleus accumbens, which is intensely pleasurable. The varying effects of opioids may therefore be related to varying degrees of affinity for each receptor type.

Opioids may, to varying degrees, antagonise N-methyl-D-aspartate (NMDA) receptors, activating the descending serotonin and noradrenaline pain pathways from the brain stem. Stimulation of these same NMDA receptors may result in neuropathic pain and the development of tolerance. The location of endogenous opioids (endorphins) in the CNS was discovered in 1973 [3], and the first endogenous opioid (enkephalin) was discovered in 1975 [4]. Their location in the CNS allows them to function as neurotransmitters, and they

Fig. 8.1 Seven transmembrane structures of opioid G-protein-coupled receptor. Receptor activation by opioid receptor ligands leads to initiation of intracellular transduction pathways that include stimulation of potassium efflux, inhibition of VSCCs, and inhibition of adenylyl cyclase. In this diagram the G protein is denoted α, β, γ, but the α-subunit interacts with K^+/Ca^{2+} channel and adenylate cyclase

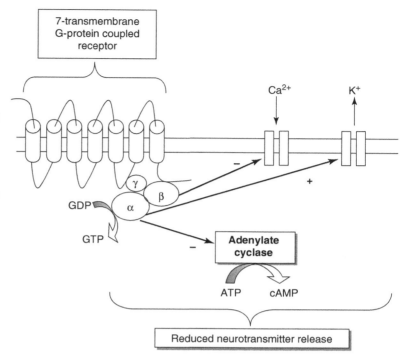

may play a role in hormone secretion, thermoregulation, and cardiovascular control.

Enkephalins are derived from pro-enkephalin and are relatively selective δ ligands. Endorphins are derived from pro-opiomelanocortin (also the precursor for ACTH and MSH) and bind to the μ receptor. Dynorphins are derived from pro-dynorphins and are highly selective at the μ receptor.

Nociceptins (nociceptin/orphanin FQ [N/OFQ]) (orphanin), identified in 1995, may have potent hyperalgesic effects. They have little affinity for the μ, δ, or κ receptors, and their receptors are now being called ORL-1 ("opioid-receptor-like"). Nociceptin antagonists may be antidepressants and analgesics. Pure opioid agonists (e.g., morphine, hydromorphone, and fentanyl) stimulate μ receptors and are the most potent analgesics. As the dose is increased, analgesia theoretically occurs in a log-linear fashion; the degree of analgesia induced is limited only by intolerable dose-related adverse effects. In contrast, opioid agonists/antagonists and opioid partial agonists (buprenorphine, pentazocine, nalbuphine, butorphanol, nalorphine)

exhibit a ceiling effect on the degree of analgesia that they can produce. Opiate agonist/antagonists and partial agonists can precipitate opioid withdrawal reactions. The respiratory depressant effects of partial agonists are not completely reversed with naloxone (Table 8.2).

Drug Absorption

Most opioids are well absorbed from GI tract apart from the fentanyl group of drugs. The oral route is generally preferred and they are usually well absorbed orally. All opioids undergo first-pass metabolism which in some cases leads to the production of active metabolites (as for morphine and codeine).

Distribution

Distribution of opioids is dependent on their lipid solubility. Fentanyl which has a high lipid solubility is distributed throughout the fat stores and

Table 8.2 Pharmacokinetics of opioids

Drug	Structure	Half-life (h)	Volume of distribution (L/kg)	Clearance (L/h)	Mechanism of clearance
Codeine		3.5	5	101	*Phase I* CYP2D6
Tramadol		6	4.1	5.6	*Phase I* CYP3A4
Morphine		2.5	4	63	*Phase II* Glucuronidation
Hydromorphone		3	4	1.66	*Phase II* Glucuronidation
Oxycodone		3	4	48.6	*Phase I* CYP3A4
Buprenorphine		22.5	4.1	54	*Phase I* CYP3A4 CYP3A5 CYP3A7
Methadone		15	6	8.3	*Phase I* CYP3A4 CYP2B6
Fentanyl		7	4	35	*Phase I* CYP3A4
Alfentanil		1.5	0.7	21	*Phase I* CYP3A4 CYP3A5
Pethidine		4.5	5.7	67.9	*Phase I* CYP2B6 CPY3A4 CYP2C19
Tapentadol		4.3	7.5	5.9	*Phase II* Glucuronidation

so has a higher volume of distribution. Similarly, drugs like morphine, which are hydrophilic, have a smaller volume of distribution. The metabolites of the drugs will usually have a smaller volume of distribution compared to the parent compound, as metabolism renders the drug more water soluble.

Metabolism

Metabolism is the transformation that drugs undergo, enabling them to be excreted from the body. Some drugs have metabolites that are pharmacologically active. Altered metabolism may result in a drug having either a very profound effect or very little efficacy depending on the capacity of the metabolic pathway.

Most opioids undergo first-pass metabolism in the liver before they enter the systemic circulation. This reduces the bioavailability of the drug. Opioid metabolism takes place primarily in the liver, which produces enzymes for this purpose. The enzymes promote two forms of metabolism: phase1 (modification) reactions and phase 2 (conjugation).

Phase 1 involves typically either hydrolysis or oxidation, involving the cytochrome P450 (CYP) enzymes. These enzymes facilitate the following reactions:
N-, O-, and S-dealkylation
Aromatic, aliphatic, or N-hydroxylation
N-oxidation
Sulfoxidation
Deamination
Dehydrogenation
Phase 1 reactions of opioids are catalysed by:
CYP3A4 catalyses more than 50 % of drugs, so there is a higher chance of drug interactions.
CYP2D6 catalyses a smaller number of drugs, so it has a smaller chance of drug interactions.
Phase 2 metabolism involves conjugation of the drug to hydrophilic substances so making it

easier for them to be eliminated. Examples of conjugates are:
Glucuronic acid
Sulphate
Glycine
Glutathione
Glucuronidation is the most important phase two reaction, catalysed by the enzyme uridine diphosphate glucuronosyltransferase (UGT), namely, UGT2B7. Drugs like morphine, oxymorphone, and hydromorphone are metabolised by this pathway.

Active Metabolites

Several drugs which undergo metabolism produce active metabolites. In some instances, the metabolites have significant analgesic activity. When several metabolites are formed, it is possible that the altered metabolism, be it due to medical comorbidities, genetic factors, or drug interactions, may change the balance of the metabolites, so affecting the efficacy and/or tolerability of the drug.

Drug Elimination

This usually follows from metabolism, where drugs which are rendered more water soluble are excreted in urine. Therefore, renal dysfunction is an important factor in the toxicity of these drugs. Some drugs (e.g., buprenorphine) are excreted in bile and so are useful in patients with decreased renal function (Table 8.3).

Codeine

Codeine, a methylated morphine derivative, was first isolated in 1832. It is a naturally occurring weak opiate, recommended for stage two of the

Table 8.3 Adverse effects of opioid therapy

Central nervous system
  Euphoria
  Drowsiness, sedation, and sleep disturbance
  Hallucinations
  Dysphoria and agitation
  Dizziness and seizures
  Aberrant behaviour
  Hyperalgesia
Respiratory system
  Respiratory depression
Ocular system
  Constriction of the pupil of the eye
Gastrointestinal system
  Constipation, nausea, and vomiting
  Delayed gastric emptying
Genitourinary
  Urinary retention
Endocrine
  Hormonal and sexual dysfunction
Cardiovascular
  Decreased blood pressure
  Slowed heart rate
  Peripheral edema (swelling)
Musculoskeletal system
  Muscle rigidity and contractions
  Osteoporosis
Immune system
  There have been reports suggesting that some
opioids tend to promote proliferation and growth of
tumour cells. However, the clinical significance of this
is yet to be established.

WHO pain ladder. It is absorbed following oral administration, with peak plasma concentrations within 1 h. It has a large volume of distribution (5 L/kg) and has a plasma half-life of 3–4 h. Codeine is metabolised by O- and N-demethylation in the liver to morphine, norcodeine, and codeine-6-glucuronide – thought to be the major active metabolite [5]. Therefore, some individuals that have a deficiency of the enzyme, CYP2D6, will have a reduced response to the drug [6]. This is so for approximately 8 % of the Caucasian population, 2 % of Asians, and 1 % of Arabs, who are described as poor metabolisers. Eighty-six percent of the drug is excreted in urine, 40–70 % as free or conjugated codeine, and 10–20 % as free or conjugated norcodeine.

Tramadol

Tramadol is a synthetic 4-phenylpiperidine analogue of codeine. It is a central analgesic with a low affinity for opioid receptors. Its selectivity for mu receptors has recently been demonstrated, and the M1 metabolite of tramadol, produced by O-demethylation in the liver, shows a higher affinity for opioid receptors than the parent drug. The rate of production of this M1 derivative (O-desmethyltramadol) is influenced by a polymorphic isoenzyme of the debrisoquine-type cytochrome P450 2D6 (CYP2D6). Nevertheless, this affinity for mu receptors of the CNS remains low, being 6,000 times lower than that of morphine. Moreover, and in contrast to other opioids, the analgesic action of tramadol is only partially inhibited by the opioid antagonist naloxone, which suggests the existence of another additional mechanism of action. This mechanism was demonstrated by the discovery of monoaminergic activity, which inhibits noradrenaline (norepinephrine) and serotonin (5-hydroxytryptamine; 5-HT) reuptake, making a significant contribution to the analgesic action by blocking nociceptive impulses at the spinal level. (+/−)-Tramadol is a racemic mixture of 2 enantiomers, each one displaying differing affinities for various receptors. (+/−)-Tramadol is a selective agonist of mu receptors and preferentially inhibits serotonin reuptake, whereas (−)-tramadol mainly inhibits noradrenaline reuptake. The action of these 2 enantiomers is both complementary and synergistic and results in the analgesic effect of (+/−)-tramadol [7]. After oral administration, tramadol demonstrates 68 % bioavailability, with peak serum concentrations reached within 2 h. The elimination kinetics can be described as 2 compartmental, with a half-life of 5.1 h for tramadol and 9 h for the M1 derivative after a single oral dose of 100 mg.

Tramadol is 20 % protein bound and is mainly (90 %) eliminated in the urine with the remaining 10 % being eliminated in the bile. Tramadol is metabolised by the CYP2D6 group of enzymes to O-desmethyltramadol (M1) which is an active metabolite with an affinity for mu receptors which is 300 times greater than the parent compound. The only other active metabolite is O,N- didesmethyltramadol (M5), which has weak analgesic activity [8]. The metabolites are renally excreted.

Serotonin syndrome has been reported in patients taking selective serotonin reuptake inhibitors (SSRIs) in conjunction with tramadol. This is usually with significant doses of SSRIs with tramadol [9].

Morphine

This is the prototype analgesic for the management of cancer pain [10]. There has been extensive clinical experience with this drug and various routes of administration available as well as the availability of modified release preparations. Morphine, a phenanthrene derivative and a pure agonist at the mu receptor, is the most abundant opiate found in the sap of the poppy plant *P. somniferum*.

Morphine is a hydrophilic drug, with low protein binding (36 %) and a low volume of distribution (2–4 L/kg) due to its water solubility. Morphine is readily absorbed from the GI tract with 25 % bioavailability with peak levels appearing 45mins after the oral administration of a dose of immediate-release morphine sulphate.

Morphine is metabolised in the liver, by glucuronidation to two major metabolites: morphine-6-glucuronide and morphine-3-glucuronide. Other minor routes of metabolism include N-demethylation to normorphine, or normorphine-6-glucuronide, diglucuronidation to morphine-3, 6-diglucuronide, and formation of morphine ethereal sulphate. A small proportion is transformed to hydromorphone [11]; however, there is no evidence that this produces a clinically significant effect.

M6G, like morphine, is an agonist at the mu receptor with a lower affinity for the mu2 subtype as opposed to the mu1 subtype of this receptor. Mu1 is thought to mediate analgesia, while mu2 is thought to be responsible for the adverse effects of the mu receptor agonists, viz., sedation, respiratory depression, and the GI side effects.

As described above, the elimination of morphine is by glucuronidation in the liver. The elimination of both major metabolites is via the renal route. M6G, an active metabolite in terms of analgesia, is via the kidney, and it is accumulation of this metabolite that is probably responsible for the respiratory depression seen in renal dysfunction [12]. M3G has no analgesic activity and may have neuroexcitatory actions.

Hydromorphone

Hydromorphone is a semisynthetic compound, made from morphine by a process of catalytic hydrogenation in which a hydrogenated ketone is added to the morphine molecule. It is a pure agonist at the mu receptor. It has good oral bioavailability due to its high lipid solubility, with a large volume of distribution.

Hydromorphone is metabolised to several metabolites, some of which are active. The main metabolite is hydromorphone-3-glucuronide which has neuroexcitatory potential similar to that of M3G [13].

Oxycodone

This is a phenanthrene class of opioid receptor, which acts as an agonist at the mu receptor and other receptors, including the kappa receptor. It was first produced by Freund and Speyer in 1916. They looked at thebaine derivatives in an attempt to find a safer alternative to diamorphine, with the analgesic effects and low-dependence potential. However, since its launch, oxycodone has become a frequently abused drug.

High oral absorption with low first-pass metabolism results in 85 % drug bioavailability after an oral dose of the immediate-release preparation. There is a biphasic absorption pattern. The volume of distribution is low at 2.6 L/kg. Oxycodone undergoes extensive metabolism in the liver to noroxycodone by CYP3A4 and to oxymorphone by CYP2D6. Oxymorphone is a weaker opioid agonist than oxycodone; however, its contribution to analgesia is thought to be negligible [14].

Buprenorphine

Buprenorphine is a synthetic opioid which was first produced in the 1970s. It is a partial agonist at the mu receptor and an antagonist at the kappa receptor. A ceiling effect has been described, however, this is at high doses (15 mg) not used in clinical practice. Due to its low bioavailability following oral administration, buprenorphine is administered sublingually; this has the advantage of being useable in patients who are not able to take drugs orally. It may also be used parenterally. More recently, buprenorphine has been available as a transdermal formulation which can be administered every 3 days (Transtec) or every 7 days (BuTrans). The BuTrans patch comes in low doses starting at 5 mcg/h. This may be a more convenient method of administering these drugs for patients with long-term stable pain. Breakthrough analgesia may then be provided using buprenorphine sublingual tablets or morphine.

Buprenorphine is metabolised via CYP3A4 to the active metabolite, norbuprenorphine [15]. Both buprenorphine and norbuprenorphine undergo glucuronidation. As buprenorphine is mainly excreted in bile, it is the agent of choice for patients with renal dysfunction.

Buprenorphine may precipitate withdrawal in patients who are dependent on strong opioids. The reversal of the respiratory depression caused by buprenorphine may require relatively large doses of naloxone [16].

Buprenorphine has for nearly 10 years been used as an alternative to methadone in drug rehabilitation programs. It is available in oral or sublingual tablets (Subutex).

Methadone

Methadone is a synthetic opioid which is a racemic mixture of the dextrorotatory (S-methadone) and the levorotatory (D-methadone) isomers. Methadone, the D-methadone isomer, is an agonist at the mu, kappa, and delta receptors, while both isomers are antagonistic at the NMDA receptors. The S-methadone isomer inhibits serotonin and noradrenaline uptake in the CNS. In high doses, it blocks potassium channels, which can cause ventricular arrhythmias in high doses.

Methadone is a highly lipophilic drug with a volume of distribution of 5 L/kg. With repeated dosing, it accumulates in brain, liver, heart, kidney, gut, and muscle, due to its high affinity for these tissues. As it is slowly released from these tissues, it has a long half-life. Although the half-life is usually quoted as being 24 h, there is a wide range, from 8 to 120 h.

Methadone has a bioavailability of between 70 and 90 % following oral administration.

Methadone is mainly metabolised by N-demethylation via CYP3A4, CYP2B6, CYP1A2, and CYP2D6 to a much lesser extent. Excretion is mainly in the feces but also via the kidney (depending on the urine pH). Methadone does not accumulate in renal failure and is also not removed in dialysate.

Methadone, due to its complex pharmacokinetics, drug interactions, and possible QT prolongation [17], is difficult to use, and it is best reserved for use by physicians experienced in its use.

Fentanyl

Fentanyl was first synthesised in Belgium by Dr Janssen in 1959. It is a piperidine derivative which is very lipid soluble and highly protein bound (80–85 %). The free fraction (pharmacologically active) is increased with acidosis. The main binding protein is alpha-1-acid glycoprotein as well as albumin and lipoproteins to a lesser extent.

It was initially available for anesthesia and sedation, usually used intravenously. However, it has over the past 20 years become available for use as transdermal and buccal preparations. When used buccally, there is rapid absorption of 25 % of dose with the remaining 75 % being swallowed and slowly absorbed from the gastrointestinal tract. About 25 % of the total dose of fentanyl escapes hepatic and intestinal first-pass metabolism. The absolute bioavailability is approximately 50 % compared to intravenous fentanyl, divided equally between the rapid oromucosal and slower gastrointestinal absorption.

Fentanyl is metabolised in the liver and intestinal mucosa to norfentanyl via the CYP3A4 isoform [18]. Norfentanyl is not pharmacologically active. Less than 7 % of the dose is excreted unchanged in the urine and 1 % unchanged in feces. The metabolites are mainly excreted in urine, with faecal excretion being of secondary importance.

Alfentanil

Alfentanil, like fentanyl, is a synthetic piperidine derivative. It has a lower potency and a shorter duration of action. The volume of distribution is 0.5–1 L/kg, indicating that this drug is not distributed in the tissues. Alfentanil is 92 % protein bound, mainly to alpha-1-acid glycoprotein.

The major metabolite is noralfentanil, produced by N-dealkylation of the piperidine nitrogen via CYP3A4 [19, 20]. The other metabolite is N-phenylpropanamide, formed by N-dealkylation of the amide nitrogen. Only 0.4 % of the dose administered is recovered in the urine.

Although alfentanil has been shown to have more cardiovascular stability, it produces more respiratory depression compared to fentanyl. The half-life is prolonged in the elderly.

Pethidine

Pethidine was the first opioid to be synthesised in 1932. It was initially produced as an antispasmodic. Pethidine has local anaesthetic (acting on the sodium channels), opioid, and antimuscarinic actions due to its structural similarity to tropane alkaloids.

Pethidine has a short duration of action, fast onset, and high incidence of euphoria, making it especially likely to have the potential for addiction [21].

Pethidine 30–50 % bound to plasma proteins. The half-life is 3–6 h. Pethidine is metabolised via three pathways in the liver:

By liver carboxyesterases to pethidinic acid which is inactive

By glucuronidation of pethidine, norpethidine, and pethidinic acid

By CYP2B6, CYP3A4, and CYP2G9 to norpethidine which is neurotoxic. Norpethidine is excreted in the urine and can accumulate in renal failure, causing neuroexcitatory effects [22]

Diamorphine

Diacetylmorphine, the 3,6 diacetyl ester of morphine, is a synthetic compound. In man, diamorphine has a half-life of 2–3 min being hydrolyzed to monoacetylmorphine which crosses the blood–brain barrier more readily than morphine. This explains the faster onset of action of diamorphine as compared to morphine. Monoacetylmorphines are more slowly hydrolyzed to morphine in the blood. Morphine undergoes glucuronidation in the liver, and its glucuronides are largely eliminated in the urine, with 7–10 % being eliminated in feces.

Tapentadol

This is a new drug with a structure that is related to tramadol. It is an opioid, with two analgesic mechanisms [23]:

Agonist at the mu receptor with 50 times less affinity as compared to morphine

Inhibition of noradrenaline uptake

The bioavailability is 30 % after oral administration. The drug is metabolised in the liver by conjugation to glucuronide and sulphate and eliminated in the urine, with 1 % faecal excretion. It is indicated for inflammatory and neuropathic pain [24].

The WHO Pain Ladder

The WHO pain ladder was first publicised in 1986, to provide a simple method of providing pain relief for cancer patients. The principles were that pain relief should be given by:

• The clock
• The ladder
• Mouth
• The individual's response
• Paying attention to detail

When these principles were followed, between 70 and 95 % of patients would achieve control of their pain. The initial guidance was expanded to include adjuvants like NSAIDS, antidepressants, and anticonvulsants.

The use of step-two drugs has been questioned. However, they are still valuable for patients with moderate pain because the use of codeine or tramadol will delay the start of strong opioids (like morphine) which have been shown to have a higher incidence of side effects [25].

The use of opioid analgesics in cancer pain (step3) is well recognised in the early stages, i.e., at diagnosis and during the initial treatment, be it surgery or chemotherapy. As these treatments have become more effective in controlling the disease process, there may be a prolonged period of remission. During this phase of the disease, the use of opioids may be both unnecessary and undesirable, as the persisting pain due to surgery or chemotherapy may be neuropathic and not very responsive to opioids. Furthermore, there has been some evidence that the use of strong opioids may reduce immunity and possibly promote metastases [26]. In the late stages of cancer treatment and palliative care, the use of strong opioids is again an essential part of the effective management of the pain and symptoms that cancer patients experience towards the end of life; nonetheless, recent publication has stressed the need for rigours evidence-based research in the use of opioids in cancer pain in its different complexity [27].

Despite the fact that the WHO guidelines were published 25 years ago and the fact that opiates have been used in various parts of the world for millennia, it is disappointing that opioids are still not available to nearly 80 % of the world's population and there are still large areas of the world where access to strong opioids for the management of cancer pain is still very limited [28]. The reasons cited for this in a recent report by the WHO are:

- Regulatory impediments which restrict the prescription of opioids
- Insufficient education, training, and support of a specialised pain service
- Economic and procurement factors

The use of opioid rotation is only indicated where patients are experiencing significant side effects. If side effects are severe, the use of the epidural or intrathecal route may be considered, as this will allow the use of a smaller dose of the opioid along with local anaesthetics and clonidine.

The elderly and patients with decreased liver and renal function may be more sensitive to opiates, and suitable adjustments of dose and duration will be required, as recommended in the WHO ladder.

While there are newer drugs available for the management of pain, opioids are likely to remain pivotal compounds in the control of pain in cancer. An improved understanding of their molecular mechanisms, genetics, and pharmacokinetic differences between opioids as well as an appreciation of the complexity of cancer pain will, hopefully, lead to a more rational and selective use of drugs with a better side effect profile.

References

1. Lewin L. Phantastica. New York: Dutton; 1931. p. 35.
2. Pasternak GW. Molecular insights into mu opioid pharmacology: from the clinic to the bench. Clin J Pain. 2010;26 Suppl 10:S3–9.
3. Pert CB, Snyder SH. Opiate receptor: its demonstration in nervous tissue. Science. 1973;179:1011–4.
4. Hughes J, Smith T, Kosterlitz H, Fothergill L, Morgan B, Morris H. Identification of two related pentapeptides from the brain with potent opiate agonist activity. Nature. 1975;258:577–80.
5. Lotsch J, Skarke C, Schmidt H, Rohrbacher M, Hofmann U, Schwab M, et al. Evidence of morphine-independent central nervous opioid effect after administration of codeine: contribution of other codeine metabolites. Clin Pharmacol Ther. 2006;79:35–48.
6. Susca MT, Murray-Carmichael E, de Leon J. Response to hydrocodone, codeine and oxycodone in a CYP2D6 poor metabolizer. Prog Neuropsychopharmacol Biol Psychiatry. 2006;30(7):1356–8.
7. Raffa RB, Friderichs E, Reimann W, Shank RP, Codd EE, Vaught JL, et al. Complementary and synergistic antinociceptive interaction between the enantiomers of tramadol. J Pharmacol Exp Ther. 1993;267:331–40.
8. Gillen C, Haurand M, Kobelt DJ, Wnendt S. Affinity, potency and efficacy of tramadol and its metabolites

at the cloned human μ-opioid receptor. Naunyn Schmiedebergs Arch Pharmacol. 2000;362:116–21.

9. Gnanadesigan N, Espinoza RT, Smith R, Israel M, Reuben DB. Interaction of serotonergic antidepressants and opioid analgesics: is serotonin syndrome going undetected? J Am Med Dir Assoc. 2005;6(4):265–9.

10. Flemming K. The use of morphine to treat cancer-related pain: a synthesis of quantitative and qualitative research. J Pain Symptom Manage. 2010;39:139–54.

11. McDonough PC, Levine B, Vorce S, Jufer RA, Fowler D. The detection of hydromorphone in urine specimens with high morphine concentrations. J Forensic Sci. 2008;53(3):752–4.

12. Angst MS, Bührer M, Lötsch J. Insidious intoxication after morphine treatment in renal failure: delayed onset of morphine-6-glucuronide action. Anesthesiology. 2000;92(5):1473–6.

13. Smith MT. Neuroexcitatory effects of morphine and hydromorphone: evidence implicating the 3-glucuronide metabolites. Clin Exp Pharmacol Physiol. 2000;27(7):524–8.

14. Lalovic B, Kharasch E, Hoffer C, Risler L, Liu-Chen LY, Shen DD. Pharmacokinetics and pharmacodynamics of oral oxycodone in healthy human subjects: role of circulating active metabolites. Clin Pharmacol Ther. 2006;79(5):461–79.

15. Cone EJ, Gorodetzky CW, Yousefnejad D, Buchwald WF, Johnson RE. The metabolism and excretion of buprenorphine in humans. Drug Metab Dispos. 1884;12:577–81.

16. Gal TJ. Naloxone reversal of buprenorphine-induced respiratory depression. Clin Pharmacol Ther. 1989;45:66–71.

17. Krantz MJ, Lewkopwiez L, Hays H, Woodrooffe MA, Robertson AD, Mehler PS. Torsade de pointes associated with very high doses of methadone. Ann Intern Med. 2002;137:501–4.

18. Feierman DE, Lasker JM. Metabolism of fentanyl, a synthetic opioid analgesic, by human liver microsomes. Role of CYP3A4. Drug Metab Dispos. 1996;24: 932–9.

19. Kharasch ED, Russell M, Mautz D, Thummel KE, Kunze KL, Bowdle TA, et al. The role of cytochrome P450 3A4 in alfentanil clearance. Implications for interindividual variability in disposition and perioperative drug interactions. Anesthesiology. 1997;87:36–50.

20. Labroo RB, Thummel KE, Kunze KL, Podoll T, Trager WF, Kharasch ED. Catalytic role of cytochrome P4503A4 in multiple pathways of alfentanil metabolism. Drug Metab Dispos. 1995;23:490–6.

21. Latta KS, Ginsberg B, Barkin RL. Meperidine: a critical review. Am J Ther. 2002;9(1):53–68. Philadelphia: Lippincott Williams & Wilkins.

22. Ramirez J, Innocenti F, Schuetz EG, Folckhart DA, Relling MV, Santucci R, et al. CYP2B6, CYP3A4 and CYP2C19 are responsible for the in vitro N-demethylation of meperidine in human liver microsomes. Drug Metab Dispos. 2004;32(9): 930–6.

23. Tzschentke TM, Jahnel U, Kogel B, Christoph T, Englberger W, De Vry J, et al. Tapentadol hydrochloride: a next-generation, centrally acting analgesic with two mechanisms of action in a single molecule. Drugs Today (Barc). 2009;45(7):483–96. Erratum in: Drugs Today (Barc). 2009;45(9):711.

24. Schiene K, De Vry J, Tzschentke TM. Antinociceptive and antihyperalgesic affects of tapentadol in animal models of inflammatory pain. J Pharmacol Exp Ther. 2011;339(2):537–44.

25. Wilder-Smith CH, Schimke J, Osterwalder B, Senn HJ. Oral tramadol, a mu-opioid agonist and monoamine reuptake blocker, and morphine for strong cancer-related pain. Ann Oncol. 1994;5(2):141–6.

26. Afsharimani B, Cabot P, Parat MO. Morphine and tumour growth and metastasis. Cancer Metastasis Rev. 2011;30(2):225–38.

27. Caraceni A, Hanks G, Kaasa S, et al. Evidence-based guidelines for the use of opioid analgesics in the treatment of cancer pain: the 2012 EAPC recommendations. Lancet Oncol. 2012;13(2):e58–68. doi:10.1016/S1470-2045(12)70040-2.

28. WHO. WHO policy guidelines ensuring balance in national policies on controlled substances, guidance for availability and accessibility for controlled medicines. Geneva, WHO. 2011. Available from: www.who.int/medicines/areas/quality_safety/guide_nocp.

Zbigniew (Ben) Zylicz

Abstract

Breakthrough (episodic) pain (BTP) is a term used to describe a transient exacerbation of pain that occurs either spontaneously or in relation to a specific trigger, despite relatively stable and adequately controlled background pain. There are two main types of BTP: predictable and unpredictable. Because the definition remains a bit vague and the pain is hard to measure objectively, authors differ in their prevalence estimates. Each of the BTPs needs to be carefully assessed and observed. There is no generic treatment of all BTPs. Morphine given either orally or subcutaneously is a reasonable treatment in many but not all cases. Some pains with a very fast onset can be treated with rapidly absorbing transmucosal fentanyls. However, the use of these products is not yet established independently, and the costs of such a treatment may be high.

Keywords

Breakthrough pain • Episodic pain • Pain diagnosis • Morphine • Transmucosal fentanyl

Introduction

Breakthrough (episodic) pain (BTP) is a term used to describe a transient exacerbation of pain that occurs either spontaneously or in relation to a specific trigger, despite relatively stable and adequately controlled background pain [1–3]. This definition excludes patients with poorly relieved background pain, and pain recurring shortly before the next dose of regular analgesic is due (known as "end-of-dose pain"). However, these two types of pain will be discussed here in more detail in order to differentiate them from BTP. Procedure pain is included in this definition and will be discussed here also.

Thus, there are two main types of BTP:

- Predictable (incident) pain which is an exacerbation of pain caused by weight-bearing and/or activity (including swallowing, defecation, coughing, nursing/medical procedures), which may or may not be at the same location as the background (controlled) pain.

Z. Zylicz, MD, PhD
Department of Research and Education,
Hildegard Hospiz, St. Alban Ring 151,
Basel 4020, Switzerland
e-mail: ben.zylicz@hildegard-hospiz.ch

M. Hanna, Z. Zylicz (eds.), *Cancer Pain*,
DOI 10.1007/978-0-85729-230-8_9, © Springer-Verlag London 2013

- Unpredictable (spontaneous) pain, unrelated to movement or activity – e.g., a colic, stabbing pain associated with nerve injury.

Both predictable and unpredictable BTP may or may not be at the same location as the background (controlled) pain.

Unfortunately, in practice, BTP is often inadequately assessed and poorly differentiated from other types of pains [4]. This chapter will summarise the basic knowledge about BTP and its assessment and differentiation from other types of pain exacerbation and will propose rational treatment.

Epidemiology and Clinical Characteristics of BTP

The epidemiology of BTP has been extensively studied [1, 5–7]. The pain tends to have a rapid onset (median of 3, ranging from 1 to 30 min) and relatively short duration (median 30, ranging from 1 to 180 min) [6–8].

The prevalence of BTP varies between studies in part because of the use of different definitions, reflecting the lack of a universally agreed gold standard [9]. Nonetheless, BTP appears to be common in both cancer patients (according to some sources up to 90 %) and noncancer patients (up to 75 %) receiving opioid medication for persistent pain [10]. BTP is often a resurgence of background pain and thus may be either functional (e.g., tension headache) or pathological and either nociceptive (associated with tissue distortion or injury) or neuropathic (associated with nerve compression or injury) or a mixture of these two [10]. Patients may experience more than one type of BTP, and these may have different causes. BTP may result in a number of negative complications that can contribute to poor quality of life [2]. They can be physical (e.g., immobility, insomnia), psychological (e.g., anxiety, depression), spiritual (e.g., hopelessness), and social (e.g. unemployment, isolation).

Pain on movement is one of the most common types of BTP [3]. It may be caused by increasing pressure on the inflamed bone tissue or nerves, but it may also reflect increased central sensitisation [11]. Axial pain on movement is frequently caused by the compression of structures between vertebrae. This type of pain is usually classified as mixed nociceptive and neuropathic pain.

BTP may be visceral in origin, e.g., esophageal and bladder spasm or biliary and ureteric colic. These pains involve the smooth muscle in organs innervated by vagal nociceptive afferents. The pain may be accompanied by other vagal effects such as bradycardia, hypotension, pallor, and nausea and vomiting. Antimuscarinic drugs are the mainstay of the treatment for this type of BTP. In some circumstances (e.g., biliary colic), opioids may paradoxically increase the intensity and duration of the pain by causing contraction of the sphincter of Oddi and increased pressure in the biliary tree.

Many patients with cancer cachexia and tissue wasting may experience nerve compression or myofascial pain due to debility. This can result in pain that can be severe and exacerbated by movement. Whenever possible, specific treatment that addresses the underlying cause should be considered. For example, painful muscle cramps may result from hypocalcemia and/or hypomagnesemia, and consequently, replacement therapy would be an appropriate treatment [12].

Certain phenomena involved in BTP may have a circadian rhythm with different patterns seen between day and night [13, 14]. For example, factors which may result in more pain being experienced at night include:

- Positional, e.g., lying recumbent may result in greater compression of the celiac plexus in patients with pancreatic cancer.
- Cognitive, e.g., impairment tends to be worse in the evening/nighttime [14].
- Pharmacokinetic, e.g., the metabolism of analgesics may differ over the course of 24 h; this may be partly related to variation in renal function and can worsen in patients with compensated heart failure [15–17].

Evaluation of BTP

BTP is often inadequately assessed. This can lead to inappropriate management strategies. The assessment of the pain depends primarily on the taking of a meticulous pain history (see Table 9.1) and performing physical examination including palpation of painful sites in order to induce pain exacerbation (e.g., in nerve compression), passive and active movements, and the examination of skin sensitivity (hyperalgesia or allodynia) which would suggest the neuropathic nature of the pain and its precise localisation (root compression or discrete peripheral nerve compression). The

Table 9.1 Questions about the breakthrough pain

Is the background pain well controlled? Is there any residual pain?
Does the pain have the character of acute exacerbations?
Time of onset? Duration? Intensity? Frequency?
Localisation of pain exacerbations?
What character does the pain have?
Is the pain similar to the "background pain"?
What is the relationship to the administration of analgesics?
Is radiation treatment a factor? What are the accompanying symptoms?
What are the exacerbating factors?
Is the pain predictable?
Is the pain related to movements? Are those movements volitional or non-volitional?
What are the relieving factors: drugs, interventions, etc.?
Does the pain interfere with normal daily activity? Does the pain interfere with the patient's sleep?

results of an examination may also suggest the most suitable imaging technique, which may lead to precise diagnosis and treatment (Table 9.1).

BTP should be differentiated from the end-of-dose pain, where an increase in the dose/frequency of regular background analgesia (e.g., a modified-release strong opioid, by mouth or transdermal patch) is indicated. Such increases can continue as long as effective and tolerated. Short-term benefit requiring frequent dose escalation, particularly when accompanied by hyperalgesia or allodynia, should arouse suspicion of opioid-induced hyperalgesia (see Chap. 10).

Management of BTP

When designing a management strategy before changing the pharmacological treatment, it should not be forgotten that even in advanced cancer, there may be treatments for the underlying cancer (e.g., radiotherapy) or precipitating factors, (e.g., cough, constipation) that may cause BTP. Nondrug approaches (e.g., surgical fixation of a long bone, vertebroplasty) can also be important.

Common drug approaches are outlined below.

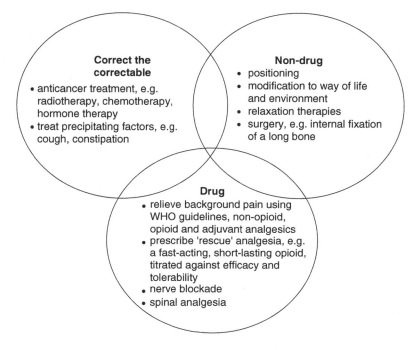

Fig. 9.1 Multimodal approach to managing breakthrough (episodic) pain

Morphine

BTP can be treated with oral morphine [18–20]. When the onset of pain is rapid, the SC or IV route may be considered [21, 22], although this is not always practical or acceptable at home. For home care, morphine administered intranasally may be a promising alternative [23, 24].

Despite the lack of evidence, morphine remains the gold standard for the treatment of pain exacerbations [25]. Most often, doses equal to 1/6–1/10 (the so-called 4-h's dose) of the daily dose of morphine are used. However, patient requirements vary widely, usually between 5 and 20 % of the daily dose. In general, individual dose titration may be required [18, 19]. One study suggests that there is no relationship between the most effective dose of oral morphine for BTP and the background morphine dose [26].

The practice of using the 4-h's dose for all other opioids is not supported by research and should be avoided, as it has been found that the rescue dose of fentanyl needed for optimal treatment of BTP is independent of the background opioid dose [26–28]. Similarly, the oral morphine rescue dose in a patient using transdermal fentanyl or buprenorphine cannot be calculated with certainty but needs to be titrated; the first dose should be as low as 5 or 10 mg, adjusted to specific patient needs and taking adverse effects into consideration. The analgesic response to this dose should be carefully recorded. Time to onset of analgesia, time and extent of peak analgesia, and analgesia duration are important factors in order to assess the effect and to plan further treatment. It is not unusual for a patient treated with 200 mcg/h of transdermal fentanyl and still presenting with BTP to respond well to 10 mg of oral morphine. The calculation of the dose (using tables and oral morphine equivalents) may massively overestimate the needed dose and increase the danger of toxicity.

Opioid Combinations

Until recently, opioids were seen as a group of similar drugs, and their differences from the clinical point of view were rarely addressed. For many years, it was advisable to use the same opioid for treating both breakthrough pain and background pain. However, many clinicians observed that switching from one opioid to another may improve analgesia and reduce adverse effects [29, 30]. It follows that the combination of two opioids (one for the background and another for the breakthrough treatment) may produce better effects [31]. Unfortunately, the prevalence of the previous paradigm ("all opioids are the same") resulted in few formal studies of the combinations of opioids [32]. From the clinical point of view, the treatment of BTP with combinations of morphine and oxycodone, morphine with methadone, and fentanyl and morphine attracted the most attention, but formal clinical studies are still missing.

Different Opioids in BTP

Besides orally administered morphine or SC/IV, as alluded to above, oxycodone, orally and SC/IV, can be useful [33]. Sublingual methadone has been proposed recently as it has different pharmacokinetic properties [34], as methadone seems to be effective in some cases of opioid-resistant pain [35]. By far the most well known and the drug most pushed by the pharmaceutical companies is fentanyl for the treatment of BTP.

Originally, fentanyl drops, drawn from ampoules for parenteral use, were administered sublingually for this purpose [36]. This cheap, successful but unreliable-in-practice method has been redeveloped by the pharmaceutical industry to considerable hype in the early twenty-first century. We have devoted a separate heading to these preparations at the end of the chapter.

Other Drugs and Procedures

Ketamine

Ketamine is a well-known and safe anaesthetic, used in everyday practice of pain control. The use of ketamine either orally or parenterally in the treatment of BTP together with background opioid(s) had been proposed [37, 38]. Here too, the doses should be titrated according to the outcome and pattern of adverse effects. Data from high-quality clinical trials are lacking. The use of the extremely expensive S-ketamine is probably not justified, as in many cases, good effects can be achieved with ketamine racemate at low doses without toxicity. However, the long-term use of ketamine may cause considerable liver damage [39]. Oral ketamine acts more potently than after parenteral administration [40– 43]. This is probably due to the higher concentrations of the active metabolite norketamine after oral administration. Other than a number of anecdotal reports, oral or transmucosal ketamine has not been formally studied.

Infiltration with Local Anaesthetic with or Without Corticosteroids

Occasionally, pain on movement may be difficult to control. In some patients, topical corticosteroids injected into the painful site may help. This kind of infiltration, usually using methylprednisolone or triamcinolone acetonide combined with bupivacaine, may be highly effective even for a period of up to 2 months [44–46] (see Chap. 14).

Systemic Corticosteroids

Systemic corticosteroids, such as dexamethasone, at a starting dose of 12 mg od, may be helpful where local injection of corticosteroids is not feasible. Dexamethasone should ideally be supplemented by proton pump inhibitors to prevent gastric complications. Dexamethasone of sufficient dose, if not successful within 24–48 h, should be discontinued promptly, as it may later cause a number of complications, including proximal muscle dystrophy and adrenal insufficiency, and can considerably harm a patient's well-being.

Anaesthesiological Techniques

Nerve blocks and other neuroablative procedures are sometimes necessary and effective (see Chap. 18). However, for some patients with advanced cancer, they may be too late to perform. These procedures need to be performed in highly specialised centres that tend to cover patients from large catchment areas in order to maintain their experience. The pain and discomfort of the transportation to these centres may be an important threshold, making these procedures unavailable to many patients. Spinal or epidural administration of morphine together with local anaesthetics and/or clonidine may be helpful [47]. This method was very popular until late the 1990s, but despite its high efficacy, it lost its popularity because of its many severe complications, especially in patients with reduced immunity in the advanced stages of a disease [48].

Specific Issues with the BTP Related to Movement

Most movements are under voluntary control, and the patient is able to predict the painful moment and, if possible, avoid it [2, 8, 49]. However, many movements and reflexes are beyond or under only partially voluntary control. Coughing, laughing, sneezing, hiccuping, eating, defecating, and micturition can all precipitate BTP. Occasionally, these movements may generate a Valsalva manoeuvre, and this in turn may cause transient elevation of intracranial pressure [50]. In patients with brain tumours, such an increase in intracranial pressure may cause short-lasting severe headache, nausea, vomiting, photophobia, lethargy, and neurological deficit [51]. The movements may be associated with friction from fractured bones or increased muscle tension and increased pressure/tension on the entrapped nerve. For example, a persistent cough may elicit rib fracture and pain, and defecation may precipitate an intensive pain when a tumour infiltrates the sacral nerves. Withholding cough and voiding urine or defecation may have serious consequences, which is why the cause of withholding should be identified and treated.

Pain on movement which is only under partial volitional control should be treated vigorously. However, this treatment is usually indirect. If the patient is experiencing pain when coughing, the cough may be inhibited by codeine. However, some types of cough, especially dry, nonproductive ones, may be insensitive to codeine [52]. In these cases, paroxetine or other SSRIs may be tried [53]. Esophageal cramp may respond to calcium antagonists [54]. Increasing gastric pH by using proton pump inhibitors may be successful if reflux esophagitis is present. Gastric pain should be treated primarily with specific antacid drugs.

However, most often, severe abdominal pain associated with involuntary movement is experienced because of the traction of the intra-abdominal adhesions of a tumour infiltrating the peritoneum.

Adhesiolysis, even laparoscopic, is not practical in the terminally ill. It has proved to be of no value even in patients with better performance status [55]. In this type of pain, exacerbated by constipation, laxatives may be helpful. Indwelling catheters in pleura or the peritoneum as well as nasogastric tubes may occasionally cause severe pain. Their removal should be carefully considered by the multidisciplinary team, as there may be few alternatives left.

Entonox

A 50/50 mixture of nitrous oxide and oxygen (Entonox) had been applied in the treatment of predictable pain, mainly due to procedures [56–58]. Theoretically, because of its rapid onset and short duration of analgesia, Entonox could be used many times a day for the treatment of all kinds of BTP. However, there is little evidence of the effects of Entonox outside the hospital setting, and its use in the community is not validated [59]. And most importantly, repetitive use of Entonox may be toxic, and patients complain of somnolence, nausea, and vomiting [60].

BTP Other Than Background Pain

Many patients experience BTP other than background pain. Frequently, but not always, it is of a neuropathic origin. This pain may be either "invisible" and thus undiagnosed during the earlier analysis or exacerbated, for example, by opioid-induced hyperalgesia (see Chap. 10). This pain may become a problem when the main pain is adequately controlled. These pains are clearly distinguishable in localisation and character from the background/main pain. Frequently, these kinds of pain are insensitive to the administered analgesic, and not infrequently, they respond to the treatment of neuropathic pain. This neuropathic pain can be dysesthetic in nature (allodynia, hyperalgesia) (see Chap. 13). The pain may also be shooting and radiating due to nerve compression or damage. Neuropathic pain may also be experienced spontaneously, but it is usually initiated or exacerbated by movement. The pain may or may not be related to cancer (see Chap. 14). In acute and severe exacerbations of neuropathic BTP, clonazepam

injections 0.5–1 mg may be useful. For a review of therapy for neuropathic pain, please see Chap. 13.

Procedure Pain

In palliative care, the necessity for performing painful procedures is kept to a minimum. Many invasive, and painful, methods are seen as inappropriate or even contraindicated. None the less, more than 20 % of terminally ill patients need to have their wound dressings regularly changed [61]. Other painful procedures are the digital rectal evacuation, abscess incisions, or insertion of the IV cannulas. As this type of pain is predictable, treatment can be planned. Local anaesthetic injected into the painful site, or put on the wound or the skin as anaesthetic gel prior to procedure, may help [62–64]. This is especially useful with children. Ketamine can also be administered orally or parenterally before the procedure, usually with midazolam. Rapidly absorbed fentanyls may be a good choice [65].

Transmucosal Fentanyls

Fentanyl is a strong μ-opioid receptor agonist. It has a relatively low molecular weight and (unlike morphine) is highly lipophilic. This makes it suitable for transdermal and transmucosal administration. Several formulations are licensed for the treatment of breakthrough (episodic) cancer pain, with others on the way, e.g., a buccal soluble film. These include:
- Lozenge on a stick (Actiq®)
- SL (Abstral®) or buccal/SL (Effentora®) tablet
- Nasal spray (Instanyl®, PecFent®)

Formulations range from an aqueous solution of fentanyl (Instanyl®) to combinations with bioadhesive substances, e.g., croscarmellose (Abstral®), pectin (PecFent®). Thus, the pharmacokinetic characteristics of the products vary, and they are not interchangeable. Fentanyl is readily absorbed transmucosally, and these modifications tend to slow the rate of absorption. Various justifications are given (e.g., to aid mucosal adherence, to attenuate the peak plasma concentration), but the fact that a novel delivery system can be patented (although not fentanyl itself) is also relevant (Table 9.2).

Table 9.2 Selected characteristics and pharmacokinetic data for transmucosal fentanyl products[a,b]

	Abstral®	Actiq®	Effentora®[c]	Instanyl®	PecFent®
Formulation	SL tablet	Buccal lozenge	Buccal/SL tablet	Nasal spray	Nasal spray
Dose range (µg per dose)	100, 200, 300, 400, 600, 800; different shapes and coloured code, packs of 10 or 30	200, 400, 600, 800, 1,200, 1,600; on a stick, marked with dose, in colour-coded cartons, in packs of 3 or 30	100, 200, 400, 600, 800 (100 s smaller in size) embossed 1, 2, etc., in packs of 4 or 28	50, 100, 200 (in 100 µl); dose repeated once after 10 min. P.R.N.; colour code and in 10 and 20 dose bottles	100, 200, 400, 800 given as 1 or 2 doses of 100 or 400 µg/spray; colour coded and in 8 dose bottles
Maximum dose/episode	800 µg	1,600 µg	800 µg	400 µg	800 µg
Maximum frequency of use	Maximum 4 episodes/24 h, ideally ≥4 h apart (see dose and use)	Maximum 4 episodes/24 h, ideally ≥4 h apart (see dose and use)	Maximum 4 episodes/24 h, ≥4 h apart	Maximum 4 episodes/24 h, ≥ 4 h apart	Maximum 4 episodes/24 h, ≥ 4 h apart
Approximate cost/tablet or spray	£5	£6	£5	£6; >50 % of patients require 2 doses, thus average cost ≥£9	£3.8; about 50 % of patients require 200 or 800 µg dose, thus average cost=£5.7
Time to dissolution	<2 min	Applied over 15 min	Buccal 14–25 min	N/A	N/A
Onset of action[d]	10 min	15 min	10 min	5 min	10 min
Time to peak plasma conc. Median (range)	30–60 min (10–90); longer with higher strengths, but 600 and 800 µg note examined in patients	Across dose range 90 min (30–480) [66]	Pooled data 53 min (20–240) [67]	Across dose range 12–15 min (6–90) [68]	Across dose range 15–21 min (5–180) [69]
Plasma half-life (range)	Mean 5–6 h, but 600 and 800 µg not examined in patients	Median 18 h (7–49), 800 µg [66]	Median 12 h (2–44), pooled data [67]	Median 19 h (8–30); 200 µg, two doses 10 min apart [70]	Mean 15–25 h
Duration of action	≥1 h	≥1 h (≤3.5 h reported with higher doses) [71]	≥2 h	≥1 h	≥1 h
Bioavailability	70 % (estimated)	50 % (25 % transmucosal, 25 % oral) [71]	65 % (50 % transmucosal, 15 % oral)	90 %	No data
Comments		Requires continual movement around the mouth; less effective if finished <15 min as more is swallowed	Absorption not affected by mild (grade 1) mucositis [72]	Non-preserved solution, pH 6.6, osmolality ≈0.9 % saline	Preserved solution containing pectin, adjusted for pH and osmolality. C_{max} is about 1/3 of that of Instanyl. Audible click denotes dose administered; visual priming guide and dose counter, end-of-use lock

[a] The source (i.e., healthy volunteers vs. patients) and quality (e.g., small number of subjects, whole dose range was not studied, use of massage over buccal tablet) of the data varies widely

[b] Data based on venous blood sampling; with arterial sampling, a higher maximum concentration is achieved about 15 min quicker [73]

[c] Pharmacokinetics are similar for either buccal or SL placement

[d] Earliest statistically significant difference between fentanyl product and placebo in mean pain intensity difference; a clinically meaningful difference has been variably defined and generally takes longer

Table 9.3 Problems with the use of transmucosal fentanyls for the treatment of breakthrough pain

Expensive
Lack of data from independent trials
Patients used in most of the trials are 10–15 years younger and with good performance status which is significantly different from the patient population in palliative care
In some instances, the regulatory authorities expressed concerns about the amount and/or the quality of the data
The speed of action is being promoted by manufacturers. Although some patients report the first decrease of pain in 10–15 min after administration, the meaningful analgesia usually happens later
Lack of comparisons between the (many) preparations
No comparison with morphine injections
Boxes sometimes difficult to open
In the long term, patients tend to use more doses "as they like it"
May induce opioid-induced hyperalgesia

With the buccal/SL products, the amount of fentanyl absorbed directly across the mucosa or swallowed varies with formulation and route of administration. About two thirds of any swallowed fentanyl will be eliminated by intestinal or hepatic first-pass metabolism. Nonetheless, significant amounts of swallowed fentanyl are absorbed, e.g., about 25 and 15 % of the systemically available Actiq® and Effentora®, respectively, are via GI absorption [71, 72]. The effects of the GI absorption on the plasma concentration of fentanyl include producing a "double peak," maintaining high levels for longer (e.g., >2 h) and contributing to the wide range in T_{max} [67] (Table 9.3).

Conclusions

BTP is a difficult-to-treat kind of pain. Teaching how to diagnose and differentiate pain remains the primary aspect of pain control in cancer and the one that has the most potential of overall improvement. Generic treatment of the BTP with opioids, especially transmucosal fentanyls, is advisabvle only after thorough work-up.

Acknowledgments We are grateful to palliativedrugs. com for granting permission to use some of their material, including table relating to transmucosal fentanyls. The full monograph is available in Twycross R and Wilcock A (2011) Palliative Care Formulary (4e). Palliativedrugs. com, Nottingham.

References

1. Caraceni A, Martini C, Zecca E, Portenoy RK. Breakthrough pain characteristics and syndromes in patients with cancer pain. An international survey. Palliat Med. 2004;18:177–83.
2. Portenoy RK, Bruns D, Shoemaker B, Shoemaker SA. Breakthrough pain in community-dwelling patients with cancer pain and noncancer pain, part 2: impact on function, mood, and quality of life. J Opioid Manag. 2010;6:109–16.
3. Caraceni A, Hanks G, Kaasa S, et al. Use of opioid analgesics in the treatment of cancer pain: evidence-based recommendations from the EAPC. Lancet Oncol. 2012;13:e58–68.
4. Davies AN, Dickman A, Reid C, Stevens AM, Zeppetella G. The management of cancer-related breakthrough pain: recommendations of a task group of the Science Committee of the Association for Palliative Medicine of Great Britain and Ireland. Eur J Pain. 2009;13:331–8.
5. Patt RB, Ellison NM. Breakthrough pain in cancer patients: characteristics, prevalence, and treatment. Oncology (Huntingt). 1998;12:1035–46; discussion 49–52.
6. Bhatnagar S, Upadhyay S, Mishra S. Prevalence and characteristics of breakthrough pain in patients with head and neck cancer: a cross-sectional study. J Palliat Med. 2010;13:291–5.
7. Zeppetella G, O'Doherty CA, Collins S. Prevalence and characteristics of breakthrough pain in cancer patients admitted to a hospice. J Pain Symptom Manage. 2000;20:87–92.
8. Portenoy RK, Hagen NA. Breakthrough pain: definition, prevalence and characteristics. Pain. 1990;41:273–81.
9. Bennett MI. Cancer pain terminology: time to develop a taxonomy that promotes good clinical practice and allows research to progress. Pain. 2010;149: 426–7.
10. Portenoy RK, Bennett DS, Rauck R, et al. Prevalence and characteristics of breakthrough pain in opioid-treated patients with chronic noncancer pain. J Pain. 2006;7:583–91.
11. Sabato AF. Idiopathic breakthrough pain: a new hypothesis. Clin Drug Investig. 2010;30 Suppl 2:27–9.
12. Thompson PD. Muscle cramp syndromes. Handb Clin Neurol 2007;86:389–96.
13. Carney E. Managing nocturnal breakthrough pain. Nursing. 1995;25:20.
14. Gagnon B, Lawlor PG, Mancini IL, Pereira JL, Hanson J, Bruera ED. The impact of delirium on the

circadian distribution of breakthrough analgesia in advanced cancer patients. J Pain Symptom Manage. 2001;22:826–33.

15. Marchant EG, Mistlberger RE. Morphine phase-shifts circadian rhythms in mice: role of behavioural activation. Neuroreport. 1995;7:209–12.

16. Noiman R, Korczyn AD. Circadian rhythm of the pupillary response to morphine and to naloxone. Chronobiol Int. 1985;2:239–41.

17. Choi HW, Wild KD, Hubbell CL, Reid LD. Chronically administered morphine, circadian cyclicity, and intake of an alcoholic beverage. Alcohol. 1990; 7:7–10.

18. Walsh D, Doona M, Molnar M, Lipnickey V. Symptom control in advanced cancer: important drugs and routes of administration. Semin Oncol. 2000;27: 69–83.

19. Hanks GW, Conno F, Cherny N, et al. Morphine and alternative opioids in cancer pain: the EAPC recommendations. Br J Cancer. 2001;84:587–93.

20. Coluzzi PH. Cancer pain management: newer perspectives on opioids and episodic pain. Am J Hosp Palliat Care. 1998;15:13–22.

21. Mercadante S, Villari P, Ferrera P, et al. Safety and effectiveness of intravenous morphine for episodic breakthrough pain in patients receiving transdermal buprenorphine. J Pain Symptom Manage. 2006;32: 175–9.

22. Mercadante S, Villari P, Ferrera P, Casuccio A, Mangione S, Intravaia G. Transmucosal fentanyl vs intravenous morphine in doses proportional to basal opioid regimen for episodic-breakthrough pain. Br J Cancer. 2007;96:1828–33.

23. Fitzgibbon D, Morgan D, Dockter D, Barry C, Kharasch ED. Initial pharmacokinetic, safety and efficacy evaluation of nasal morphine gluconate for breakthrough pain in cancer patients. Pain. 2003;106:309–15.

24. Pavis H, Wilcock A, Edgecombe J, et al. Pilot study of nasal morphine-chitosan for the relief of breakthrough pain in patients with cancer. J Pain Symptom Manage. 2002;24:598–602.

25. Ruiz-Garcia V, Lopez-Briz E. Morphine remains gold standard in breakthrough cancer pain. BMJ. 2008;337: a3104.

26. Coluzzi PH, Schwartzberg L, Conroy JD, et al. Breakthrough cancer pain: a randomized trial comparing oral transmucosal fentanyl citrate (OTFC) and morphine sulfate immediate release (MSIR). Pain. 2001;91:123–30.

27. Portenoy RK, Taylor D, Messina J, Tremmel L. A randomized, placebo-controlled study of fentanyl buccal tablet for breakthrough pain in opioid-treated patients with cancer. Clin J Pain. 2006;22:805–11.

28. Slatkin NE, Xie F, Messina J, Segal TJ. Fentanyl buccal tablet for relief of breakthrough pain in opioid-tolerant patients with cancer-related chronic pain. J Support Oncol. 2007;5:327–34.

29. Mercadante S, Bruera E. Opioid switching: a systematic and critical review. Cancer Treat Rev. 2006;32: 304–15.

30. Quigley C. Opioid switching to improve pain relief and drug tolerability. Cochrane Database Syst Rev. 2004;CD004847.

31. Pasternak GW. Preclinical pharmacology and opioid combinations. Pain Med. 2012;13 Suppl 1:S4–11.

32. Fallon MT, Laird BJ. A systematic review of combination step III opioid therapy in cancer pain: an EPCRC opioid guideline project. Palliat Med. 2011;25:597–603.

33. Ordonez Gallego A, Gonzalez Baron M, Espinosa Arranz E. Oxycodone: a pharmacological and clinical review. Clin Transl Oncol. 2007;9:298–307.

34. Hagen NA, Moulin DE, Brasher PM, et al. A formal feasibility study of sublingual methadone for breakthrough cancer pain. Palliat Med. 2010;24:696–706.

35. Scholes CF, Gonty N, Trotman IF. Methadone titration in opioid-resistant cancer pain. Eur J Cancer Care (Engl). 1999;8:26–9.

36. Bushnaq M, Al-Shoubaki M, Milhem M. The feasibility of using intravenous fentanyl as sublingual drops in the treatment of incidental pain in patients with cancer. J Palliat Med. 2009;12:511–4.

37. Cherry DA, Plummer JL, Gourlay GK, Coates KR, Odgers CL. Ketamine as an adjunct to morphine in the treatment of pain. Pain. 1995;62:119–21.

38. Friedman R, Jallo J, Young WF. Oral ketamine for opioid-resistant acute pain. J Pain. 2001;2:75–6.

39. Noppers IM, Niesters M, Aarts LP, et al. Drug-induced liver injury following a repeated course of ketamine treatment for chronic pain in CRPS type 1 patients: a report of 3 cases. Pain. 2011;152:2173–8.

40. Furuhashi-Yonaha A, Iida H, Asano T, Takeda T, Dohi S. Short- and long-term efficacy of oral ketamine in eight chronic-pain patients. Can J Anaesth. 2002;49: 886–7.

41. Blonk MI, Koder BG, van den Bemt PM, Huygen FJ. Use of oral ketamine in chronic pain management: a review. Eur J Pain. 2010;14:466–72.

42. Grant IS, Nimmo WS, Clements JA. Pharmacokinetics and analgesic effects of i.m. And oral ketamine. Br J Anaesth. 1981;53:805–10.

43. Enarson MC, Hays H, Woodroffe MA. Clinical experience with oral ketamine. J Pain Symptom Manage. 1999;17:384–6.

44. Zylicz Z, Haijman J. Suprascapular nerve entrapment: a neglected cause of shoulder pain in cachectic patients? J Pain Symptom Manage. 2000;20:315–7.

45. Penn J, Zylicz Z. Could shoulder pain be suprascapular nerve entrapment? Eur J Pall Care. 2006;13:98–100.

46. Zylicz Z. Obturator nerve block as a clue to the diagnosis of focal spinal metastases of gastric cancer – a case report. Adv Pall Med. 2009;8:121–4.

47. Van Dongen RT, Crul BJ, De Bock M. Long-term intrathecal infusion of morphine and morphine/bupivacaine mixtures in the treatment of cancer pain: a retrospective analysis of 51 cases. Pain. 1993;55:119–23.

48. Aprili D, Bandschapp O, Rochlitz C, Urwyler A, Ruppen W. Serious complications associated with external intrathecal catheters used in cancer pain patients: a systematic review and meta-analysis. Anesthesiology. 2009;111:1346–55.

49. Portenoy RK, Payne D, Jacobsen P. Breakthrough pain: characteristics and impact in patients with cancer pain. Pain. 1999;81:129–34.
50. Suwanwela N, Phanthumchinda K, Kaoropthum S. Headache in brain tumor: a cross-sectional study. Headache. 1994;34:435–8.
51. Hayashi M, Handa Y, Kobayashi H, Kawano H, Ishii H, Hirose S. Plateau-wave phenomenon (I). Correlation between the appearance of plateau waves and CSF circulation in patients with intracranial hypertension. Brain. 1991;114(Pt 6):2681–91.
52. Eccles R. Codeine, cough and upper respiratory infection. Pulm Pharmacol. 1996;9:293–7.
53. Zylicz Z, Krajnik M. What has dry cough in common with pruritus? Treatment of dry cough with paroxetine. J Pain Symptom Manage. 2004;27:180–4.
54. Nasrallah SM. Nifedipine in the treatment of diffuse oesophageal spasm. Lancet. 1982;2:1285.
55. Swank DJ, Swank-Bordewijk SC, Hop WC, et al. Laparoscopic adhesiolysis in patients with chronic abdominal pain: a blinded randomised controlled multi-centre trial. Lancet. 2003;361:1247–51.
56. Landman J. Evaluation of nitrous oxide anesthesia for endoscopic and laparoscopic urological applications. J Urol. 2007;178:14.
57. Gudgin EJ, Besser MW, Craig JI. Entonox as a sedative for bone marrow aspiration and biopsy. Int J Lab Hematol. 2008;30:65–7.
58. Chakupurakal G, Delgado J, Nikolousis E, et al. Midazolam in conjunction with local anaesthesia is superior to Entonox in providing pain relief during bone marrow aspirate and trephine biopsy. J Clin Pathol. 2008;61:1051–4.
59. Owen J. Using Entonox in the community. Nurs N Z. 2008;14:3.
60. Doran M, Rassam SS, Jones LM, Underhill S. Toxicity after intermittent inhalation of nitrous oxide for analgesia. BMJ. 2004;328:1364–5.
61. Galvin J. An audit of pressure ulcer incidence in a palliative care setting. Int J Palliat Nurs. 2002;8:214–21.
62. Holdsworth MT, Raisch DW, Winter SS, et al. Pain and distress from bone marrow aspirations and lumbar punctures. Ann Pharmacother. 2003; 37:17–22.
63. Russell SC, Doyle E. A risk-benefit assessment of topical percutaneous local anaesthetics in children. Drug Saf. 1997;16:279–87.
64. Monk TG, Ding Y, White PF, Albala DM, Clayman RV. Effect of topical eutectic mixture of local anesthetics on pain response and analgesic requirement during lithotripsy procedures. Anesth Analg. 1994;79:506–11.
65. MacIntyre PA, Margetts L, Larsen D, Barker L. Oral transmucosal fentanyl citrate versus placebo for painful dressing changes: a crossover trial. J Wound Care. 2007;16:118–21.
66. Darwish M, Kirby M, Robertson Jr P, Tracewell W, Jiang JG. Absolute and relative bioavailability of fentanyl buccal tablet and oral transmucosal fentanyl citrate. J Clin Pharmacol. 2007;47:343–50.
67. Agency EM. Effentora: EPAR- scientific discussion. 2008.
68. Kaasa S, Moksnes K, Nolte T, Lefebvre-Kuntz D, Popper L, Kress HG. Pharmacokinetics of intranasal fentanyl spray in patients with cancer and breakthrough pain. J Opioid Manag. 2010;6:17–26.
69. Agency. EM. Assessment report of Pecfent. Procedure NoEMA/H/C001164. 2010.
70. Agency EM. Assessment report for Instanyl. Procedure NOEMA/H/959, London. 2009.
71. Lichtor JL, Sevarino FB, Joshi GP, Busch MA, Nordbrock E, Ginsberg B. The relative potency of oral transmucosal fentanyl citrate compared with intravenous morphine in the treatment of moderate to severe postoperative pain. Anesth Analg. 1999;89: 732–8.
72. Darwish M, Kirby M, Robertson P, Tracewell W, Jiang JG. Absorption of fentanyl from fentanyl buccal tablet in cancer patients with or without oral mucositis: a pilot study. Clin Drug Investig. 2007;27:605–11.
73. Darwish M, Kirby M, Robertson Jr P, Hellriegel E, Jiang JG. Comparison of equivalent doses of fentanyl buccal tablets and arteriovenous differences in fentanyl pharmacokinetics. Clin Pharmacokinet. 2006;45:843–50.

Opioid-Induced Hyperalgesia

10

Jakob Sørensen and Per Sjøgren

Abstract

Opioid-induced hyperalgesia (OIH) is defined as a state of nociceptive sensitisation caused by exposure to opioids. The condition is characterised by a paradoxical response whereby a patient receiving opioids for the treatment of pain could actually become more sensitive to certain painful stimuli. The type of pain experienced might be the same as the underlying pain or might be different from the original underlying pain.

Observational, cross-sectional, and prospective controlled trials have examined the expression and potential clinical significance of OIH in humans. Most studies have been conducted using several distinct cohorts and methodologies utilising former opioid addicts on methadone maintenance therapy, perioperative exposure to opioids in patients undergoing surgery, cancer patients on opioids, and healthy human volunteers after acute opioid exposure using human experimental pain testing.

There are several proposed mechanisms for OIH; among these mechanisms involving the central glutaminergic system, spinal dynorphins, descending facilitation, genetic mechanisms, and decreased reuptake and enhanced nociceptive response have been described as the important mechanisms.

Clinicians should suspect OIH when opioid treatment's effect seems to wane in the absence of disease progression, particularly if found in the context of unexplained pain reports or diffuse allodynia unassociated with the original pain, and increased levels of pain with increasing dosages. The treatment involves reducing the opioid dosage, tapering them off, or supplementation with NMDA receptor inhibitors.

J. Sørensen, MD
Section of Palliative Care,
Department of Oncology,
Odense University Hospital, Sdr. Boulevard 29,
DK 5000 Odense C, Denmark
e-mail: jakob.soerensen@ouh.regionsyddanmark.dk

P. Sjøgren, MDSci (✉)
Section of Palliative Medicine,
Department of Oncology,
Rigshospitalet Hospital, Blegdamsvej 9,
2100 Ø Copenhagen, Denmark
e-mail: p.sjogren@adr.dk

M. Hanna, Z. Zylicz (eds.), *Cancer Pain*,
DOI 10.1007/978-0-85729-230-8_10, © Springer-Verlag London 2013

Keywords

Consistent in preclinical studies • Decrease in pain threshold • Sparse evidence in humans • NMDA receptor activation crucial • μ-receptors might not be involved • Assembles neuropathic pain • Treatment with opioid rotation, opioid cessation, or NMDA receptor antagonists

Introduction

For many years, opioids have been the cornerstone for the treatment of cancer pain, and in the last two decades, opioids have been increasingly used for the treatment of chronic noncancer pain conditions [1]. Thus, an increase in opioid consumption has been noticed worldwide, and both cancer and chronic noncancer pain patients are being treated with consistently higher doses for longer periods. In these patients, long-term opioid treatment – apart from inducing analgesia and traditional side effects (nausea, sedation, constipation, itching, etc.) – may induce physical dependence, addiction and abuse, cognitive disorders, suppression of immune and reproductive systems, tolerance, and opioid-induced hyperalgesia (OIH).

Although clinical guidelines emphasise physician monitoring of addiction, abuse, and diversion, OIH is often overlooked as a potential complication of opioid therapy [2]. According to the literature, a growing body of observations and evidence for unintended pronociceptive consequences of long-term use of opioids is emerging, and although there exists some confusion regarding the terminology, OIH seems to be the preferred term. Hyperalgesia is described as an enhanced pain response to a noxious stimulus, whereas allodynia, which can also accompany hyperalgesia, is a pain response to an innocuous stimulus. However, OIH is broadly defined as a state of nociceptive sensitisation caused by exposure to opioids. The condition is characterised by a paradoxical response, whereby a patient receiving opioids for the treatment of pain might actually become more sensitive to certain painful stimuli. The type of pain experienced by an individual might be the same as the underlying pain or might be different from the original underlying pain,

and typically OIH produces diffuse pain, less defined in quality, which extends to other areas of distribution than the preexisting pain. Thus, the original pain type may be amplified, combined with a state of more generalised hyperalgesia/allodynia resembling neuropathic pain. However, there still exists no generally accepted operational definition of OIH among researchers in human clinical trials; hyperalgesia is defined as a decrease in either pain threshold or pain tolerance after chronic opioid exposure. Pain threshold is the first experience of pain from a given stimulus, whereas pain tolerance is the amount of pain from a given stimulus an individual can tolerate before seeking relief (e.g., the period of time before discontinuing an experimental pain procedure due to pain). Threshold and tolerance are two different constructs with, potentially, two different psychophysical mechanisms. Due to the lack of consensus regarding a definition of OIH among pain researchers, it can be difficult to compare results across studies of available literature and draw firm conclusions.

In the 1970s, animal studies demonstrated that opioids can paradoxically increase sensitivity to pain and may aggravate preexisting pain [3]. OIH in humans was first described in the peer-reviewed literature in 1943 [4] but has gained increasing attention over the latest two decades. In the beginning of the 1990s, OIH was primarily described in patients with advanced cancer receiving high doses of opioids for prolonged periods [5, 6]. However, recent studies indicate that OIH may be much more prevalent and clinically relevant, as it has been found in former addicts undergoing methadone maintenance [7], during perioperative exposure to opioids [8], and in chronic noncancer patients treated with opioids [9]. Thus, OIH has virtually been described in all the patient categories that have been treated with opioids. Therefore, a burning clinical issue is whether OIH can explain the loss of opioid efficacy in some selected cases or whether OIH has tremendous significance for many patients in long-term opioid therapy.

However, in the clinic, the decreased effectiveness of the opioid therapy raises the difficult question of whether it is a sign of tolerance development, OIH, progression of tissue injury, or a combination of these factors. In the following, we will address preclinical and clinical data, mechanisms, and future directions for the treatment of OIH.

Preclinical Data

For decades, it has been known that exposure to opioids can cause a paradox decrease in nociceptive threshold in rodents, and studies in animal models have indicated that opioid exposure can induce an increase in pain sensitivity and potentially exacerbate preexisting pain.

In 1971, Kayan et al. demonstrated that morphine produced hyperalgesia in rats receiving repeated subcutaneous injections. They used the hot plate model measuring changes in response latency, which was found between 60 and 120 min after drug administration. The administration of nalorphine did not abolish hyperalgesia but delayed the onset [3]. Ten years later Woolf showed that repeated intrathecal injections of morphine caused a similar response to systemic administration [10].

Célèrier et al. evaluated the sensitivity to nociceptive stimuli in the rat (paw-pressure vocalisation test) following four s.c. bolus injections (every 15 min) of fentanyl on immediate (for several hours) and long-term (for several days) administration. A dose-dependent effect was demonstrated, where higher doses of acute treatment with fentanyl produced a pronounced hyperalgesic response. The higher fentanyl doses used, the more pronounced fentanyl-induced hyperalgesia was demonstrated. Ketamine pretreatment, which had no analgesic effect on its own, enhanced the earlier response (analgesia) and prevented the development of long-lasting hyperalgesia [11].

In 2001, the same group demonstrated progressive enhancement of delayed hyperalgesia induced by repeated heroin administration. Further, they showed that both magnitude and duration of heroin-induced delayed hyperalgesia increased with intermittent heroin injections involving a decrease in the analgesic effectiveness of a given heroin dose. The heroin-addicted animals were sensitive to even a small dose of heroin, which triggered a delayed hyperalgesia, which could not be demonstrated after a similar dose in heroin naïve rats. The finding was interpreted as the development of central sensitisation [12].

Development of hyperalgesia following chronic exposure to opioids has also been investigated in an 8-day model, where morphine was administered by a once-daily intrathecal injection in rats. This study showed that the nociceptive threshold was reliably decreased in the morphine-treated rats compared to placebo. In association with the development of morphine tolerance, thermal hyperalgesia to radiant heat developed in these same rats. The effect lasted for at least 48 h after the last injection. These data indicated that thermal hyperalgesia develops in association with the development of morphine tolerance and that the co-activation of central NMDA and non-NMDA receptors is crucial for both the development and expression of thermal hyperalgesia in morphine-tolerant rats [13].

Intermittent administrations of opioids in experimental animal models could be explained by a mechanism of repetitive withdrawal hyperalgesia. In order to exclude this, several investigators have demonstrated a corresponding reduction in nociceptive thresholds and development of hyperalgesia in rodents following continuous exposure to opioids. Thus, two groups of rats had implanted either subcutaneous morphine pellets or subcutaneous morphine infusions by osmotic mini-pumps in order to deliver morphine continuously providing stable plasma concentrations. Seven days of continuous morphine exposure caused tactile allodynia and thermal hyperalgesia. These findings indicated that the development of OIH is a non-withdrawal phenomenon [14–16].

Development of OIH in these experiments varied not only with the period of time of opioid exposure but also with the type and dose of opioid as well as with the experimental pain model (i.e., thermal, mechanical, electrical, or chemical). Originally, the development of OIH was thought to depend solely on varying opioid-dosing regimens (including maintenance dosing, brief high doses, and brief low or ultra-low doses). Preclinical data have suggested hyperalgesia after each of these regimens; however, there still are too few studies and too many variables to explain the mechanisms of different subtypes of OIH in humans.

Human Data

The abovementioned animal experiments in combination with a growing number of anecdotal reports and few controlled clinical studies of OIH have strongly indicated that OIH exists in humans. In order to explore human data in depth, it is mandatory to select data from a variety of different clinical and experimental settings.

Opioid Naive Individuals

A number of studies have shown that acute exposure to high doses of opioids during surgery is associated with higher pain intensity and/or opioid consumption in the postoperative period [8, 17–19].

Chia et al. showed, in an RCT comparing high and low doses of fentanyl intraoperatively in females undergoing total abdominal hysterectomy, that high doses were associated with higher consumption of opioids postoperatively 17. These findings were confirmed by Guignard's group, who found significant higher postoperative opioid consumption in the high-dose group when comparing the administration of high doses of remifentanil with low doses intraoperatively [8].

Apart from confirming the abovementioned findings in an RCT in patients undergoing surgery, Joly et al. demonstrated postoperative secondary

hyperalgesia in the wound area, which was significantly larger in the group receiving high doses of fentanyl intraoperatively. Further, the researchers showed that the hyperalgesia could be prevented by a small dose of ketamine, which indicated that an NMDA receptor-mediated process was in play [18].

Crawford et al. showed higher postoperative morphine consumption after preoperatively administrated remifentanil in a paediatric population undergoing scoliosis surgery [19].

These findings from intra- and postoperative clinical settings have been supported by experimental studies in human volunteers.

Angst et al. gave a 90-min infusion of remifentanil to healthy volunteers. The researchers produced an area of hyperalgesic skin to mechanical stimulation by intradermal electrical stimulation prior to the infusion. Two stainless steel wires connected to a needle and covered with a microdialysis catheter to prevent direct contact with the skin tissue were inserted in parallel into the dermis of the left volar forearm. A current was slowly increased until the skin area surrounding the stimulation site became hyperalgesic to mechanical stimuli. The area of hyperalgesia to mechanical stimulation significantly increased after infusion of remifentanil. The mechanical hyperalgesia was abolished with co-administration of the NMDA antagonist s-ketamine [20]. In an RCT enrolling 13 volunteers, transcutaneous electrical stimulation induced acute pain, which was kept constant during the experiment. Stable areas of mechanical hyperalgesia to punctuate stimuli and touch were established. During remifentanil infusion, the participants experienced reduced pain and areas of punctuate hyperalgesia. After cessation of the infusion, both pain and hyperalgesia were significantly increased in the remifentanil group compared to controls [21].

Hood et al. confirmed these findings in a capsaicin-induced hyperalgesia model. They found reduced pain and area of hyperalgesia during remifentanil infusion and an increase in both pain and hyperalgesia up to 4 h after cessation of infusion [22].

Chronic Noncancer Pain Patients

Chu et al. prospectively assessed the development of analgesic tolerance and hyperalgesia in patients with moderate to severe chronic low-back pain before, and 1 month after, treatment with oral morphine. They used the cold pressor test (a quantitative sensory testing technique where the participant typically places their hand in painfully cold water for as long as possible) and experimental heat pain models. They found that opioid treatment was associated with significant hyperalgesia to the cold pressor test, but not to the heat pain models [9].

Recent data from Chen et al. compared three groups of patients in a cross-sectional design. A group of healthy controls, a group of chronic pain patients without opioid treatment, and a group of chronic pain patients receiving opioid treatment participated. They compared pain threshold and pain tolerance to heat and cold as well as the degree of temporal summation of the second pain measured by a train of four of identical stimuli at 47°C, which were separated by a 2.2s interval between stimuli. They found that individuals with chronic pain on opioid therapy differed significantly from the other two groups by displaying decreased heat pain thresholds and enhanced temporal summation responses. The authors also noted that higher opioid doses correlated with the magnitude of these responses [23].

In a cross-sectional study comparing chronic pain patients with or without oral opioids, Ram and colleagues found no differences between the groups regarding cold pressor threshold, tolerance, or pain intensity levels. However, the magnitude of the diffuse noxious inhibitory control (DNIC, which is an assessment involving two simultaneous pain induction procedures) effect, a marker of pain inhibition, was larger for non-opioid-treated patients, when compared to those on opioids. Interestingly, men in the non-opioid group had a significantly larger DNIC effect compared to men in the opioid group, while there was no difference between women of the two groups. Furthermore, the authors also found that both opioid dosage and treatment duration negatively predicted DNIC in men on opioids [24].

Former Addicts on Methadone Maintenance

Opioid-dependent individuals on replacement therapy also show evidence of OIH as compared to healthy control patients. In a cross-sectional study of methadone-maintained patients, buprenorphine-maintained patients, and matched controls tested by the cold pressor test, Compton and colleagues found that methadone- and buprenorphine-maintained patients displayed shorter withdrawal latencies to cold water compared with matched controls [25]. Furthermore, Compton et al. examined whether gabapentin had the potential to reverse OIH in methadone-maintained patients. After a 5-week trial of daily gabapentin, they found statistically significant improvement in cold pressor pain threshold and tolerance from the baseline [26].

Doverty et al. compared nociceptive responses in 16 patients on stable, once-daily methadone with 16 matched controls. They used electrical stimulation and the cold pressor test. The methadone group was tested at the time of trough plasma methadone concentration (time 0) and 3 h after daily dose (time 3~peak concentration). Controls were tested 3 h apart. Using electrical stimulation, the methadone group had lower pain tolerance than controls at time 0 but significantly higher pain tolerance at time 3. No differences in pain detection values were found. Regarding the cold pressor test, methadone patients both had shorter withdrawal latencies to cold water and substantially less pain tolerance than controls [7].

Pud and colleagues also found evidence for OIH using the cold pressor test in opioid addicts and found that the alterations in pain perception lasted at least for 1 month after completing a detoxification program. They suggested that either the modulation of the nociceptive system was a phenomenon, which is present to a higher degree in individuals who are disposed to addiction, or the findings may be due to a long-lasting sensitisation of the nervous system [27].

In 2009, Hay et al. compared former addicts on methadone maintenance and chronic pain patients on morphine treatment with a control group. Cold pressor tolerance was significantly lower in the opioid-treated groups than in the controls; however, there was no difference between chronic pain patients and the methadone maintenance group. Furthermore, there was no difference in electrical stimulation test between the groups [28].

Cancer Patients

Sjøgren et al. published a small series of eight cancer patients, who all developed severe hyperalgesia and myoclonus receiving treatment with continuous i.v. morphine infusion [6]. Quantitative sensory testing was not performed in this study. Since then, no series has been published with focus on OIH in the cancer patient population; however, case reports have described the development of OIH during treatment with different types of opioids and administration forms.

Interestingly, De Conno and colleagues described a case of hyperalgesia and myoclonus in a patient treated with high doses of intrathecal (IT) administered morphine. The patient suffered from refractory thoracic pain due to a carcinoma of the right lung, and a totally implanted IT pump system was inserted. The IT dose of morphine gradually increased to 80 mg/day, and at this dose, the patient experienced spontaneous hyperesthesia and allodynia in the lower extremities with a dermatomal distribution completely different from the preexisting pain. The pain sensation was accompanied by myoclonic jerks of different muscle groups of the lower extremities. After lowering of the intrathecal morphine dose, the segmental OIH and myoclonus were significantly reduced [5].

Mercadante et al. described two cases of OIH following rapid opioid dose escalation. In the first case, a patient suffered OIH, which was relieved primarily by switching from morphine to methadone, and later in the course by changing from oral to epidural administration. In the second case, the OIH was reversed by IT administered bupivacaine in combination with small doses of morphine [29].

In 2003, Wilson et al. published a case report where a patient with metastatic testicular cancer in severe pain received huge doses of opioids orally, intravenously, and intrathecally. A metastatic destruction of L-2 involved rapidly increasing doses of oral and intravenous opioids. In order to obtain pain control, an epidural and later an IT infusion of opioids combined with bupivacaine and clonidine was established. The IT infusion was rapidly increased to huge doses of morphine (900 mg/day) without achieving pain control. At this stage, the clinicians considered the possibility of OIH and decreased the IT opioid doses to 19 mg/day. The patient achieved substantial pain relief and remained pain-free until death 6 weeks later [30].

In a case report, a patient experienced increasing, generalised burning pain and an exquisite sensitivity to light touch on huge oral doses of oxycodone (2.500–3.000 mg/daily). Switching the patient to oral methadone in a lower equipotent dose, the pain was decreased to moderate levels [31].

Vorobeychik and colleagues reported a case of OIH, where a patient with recurrent squamous cell lung carcinoma achieved a substantial pain relief after oral hydromorphone doses were reduced by 40–50 % and additional therapy with small doses of oral methadone was introduced [32].

Mechanisms

OIH is a state of sensitisation of the nociceptive nervous system caused by the exposure to opioids due to modulation of the CNS. Several mechanisms for the development of OIH have been suggested in the literature based on animal data, and especially the NMDA receptors seem to be crucial for the development of OIH. When the activated NMDA receptors are inhibited, the development of tolerance and OIH can be prevented. This has been studied in animal models by several groups using NMDA antagonists, which could prevent the development of tolerance as well as thermal hyperalgesia after repeated injections of opioids [13, 33, 34]. However, a number of alternative mechanisms for the development of OIH have contemporarily been proposed in the literature, and earlier studies indicated that cross talk of neural mechanisms of pain and tolerance may exist [35, 36].

Inhibition of the glutamate transporter system will increase the amount of available glutamate for the NMDA receptors. Mao showed that chronic exposure to opioids induced a dose-dependent downregulation of glutamate transporters in the dorsal horn. This downregulation exhibited a temporal correlation with the development of opioid tolerance and thermal hyperalgesia. The development of tolerance as well as thermal hyperalgesia was potentiated by a glutamate transporter inhibitor and reduced by a positive glutamate transporter regulator. These effects were at least in part mediated by the NMDA receptor, as the NMDA antagonist MK 801 blocked both tolerance and hyperalgesia potentiated by the glutamate transporter inhibitor in rodents [37].

The Ca^{++}-regulated intracellular protein kinase C (PKC) is probably a cellular link involved in the development of both tolerance and OIH. Mao demonstrated that intracellular PKC activation plays a critical role in the development of thermal hyperalgesia in opioid-tolerant rats [13]. Narita et al. treated mice with a μ-receptor agonist (DAMGO) intrathecally and demonstrated that PKC, especially the PKCγ isoform, played a role in uncoupling of the spinal μ-opioid receptor from G proteins, which could be of importance in the development of μ-receptor-mediated tolerance [38]. Zeitz et al. confirmed this finding by using PKCγ mutant mice, which exhibited decreased development of tolerance [39].

Prolonged morphine exposition can induce NMDA receptor-mediated neurotoxicity, which may involve apoptotic cell death in the dorsal horn. This morphine-induced neuronal apoptosis can be blocked by caspase inhibitors, leading to the assumption that opioid-induced neurotoxic effects can be regulated by the NMDAR-caspase pathway [40].

These mechanisms may involve sensitisation of dorsal horn neurons, which is believed to drive enhanced nociception in opioid-induced abnormal pain. The presence of NMDA receptors on central terminals of primary afferent fibres has been demonstrated, and since these sites also contain μ-opioid receptors, NMDA and opioid receptor activity may serve to counterbalance each other's effects [41]. Célèrier postulated an equilibrium state between the opioid-dependent analgesic systems and the NMDA-dependent pronociceptive systems, which after opioid exposure could involve a new high-level balance between the systems enhancing pain vulnerability [12].

Dynorphin is an endogenous opioid peptide with affinity to the κ-receptor system, which is widely distributed in the CNS. The spinal content of dynorphin is increased after opioid administration [42, 43], and it might have importance in sustaining the abnormal pain perception by reducing the antinociceptive effect of spinal opioids [14]. Furthermore, animal data suggest that dynorphin also has a pronociceptive action and promotes the conduction of nociceptive impulses [42]. The role of other endogenous opioids has been discussed, but a recent study has indicated that the endogenous opioid system may not be involved in modulation of OIH [44]. The investigators used the μ-receptor antagonist, naloxone, which has little or no binding on the κ-receptor agonists leaving the role of dynorphin questionable.

Modulation of pain impulses in the dorsal horn is influenced by descending facilitating and inhibiting impulses primarily generated in the rostral ventromedial medulla (RVM). Subsets of neurons in RVM have characteristic and different roles in nociceptive processing [45, 46]. "ON" cells have been proposed to permit or facilitate nociceptive transmission, and "OFF" cells to inhibit the transmission. These cells respond differently when systemic morphine is administrated. "ON" cells will be inhibited and "OFF" cells will become continuously active, which will modulate the perception of nociceptive input [47]. Vanderah showed that hyperalgesia developed in animals by continuous administration of opioids could be reversibly blocked by the microinjection of lidocaine into the RVM [48].

Lesioning the descending pathway from RVM prevents the increase of neurotransmitter peptides such as substance P and calcitonin gene-related peptide (CGRP) with opioid exposure [49]. Substance P preferentially binds to NK-1 receptors in the dorsal horn, and King et al. showed morphine-induced hyperalgesia was reversed by spinal administration of an NK-1 receptor antagonist [50]. Newer studies have emphasised the importance of chemokines and stromal-derived factor. Opioids acting via the μ-opiate receptors can modulate the expression of chemokines and their receptors on immune cells, and a similar action in the nervous system is suggested as an important messenger in the development and maintenance of OIH [51].

Genetic research has found a specific μ-receptor isoform (6TM MOR1K) that might be responsible for the development of OIH in humans by facilitating excitatory effects; however, the clinical importance of this is still unknown [52].

All these suggested mechanisms involve the NMDA and/or μ-receptors as mediators for the development of OIH. Lately, two experiments have suggested that OIH may be a non-opioid receptor phenomenon. Knockout mice without μ-, δ-, or κ-opioid receptors developed thermal hyperalgesia after acute and chronic (6 days) exposure to fentanyl [53]. This hyperalgesia could be blocked by NMDA antagonist MK-801. In an additional experiment from the same lab, the administration of morphine-6-glucuronide (a metabolite of morphine with μ-receptor agonist activity) produced hyperalgesia in knockout mice and wild-type mice treated concurrently with the opioid receptor antagonist naloxone [54]. These experiments suggest that some opioid metabolites or other endogenous substances without opioid receptor-binding properties may cause OIH through opioid receptor-independent mechanisms.

In the first series of OIH in cancer patients described by De Conno et al. [5] and Sjøgren et al. [6], a mechanism induced by the morphine metabolite morphine-3-glucoronide (M3G) was suspected. This mechanism has recently gained recurrent interest as the intrathecal or intraventricular injection of M3G in animals produced serious hyperalgesia. Juni et al. found this unrelated to prior opioid receptor activity and tolerance [55], and Lewis proposed that M3G acts through activation of microglia to produce interleukin-1, which could be blocked or reversed by IL-1 receptor antagonist. They found that the expression was mediated by a toll-like receptor-4 (TLR4), which is predominantly expressed by microglia in the spinal cord [56].

Clinical Implications and Diagnosis

Lack of effectiveness might be seen with the administration of opioids for cancer and chronic noncancer pain more commonly than anticipated and reported. Common traditional solutions to this include opioid rotation, reduction of the administered dose, or detoxification to manage OIH. However, a major dilemma faces the pain clinician in diagnosing OIH and differentiating it from tolerance as opioid rotation and reduction of dose may be risky and complicated in patients with complex pain conditions on high doses of opioids. First of all, the clinician must be able to distinguish OIH from progression of the disease. Features exist that differentiate OIH from increases in preexisting pain due to disease progression and/or pharmacologic tolerance development. Typically OIH produces diffuse pain, less defined in quality, which extends to other areas of distribution from preexisting pain. However, some reports contemporarily describe a worsening of the original underlying pain induced by dose increase [6]. Secondly, OIH has been demonstrated clinically by inducing changes in pain threshold, tolerability, and distribution pattern in methadone-maintained addicts [25], although it should noticed that quantitative sensory testing methodology has not yet been sufficiently developed and tested to diagnose and identify OIH. Therefore, clinical assessment is still the only feasible way forward in diagnosing OIH. Thus, if the preexisting pain is undertreated or pharmacologic tolerance exists, an increase in opioid dose will result in the reduction of pain. Conversely, OIH would be worsened with increasing opioid dosage.

Based on the abovementioned shortcomings regarding diagnosing OIH, it is understandable that OIH often is confused with opioid tolerance and withdrawal-associated hyperalgesia. These syndromes can manifest similar symptoms but may need to be clinically differentiated from OIH due to different effective interventions. Patients who develop opioid tolerance have no increase in baseline pain sensitivity but require increasing doses of opioids to maintain the same level of analgesia previously achieved with lower doses. In contrast, patients with OIH exhibit an increase in pain sensitivity defined by a lower nociceptive threshold and an increase in pain perception at all levels of sensory stimulation. Distinguishing OIH from tolerance in the individual patient might require a clinical demonstration of reduced pain sensitivity after opioid detoxification [57]. Physical dependence is characterised and defined by the appearance of withdrawal symptoms when the opioid dose is reduced or abruptly discontinued and may occur within a few days of continuous use. Withdrawal-associated hyperalgesia is the experience of diffuse joint pain, abdominal cramps, and other body aches, which occur when detoxifying from chronic opioid use or skipping/missing scheduled doses; it is time-limited and can be treated with NSAIDs, clonidine, benzodiazepines, and/or a controlled weaning-off opioid-dosing schedule.

Treatment Suggestions

From the first anecdotal reports on OIH, a dose reduction or switch to other opioids has been suggested as an effective remedy in cancer patients [32, 58, 59].

Most of the successful opioid rotation/switching, which has been described in the cases, has been from morphine to methadone with a considerable dose reduction as a result [60]. The rotation/switching has not only abolished the OIH but also substantially reduced other opioid toxicities. The beneficial rotation to methadone has most frequently been explained by the assumption that methadone has a week NMDA receptor antagonism, which could explain the effect [59, 61–63].

The potential involvement of the NMDA receptors in a generation of OIH has promoted the use of more specific NMDA receptor-blocking agents. The most powerful of these available is ketamine, which has been used in several settings to treat OIH in experimental settings.

The use of ketamine to reduce OIH has been demonstrated both in animal models [11, 64, 65] and in humans [18, 20, 21, 66].

In the study from 2003 on human volunteers, Koppert et al. described that the remifentanil-induced hyperalgesia was abolished by an infusion of s-ketamine of 5 µg/kg/min, suggesting a mechanism of activating the NMDA receptor. In the same study, an α-2 adrenergic agonist, clonidine, did not attenuate pain or areas of hyperalgesia [21].

In the study previously described by Angst et al. from 2003, they showed that remifentanil-induced hyperalgesia in volunteers was abolished by the co-administration of s-ketamine [20].

Joly et al. demonstrated in a clinical randomised trial that a small dose of ketamine given just after the induction of anaesthesia could prevent high-dose remifentanil-induced hyperalgesia in a population of surgical patients [18].

Forero described in a case report reversal of hyperalgesia and myoclonus with low-dose ketamine infusion. The patient, who had a long history of low-back pain and several unsuccessful treatment attempts, received a totally implanted IT catheter system, and an infusion with hydromorphone was started. The dose was increased several times to a level of 12 mg/day. He underwent surgery for examining the pump system, and postoperatively, he received intravenous patient-controlled analgesia with hydromorphone. In this period, the patient experienced severe painful spasms in his lower back that radiated to the lower extremities. I.v hydromorphone and morphine did not relieve the pain. The authors suspected opioid toxicity on top of pre-existing OIH and gave a bolus of 15 mg ketamine, which in 1 min resolved the spasms and made the patient pain-free. A maintenance infusion of ketamine was started, and the intrathecal dose of hydromorphone could be reduced to 2.5 mg/day [67].

As the pain type in OIH resembles some of the pain qualities originating from neuropathic pain conditions, the use of the adjuvant analgesics commonly used for these conditions has been suggested. Gabapentin is an anticonvulsant, which is widely used in the treatment of neuropathic pain. In an animal setting, it has been demonstrated that gabapentin prevented delayed and long-lasting hyperalgesia induced by fentanyl in rats [67].

Compton et al. have in humans demonstrated that cold pressor pain responses were decreased by the use of gabapentin in methadone-maintained addicts [26].

Conclusions and Future Directions

OIH has been reliably demonstrated to exist in the preclinical literature, and it is most often in this context defined as a decrease in pain threshold due to opioid exposure. The NMDA receptor activation seems to be crucial for the development of OIH, and opioid receptors may not exclusively be involved in the development of OIH. Although evidence is sparse, OIH in humans appears to pose a clinical challenge in acute, chronic, and cancer pain settings. However, a major challenge is to find diagnostic tools which can reliably identify the appearance of OIH. Although QST assessing patients' pain sensitivity before and during opioid therapy has been used as tools for monitoring the onset and extent of OIH in studies, there exists neither consensus nor clear evidence for their clinical relevance. Thus, in the future, OIH may emerge as a distinct, definable, and characteristic phenomenon in some cases; however, OIH may also turn out to be much more prevalent and of tremendous significance for opioid therapy in general.

Due to the vague definitions, characteristics and mechanisms of OIH-targeted treatments are not yet available, and the major remedies are opioid reduction, rotation, and adjuvant drugs (NMDA antagonists and other adjuvant analgesics). More experimental studies as well as well-designed prospective clinical trials assessing QST and other experimental pain modalities in healthy controls as well as in patients with pain before and after opioid therapy would be of interest in order to establish further knowledge of OIH. The next decade will hopefully bring more explanations regarding the mechanisms of OIH and open the field for studies of targeted treatments.

References

1. Eriksen J, Sjøgren P, Bruera E, Ekholm O, Rasmussen NK. Critical issues on opioids in chronic non-malignant pain: an epidemiological study. Pain. 2006; 125:172–9.
2. Chou R, Fanciullo GJ, Fine PG, Miaskowski C, Passik S, Portnoy RK. Opioids for chronic noncancer pain: prediction and identification of aberrant drug-related behaviors: a review of the evidence for an American Pain Society and American Academy of Pain Medicine clinical practice guideline. J Pain. 2009;10(2):131–46.
3. Kayan S, Woods LA, Mitchell CL. Morphine-induced hyperalgesia in rats tested on the hot plate. J Pharmacol Exp Ther. 1971;177(3):509–13.
4. Andrews HL. The effect of opiates on the pain threshold in post-addicts. J Clin Invest. 1943;22:511–6.
5. De Conno F, Caraceni A, Martini C, Spoldi E, Salvetti M, Ventafridda V. Hyperalgesia and myoclonus with intrathecal infusion of high-dose morphine. Pain. 1991;47:337–9.
6. Sjøgren P, Jonsson T, Jensen NH, Drenck NE, Jensen TS. Hyperalgesia and myoclonus in terminal cancer patients treated with continuous intravenous morphine. Pain. 1993;55:93–7.
7. Doverty M, White JM, Somogyi AA, Bochner F, Ali R, Ling W. Hyperalgesic responses in methadone maintenance patients. Pain. 2001;90:91–6.
8. Guignard B, Bossard AE, Coste C, et al. Acute opioid tolerance: intraoperative remifentanil increases postoperative pain and morphine requirement. Anesthesiology. 2000;93:409–17.
9. Chu LF, Clark DJ, Angst MS. Opioid tolerance and hyperalgesia in chronic pain patients after one month of oral morphine therapy: a preliminary prospective study. J Pain. 2006;7:43–8.
10. Woolf CJ. Intrathecal high dose morphine produces hyperalgesia in the rat. Brain Res. 1981;209(2):491–5.
11. Cérèlier E, Rivat C, Jun Y, et al. Long lasting hyperalgesia induced by fentanyl in rats. Anesthesiology. 2000;92:465–72.
12. Célèrier E, Laulin J-P, Corcuff J-B, Le Moal M, Simonnet G. Progressive enhancement of delayed hyperalgesia induced by repeated heroin administration: a sensitization process. J Neurosci. 2001;21(11):4074–80.
13. Mao J, Price DD, Mayer DJ. Thermal hyperalgesia in association with the development of morphine tolerance in rats: roles of excitatory amino acid receptors and protein kinase c. J Neurosci. 1994;14(4):2301–12.

14. Vanderah TW, Ossipov MH, Lai J, Malan Jr TP, Porreca F. Mechanisms of opioid-induced pain and antinociceptive tolerance: descending facilitation and spinal dynorphin. Pain. 2001;92:5–9.

15. Li X, Angst MS, Clark JD. A murine model of opioid-induced hyperalgesia. Mol Brain Res. 2001;86:56–62.

16. Li X, Angst MS, Clark JD. Opioid-induced hyperalgesia and incisional pain. Anesth Analg. 2001;93:204–9.

17. Chia Y-Y, Liu K, Wang J-J, Kuo M-C, Ho S-T. Intraoperative high dose fentanyl induces postoperative fentanyl tolerance. Can J Anaesth. 1999;46(9):872–7.

18. Joly V, Richebe P, Guignard B, Fletcher D, Maurette P, Sessler DI, et al. Remifentanil-induced postoperative hyperalgesia and its prevention with small-dose ketamine. Anesthesiology. 2005;103:147–55.

19. Crawford MW, Hickey C, Zaarour C, Howard A, Naser B. Development of acute opioid tolerance during infusion of remifentanil for pediatric scoliosis surgery. Anesth Analg. 2006;102:1662–7.

20. Angst MS, Koppert W, Pahl I, Clark DJ, Schmelz M. Short-term infusion of the µ-opioid agonist remifentanil in humans causes hyperalgesia during withdrawal. Pain. 2003;106:49–57.

21. Koppert W, Sitti R, Scheuber K, Alsheimer M, Schmelz M, Schüttler J. Differential modulation of remifentanil-induced analgesia and postinfusion hyperalgesia by s-ketamine and clonidine in humans. Anesthesiology. 2003;99:152–9.

22. Hood DD, Curry R, Eisenach JC. Intravenous remifentanil produces withdrawal hyperalgesia in volunteers with capsaicin-induced hyperalgesia. Anesth Analg. 2003;97:810–5.

23. Chen L, Malarick C, Seefeld L, Wang S, Houghton M, Mao J. Altered quantitative sensory testing outcome in subjects with opioid therapy. Pain. 2009;143:65–70.

24. Ram KC, Eisenberg E, Haddad M, Pud D. Oral opioid use alters DNIC but not cold pain perception in patients with chronic pain – new perspective of opioid-induced hyperalgesia. Pain. 2009;139:431–8.

25. Compton P, Charuvastra VC, Ling W. Pain intolerance in opioid-maintained former opiate addicts: effect of long-acting maintenance agent. Drug Alcohol Depend. 2001;63:139–46.

26. Compton P, Kehoe P, Sinha K, Torrington MA, Ling W. Gabapentin improves cold-pressure pain responses in methadone-maintained patients. Drug Alcohol Depend. 2010;109:213–9.

27. Pud D, Cohen D, Lawental E, Eisenberg E. Opioids and abnormal pain perception: new evidence from a study of chronic opioid addicts and healthy subjects. Drug Alcohol Depend. 2006;82:218–23.

28. Hay JL, White JM, Bochner F, Somogyi AA, Semple TJ, Rounsefell B. Hyperalgesia in opioid-managed chronic pain and opioid-dependent patients. J Pain 2009;10(3): 316–22.

29. Mercadante S, Ferrera P, Villari P, Arcuri E. Hyperalgesia: an emerging iatrogenic syndrome. J Pain Symptom Manage. 2003;26(2):769–75.

30. Wilson GR, Reisfield GM. Morphine hyperalgesia: a case report. Am J Hosp Palliat Care. 2003;20:459–61.

31. Davis MP, Shaiova LA, Angst MS. When opioids cause pain. J Clin Oncol. 2007;25(28):2297–8.

32. Vorobeychik Y, Chen L, Bush MC, Mao J. Improved opioid analgesic effect following opioid dose reduction. Pain Med. 2008;9(6):724–7.

33. Trujillo KA, Akil H. Inhibition of morphine tolerance and dependence by the NMDA receptor antagonist MK-801. Science. 1991;251:85–7.

34. Marek P, Ben Eliyahu S, Gold M. Excitatory amino acid antagonists (kynurenic acid and MK-801) attenuate the development of morphine tolerance in the rat. Brain Res. 1991;547:81–8.

35. Mao J, Price DD, Mayer DJ. Experimental mononeuropathy reduces the antinociceptive effects of morphine: implications for common intracellular mechanisms involved in morphine tolerance and neuropathic pain. Pain. 1995;61:353–64.

36. Mao J. NMDA and opioid receptors: their interactions in anti-nociception tolerance and neuroplasticity. Brain Res Rev. 1999;30:289–304.

37. Mao J, Sung B, Ji RR, Lim G. Chronic morphine induces downregulation of spinal glutamate transporters: implications in morphine tolerance and abnormal pain sensitivity. J Neurosci. 2002;22:8312–23.

38. Narita M, Mizoguchi H, Nagase M, Suzuki T, Tseng LF. Involvement of spinal protein kinase C gamma in the attenuation of opioid-mu-receptor mediated G-protein activity after chronic intrathecal administration of [D-Ala2, N-Mephe4, Gly-Ol5] enkephalin. J Neurosci. 2001;21:3715–20.

39. Zeitz KP, Malmberg AB, Gilbert H, Basbaum AL. Reduced development of tolerance to the analgesic effect of morphine and clonidine in PKC gamma mutant mice. Pain. 2002;94:245–53.

40. Mao J, Sung B, Ru Rong J, Grewo L. Neuronal apoptosis associated with morphine tolerance: evidence for an opioid-induced neurotoxic mechanism. J Neurosci. 2002;22:7650–61.

41. Ossipov MH, Lai J, King T, Vanderah TW, Porreca F. Underlying mechanisms of pronociceptive consequences of prolonged morphine exposure. Biopolymers. 2005;80:319–24.

42. Vanderah TW, Gardell LR, Burgess SE, Ibrahim M, Dogrul A, Zhong CM, et al. Dynorphin promotes abnormal pain and spinal opioid antinociceptive tolerance. J Neurosci. 2000;20:7074–9.

43. Campillo A, González-Cuello A, Cabañero D, Garcia-Nogales P, Asunción R, Milanés MV, et al. Increased spinal dynorphin levels and phosphor-extracellular signal-regulated kinases 1 and 2 and c-fos immunoreactivity after surgery under remifentanil anesthesia in mice. Mol Pharmacol. 2010;77(2):185–94.

44. Chu LF, Dairmont J, Zamora AK, Young CA, Angst MS. The endogenous opioid system is not involved in modulation of opioid-induced hyperalgesia. J Pain. 2011;12(1):108–11.

45. Barbaro NM, Heinricher MM, Fields HL. Putative pain modulating neurons in the rostral ventral medulla:

reflex-related activity predicts effects of morphine. Brain Res. 1986;366:203–10.

46. Heinricher MM, Morgan MM, Fields HL. Direct and indirect actions of morphine on medullary neurons that modulate nociception. Neuroscience. 1992;48:533–43.

47. Morgan MM, Heinricher MM, Fields HL. Circuitry linking opioid-sensitive nociceptive modulatory systems in periaqueductal gray and spinal cord with rostral ventromedial medulla. Neuroscience. 1992;47(4):863–71.

48. Vanderah TW, Suenaga NMH, Ossipov MH, Malan Jr TP, Lai J, Porreca F. Tonic descending facilitation from the rostral ventromedial medulla mediates opioid-induced abnormal pain and antinociceptive tolerance. J Neurosci. 2001;21(1):279–86.

49. Gardell LR, Wang R, Burgess SE, et al. Sustained morphine exposure induces a spinal dynorphin-dependent enhancement of excitatory transmitter release from primary afferent fibers. J Neurosci. 2002;22(15):6747–55.

50. King T, Gardell LR, Wang R, Vardanyan A, Ossipov MH, Malan TP, et al. Role of NK-1 neurotransmission in opioid-induced hyperalgesia. Pain. 2005;116:276–88.

51. White F, Wilson N. Opiate-induced hypernociception and chemokine receptors. Neuropharmacology. 2010;58:35–7.

52. Gris P, Gauthier J, Cheng P, Gibson DG, Gris D, Laur O, et al. A novel alternative spliced isoform of the mu-opioid receptor: functional antagonism. Mol Pain. 2010;6:33–42.

53. Waxman AR, Arout C, Caldwell M, Dahan A, Kest B. Acute and chronic fentanyl administration causes hyperalgesia independently of opioid receptor activity in mice. Neurosci Lett. 2009;462(1):68–72.

54. Van Dorp ELA, Kest B, Kowalczyk WJ, Morariu AM, Waxman AR, Arout CA, et al. Morphine-6β-glcoronide rapidly increases pain sensitivity independently of opioid receptor activity in mice and humans. Anesthesiology. 2009;110:1356–63.

55. Juni A, Klein G, Kest B. Morphine hyperalgesia in mice is unrelated to opioid activity, analgesia, or tolerance: evidence for multiple diverse hyperalgesic systems. Brain Res. 2006;1070:35–44.

56. Lewis SS, Hutchinson MR, Rezvani N, Loram LC, Zhang Y, Maier SF, et al. Evidence that intrathecal morphine-3-glucoronide may cause pain enhancement via toll-like receptor 4/MD-2 and interleukin-1β. Neuroscience. 2010;165(2):569–83.

57. Baron MJ, McDonald PW. Significant pain reduction in chronic pain patients after detoxification from high dose opioids. J Opioid Manag. 2006;2:277–82.

58. Mercadante S, Arcuri E. Hyperalgesia and opioid switching. Am J Hosp Palliat Care. 2005;22(4):291–4.

59. Okon TR, George ML. Fentanyl-induced neurotoxicity and paradoxic pain. J Pain Symptom Manage. 2008;35(3):327–33.

60. Mercadante S, Bruera E. Opioid switching: a systematic and critical review. Cancer Treat Rev. 2006;32:304–15.

61. Ebert B, Thorkildsen C, Andersen S, Christru LL, Hjeds H. Opioid analgesics as noncompetetive N-methyl_D-aspartate (NMDA) antagonists. Biochem Pharmacol. 1998;56:553–9.

62. Blackburn D, Somerville E, Squire J. Methadone: an alternative conversion regime. Eur J Palliat Care. 2002;9(3):93–6.

63. Axelrod DJ, Reville B. Using methadone to treat opioid-induced hyperalgesia and refractory pain. J Opioid Manag. 2007;3(2):113–4.

64. Richebé P, Rivat C, Laulin J-P, Maurette P, Simonnet G. Ketamine improves the management of exaggerated postoperative pain observed in perioperative fentanyl-treated rats. Anesthesiology. 2005;102:421–8.

65. Minville V, Fourcade O, Girolami J-P, Tack I. Opioid-induced hyperalgesia in a mice model of orthopaedic pain: preventive effect of ketamine. Br J Anaesth. 2010;104(2):231–8.

66. Forero M, Chan PSL, Restrepo-Garces CE. Successful reversal of hyperalgesia/myoclonus complex with low-dose ketamine infusion. Pain Pract. 2011. doi:10.1111/j.1533-2500.2011.00475.x.

67. Van Elstraete AC, Sitbon P, Mazoit J-X, Benhamou D. Gabapentin prevents delayed and long-lasting hyperalgesia induced by fentanyl in rats. Anesthesiology. 2008;108:484–94.

The Non-Pharmacological and Local Pharmacological Methods of Pain Control

11

Remigiusz Lecybyl

Abstract

There is an extensive variety of non-pharmacological and local pharmaco-logical pain management techniques available for treating cancer pain. They do not create a ladder like the pharmacological treatments, and they should be continuously available to all cancer patients. Regular reassessment should identify patients who can benefit from different non-pharmacological meth-ods during progression of the disease. Non-pharmacological methods should only be delivered in the context of holistic multidisciplinary approach. A few of the most widely accepted non-pharmacological local pharmacological methods include acupuncture, TENS, external neuromodulation, radio-fre-quency neuromodulation, APS, topical application of local anaesthetics, application of capsaicin patches, and Botox injections.

Keywords

Non-pharmacological treatment • Acupuncture • TENS • External neuro-modulation • APS • Lidocaine patch • Capsaicin patch • Botox

Introduction

The WHO pharmacotherapeutical ladder is the gold standard for cancer pain treatment [1]. The ladder consists of escalating strengths of systemic analgesic accompanied with adjuvants. Adjuvants can be systemic or local. Using local adjuvants is hindered by the multifocal or generalised topog-raphy of pain in cancer patients; however, in most cases, patient attention is drawn to one location where pain is most severe and/or most disturbing. Applying local treatment to this area can significantly contribute to overall quality of patient care. Local treatments very often produce immediate improvement with either none or min-imal systemic side effects. They produce a strong placebo effect as treatment is administrated directly to the affected area. Multifocal pain can consist of different character pains at different locations, and local treatments can address the

R. Lecybyl, MD, PhD
The Pain Management Unit,
University Hospital Lewisham,
Lewisham High Street,
SE13 6LH Lewisham, Kent, UK
e-mail: cambodja@ump.edu.pl

M. Hanna, Z. Zylicz (eds.), *Cancer Pain*,
DOI 10.1007/978-0-85729-230-8_11, © Springer-Verlag London 2013

character of pain at each location (e.g., TENS for mechanical low back pain and lignocaine patch for postherpetic neuralgia at the chest wall). One of the major barriers of wider use of local treatments is the misconception that local treatment means injections. In fact, the majority of local treatments are noninvasive (e.g., application of cold or heat, TENS, neuromodulation, mirror box, and local analgesic patches) or minimally invasive (e.g., acupuncture, trigger point treatments). In some cases, local treatments can provide diagnostic value as well.

The aim of this chapter is to present and discuss local non-pharmacological and pharmacological methods of pain control in cancer patients, where possible detailed guidelines are provided.

Acupuncture

The term "acupuncture" is poorly defined and has been used indiscriminately in literature to refer to a number of related physical therapy techniques. The following classification of therapies in acupuncture spectrum was proposed [2]:

1. Classical acupuncture – This originated in China in prehistory based on theories of meridians, energy flow, and philosophy.
2. Scientific acupuncture – This rejects, at least partially, the traditional Chinese background and is based on principles of neurophysiology and anatomy.
3. Acupuncture as a form of trigger point therapy – This is based on the concept of muscular trigger points.
4. Acupuncture with electric stimulation – This is based on passing pulse electric current through the body tissue via acupuncture needles (using pen-like topical electrodes was reported, but inclusion of this technique to acupuncture is controversial).

Acupuncture utilises multiple physical stimuli: pressure (acupressure, acupressure balls), needling (intradermal, subcutaneous, intramuscular, periosteal, intrachondral – auriculoacupuncture), electric current (electroacupuncture – needle electrode, external neuromodulation – pen-like electrode; TENS, patch electrode), and laser stimulations. Stimuli classification is further complicated by different parameters of electric and laser stimulation including intensity, frequency, and wavelength. Differing frequencies of stimulation activate different nerve fibres and can lead to distinct neurophysiological therapeutical effects.

Neurophysiological mechanisms of acupuncture have been extensively investigated. Current knowledge suggests a modulation of several endogenous analgesic mechanisms and involvement of multiple central connections and descending pain inhibitions via noradrenergic and serotonergic pathways in order to give extrasegmental pain relief [3].

Acupuncture was reported as helpful for chronic cancer pain [4]; however, the systematic review of acupuncture for the relief of cancer-related pain was inconclusive [5]. Additionally, acupuncture is increasingly used for the treatment of non-pain conditions in cancer patients including nausea, vomiting, vasomotor symptoms, xerostomia, breathlessness, and fatigue. Acupuncture is in general a very safe treatment, and any major risk related to blood-borne infections can be further reduced by employment of appropriate aseptic technique and use of disposable needles. A clinical guideline about acupuncture treatment for cancer patients was published. The aim of this guideline is to assist clinicians in making decisions and to facilitate good medical practice [6].

There is an obvious need for more formal research about acupuncture. However, due to the technical aspect of blinding, multiple philosophical concepts, and variability of applied stimuli, acupuncture is one of the most difficult fields in which to conduct formal research for the purposes of analgesia.

An example of simple classical acupuncture points selected for lumbar pain treatment is presented in Table 11.1 [7]. The location of acupuncture points is defined using the Acupuncture Unit of Measurement (AUM, human inch, cm). This unit differs from patient to patient and is defined as the distance between the two creases of the interphalangeal joints of the patient's flexed middle finger [7].

Trigger points associated with myofascial and visceral pains often lie within the areas of referred pain, but many are located at a distance from

Table 11.1   Example of simple acupuncture treatment of lumbar pain [7]

Meridian	Point	Chinese	Anatomical position
Bladder	B 23	Shen Yu	1.5 AUM lateral to inferior border of spinous process of second lumbar vertebra
Bladder	B 46	Huang Men	3 AUM lateral to inferior border of first lumbar vertebra
Bladder	B 54	Wei Chung	Exact centre of popliteal crease
Small intestine	SI 4	Wan Ku	Ulnar border of palm in a depression, proximal to fifth metacarpal
Small intestine	SI 6	Yang Lao	1 AUM above styloid process of ulna on posterior surface of forearm

Table 11.2   Electroacupuncture of right muscle trapezius trigger points

Stimulator: AWQ-104L Digital
Needles: 4 × 0.25 × 40 mm
Mode: slow/fast
Frequency: 2 Hz/100 Hz
Duration of session: 10 min

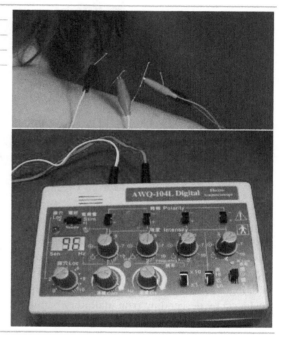

them. Furthermore, brief intense stimulation of trigger points frequently produces prolonged relief of pain [8]. Electroacupuncture of right muscle trapezius trigger points is presented in Table 11.2. Electroacupuncture can be used for neuropathic pain. An example is "Surround the dragon" [9]. The electroacupuncture technique for knee neuropathic pain is presented in Table 11.3. Acupuncture needles are inserted around hypersensitive area.

TENS

Electrical stimulation for the relief of pain has been used since ancient times, but its modern use dates from the late 1960s, following the publication of the Gate Control Theory of Pain [10]. TENS is delivered using topical flexible electrodes. Frequency of stimulation varies between 1 and 200 Hz, current intensity between 1 and 50 mA, and pulse width between 0.1 and 1 ms. The most common modalities in clinical practice are conventional TENS and acupuncture-like TENS [11, 12]. Conventional TENS uses low electric current intensity with high frequency (usually around 100 Hz) which creates a "Jaccuzi"-like sensation. Conventional TENS stimulates A-beta large-diameter afferent nerve fibres that modulate onward transmission of afferent nociceptive input in the dorsal horn of the spinal cord. Animal studies suggest that conventional TENS can increase extracellular level of gamma-aminobutyric acid in the spinal cord, reducing central sensitisation and

Table 11.3 Surround the dragon

Stimulator: AS SUPER 4
Needles: $8 \times 0.25 \times 40$ mm
Mode: slow
Frequency: 2 Hz
Duration of session: 10 min

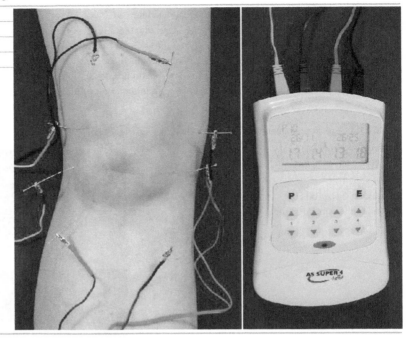

primary hyperalgesia [13]. Acupuncture-like TENS utilises high electric current intensity with low frequency (usually around 2 Hz) which creates a pinprick sensation. Acupuncture-like TENS is thought to stimulate A-delta fibres and achieve analgesia by descending pain inhibitory pathways in the spinal cord [12]. The Cohrane systematic review identified 43 studies which investigated TENS in cancer patients for pain relief. Unfortunately, only two of them met the eligibility criteria for the Cohrane systematic review. The two most common reasons for exclusion were lack of randomisation and lack of clinical data. The two randomised clinical trials included in the Cohrane review were clinically and methodologically heterogeneous, and these disparities prevented meta-analysis. The Cohrane review concluded that there is insufficient evidence available to make a decision on the use of TENS for patients with cancer pain or cancer treatment-related pain. Further research, which is specific, adequately powered, multicentred, randomised, and controlled, is needed to add to our knowledge [14]. The advantages of TENS are the possibility self-administration, its low cost, a favourable side-effect profile, and safety. The major disadvantage

of TENS is lack of proof of efficacy. An example of TENS for lumbar pain is presented in Table 11.4.

External Neuromodulation

External neuromodulation involves the application of electrical stimulation via an external nerve mapping probe connected to a pulse generator. The probe is placed within the proximity of the nerves covering the distribution of the painful areas or directly to the epicentre of the painful area (target). The stimulating ball-shaped probe (Neuro-Trace, HDC Corporation, Milpitas, California, USA; Pajunk GmbH, Geisingen, Germany) is directed at the nerves, plexuses, or target areas in patients with mainly chronic neuropathic pain syndromes. The amplitude of the devices is adjusted to a perceivable paresthesia level. Compared to TENS, external neuromodulation creates an electric field with a narrower area and a higher intensity. The external application allows the procedure to be performed on an outpatient [15] or bedside basis. Preliminary reports in the literature demonstrate evidence for

Table 11.4 TENS treatment for lumbar pain

Stimulator: TPN-EX
Mode: normal
Frequency: 100 Hz
Pulse width: 200 m
Duration of session: 30–60 min

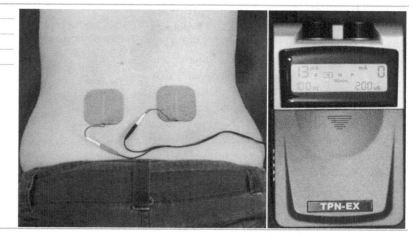

Table 11.5 External neuromodulation

Stimulator: NeuroStim
Frequency: 2 Hz
Pulse width: 1 ms
Duration of session: 10 min

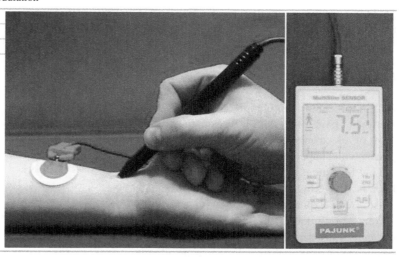

its effectiveness [16, 17]. The external neuromodulation stimulator and stimulation probe are shown in Table 11.5.

Radio-Frequency Denervation and Pulsed Radio-Frequency Neuromodulation

Radio-frequency lesioning involves passage of a very high-frequency current down a 27 G thermocouple probe; this probe is inserted through a special 22 G cannula, which is fully insulated except for its tip. When the current is passed down the thermocouple probe, it heats the surrounding tissues to a temperature for denervation usually between 72 and 85 °C, which is controlled by the operator. The diameter of the lesion is about 2–4 mm. Sensory nerves are identified by low-voltage stimulation at a frequency of 50 Hz. The cannula needs to be within 3 mm of the nerve in order to create an adequate lesion, and a maximum stimulation level of around 0.6 V would indicate this. The operator should always ensure that the cannula is not dangerously close to any motor nerve by using low-frequency

(2 Hz), low-voltage stimulation. If no muscle twitch (2 Hz) in the territory of the nerve is noted at twice the voltage strength necessary to achieve sensory stimulation (50 Hz) but at least 1 V, it can be safely assumed that there are no motor paths within 3 mm of the needle. Radio-frequency denervation can be applied to the medial branch of posterior primary ramus of spinal nerves (for facet joints denervation) (Table 11.6), peripheral nerves, sympathetic ganglia, and cervical spinal cord (percutaneous cervical cordotomy) [18].

Pulse radio-frequency neuromodulation does not produce any nerve lesion. Radio-frequency current 20 ms bursts at a repetition rate 2 Hz is delivered. The temperature of the probe is controlled to not exceed 42 °C, and radio-frequency voltage is limited to 45 V. Pulsed radio-frequency neuromodulation is used to produce pain relief predominantly by stimulation of spinal nerve roots and peripheral nerves (Table 11.7) [18].

Action Potential Stimulation

Action potential stimulation (APS) is a rare method of pain relief. APS utilises a unique concept of electrophysics: application of electric pulses with shape similar to neuro action potential but four times stronger [19]. The APS stimulator is delivering 150 Hz, monophasic square pulses with exponential decay with adjustable current amplitude. The current is delivered through transdermal electrodes. The potential advantage of electrical stimulation, as an adjunct to other pain therapies, is that this treatment modality is noninvasive and relatively safe. Such treatments have minimal side effects, assist in reduction of medication, and may improve the quality of life of the patient, permitting a return to normal working and social activities [20].

Pharmacological Local Treatments

Local anaesthetics drugs act by causing a reversible block to conduction along the nerve fibres. They can be administrated topically on skin (EMLA, Ametop, 5 % lidocaine-medicated plaster) and on mucosa (lignocaine gel) or can be

Table 11.6 L4/L5 and L5/S1 facet joints radio-frequency denervation

Target: medial branches of posterior primary rami of followed spinal nerves:
L3, L4, L5, S1
Needle is inserted under X-ray guidance, and position is confirmed by sensory stimulation:
Frequency 50 Hz
Pulse width 1 ms
Voltage <0.5 V
Proximity of motor neurons is excluded by motor stimulation:
Frequency 2 Hz
Pulse width 1 ms
Voltage double of sensory threshold and at least 1 V
RF denervation:
85 °C
1 min

Table 11.7 Pulse radio-frequency neuromodulation of greater occipital nerve

RF needle is inserted medial to the occipital artery about 2 cm lateral to the occipital protuberance.
Needle position is confirmed by sensory stimulation:
Frequency: 50 Hz
Pulse width 1 ms
Voltage up 0.5 V; If sensory threshold is higher than 0.5 V, RF needle need to be repositioned to locate nerve
Pulsed RF neuromodulation:
4 cycles 120 s each
Frequency 2 Hz
Maximal voltage 45 V
Maximal temperature 42 °C

injected. Five percent lidocaine-medicated plaster is indicated for postherpetic neuralgia but is commonly used for other focal neuropathic pains

NSAIDS – Topical NSAIDS (e.g., felbinac, ibuprofen, ketoprofen, and piroxicam) may provide some relief of pain in musculoskeletal conditions. They can be considered as an adjunctive treatment in knee or hand osteoarthritis [21].

Capsaicin is a selective agonist of TRPV1 receptor. There are two available preparations: low-concentration cream (0.025 and 0.075 %) and high-concentration patch 8 %. In hand or knee osteoarthritis, 0.025 % capsaicin cream can be considered as an adjunct [21]. The 0.075 % capsaicin cream is licensed for the symptomatic relief of postherpetic neuralgia after the lesion has healed, and for the relief of painful diabetic neuropathy [21]. Patients should apply a very small amount of capsaicin cream on the affected area four to five times per day avoiding the eyes and broken or inflamed skin and wash hands immediately after application. Application of 8 % capsaicin path results in reversible desensitisation of TRPV1-expressing cutaneous sensory nerve endings and reduction in nerve fibre density in the epidermis [22]. Capsaicin patch is licensed for the treatment of peripheral neuropathic pain in nondiabetic patients [21]. Application procedure required local analgesia (EMLA cream) due to burning pain, and patients need to be admitted to hospital for at least a few hours. The resulting pain relief is long lasting, for 12 weeks following a single patch application [23, 24]

Botox (botulinum toxin) is indicated for the symptomatic relief of blepharospasm, hemifacial spasm, and idiopathic cervical dystonia (spasmodic torticollis). Botox should only be given by physicians with appropriate qualifications and expertise in the treatment and use of the required equipment. Recently, Botox became the first treatment with labelled indication for the prophylaxis of headache in patients with chronic migraine. There is a detailed protocol for headache prophylaxis which includes injection of 31–39 precisely defined sites at head and the neck (total dose 155–195 units) [25].

Placebo Response

Placebo analgesia is a positive response to treatment which produces no specific biological effect. Deceptive use of placebos must be considered unethical; however, every health provider that treats pain patients must be aware of this important phenomenon in order to harness its huge potential [26]. Response to all analgesic treatments consists of two components: biological effect and placebo. Separated assessment of biological and placebo response is crucial for drug development. In contrast to a real clinical environment, the aim is to maximise the therapeutical effect (both the biological and placebo component). The placebo component can be very powerful: for subjects induced to believe that a potent painkiller drug has been administrated, the placebo is 56 % as effective as a

standard dose of morphine [27]. It is unethical and inappropriate to use the above data to support deceptive use of placebo instead of morphine.

Contextual effects can play a major role in the therapeutic efficacy of every treatment effort and can better explain placebo effects [28, 29]. It is essential to appreciate the contextual factors that surround all therapeutic interactions between doctors and patients, as well as other environmental factors that may affect the course of any medical condition. The contextual factors include a variety of verbal and nonverbal elements, including empathy by doctor and staff, easing of anxiety by proper diagnosis and treatment, and suggesting generic healthy regimens of diet, exercise, rest, and anxiety control [29]. Placebo response can be enhanced by continuity of care and effective interpersonal relationships [30]. Discussions between doctors and their patients should be honest and focused on positive aspects of treatment enhancing pharmacological and non-pharmacological responses to treatment and providing pain relief during that process ("make people feel better while they get better"). Clearly, this is the modern and ethical approach in using placebo in pain management.

Conclusion

Local methods of pain control in cancer patients do not create a ladder like the pharmacological approach proposed by the WHO. They can be pictured as a table full of variable options from totally noninvasive and virtually complication-free like TENS to invasive procedures accompanied by the risk of serious side effects like cordotomy. Local methods of pain control in cancer patients should always be understood as a part of holistic multidimensional pain management. In an ideal situation, all of the described techniques should be continuously available to all cancer patients, and regular reassessment should identify patients who can benefit from non-pharmacological methods of pain control. Patient can require different methods during cancer progression/regression. Invasive procedures can be recommended based on a benefit/risk ratio for a relatively small group of cancer patients (probably less than 10 %), but noninvasive and minimally invasive methods (e.g., TENS, acupuncture) can potentially be a valuable part of a multidimensional holistic approach for the majority of cancer patients. The procedure selection should be based on patient expectation, efficacy, potential side effects, and life expectancy. Patients' expectations must be carefully investigated prior to treatment, and if a patient insists on unrealistic treatment endpoints, the physician should clarify and attempt to understand the patient's expectations [25]. Clinically, the crucial point is to choose the right patient for the right treatment at the right time. More research is needed to provide data which allow defined, clear, evidence-based selection criteria for local methods of pain control.

Key Points

- All non-pharmacological methods of pain control in cancer patients will only be effective when delivered in the context of a holistic multidimensional approach.
- The basic premise of using any non-pharmacological techniques should be to choose the simplest and safest technique that is associated with the highest probability of achieving acceptable pain relief.
- Effective invasive management of pain in cancer patients depends to a large degree on proper patients' assessment and selection of treatment.

References

1. http://www.who.int/cancer/palliative/painladder/en/.
2. Filshie J, White A. Medical acupuncture – a western scientific approach. Edinburgh: Churchill Livingstone; 1998.
3. Filshie J, Thompson JW. Acupuncture. In: Doyle D, Hanks G, Cherny N, Calman K, editors. Oxford textbook of palliative medicine. Oxford: Oxford University Press; 2004. p. 410–24.
4. Alimi D, Rubino C, Pichard-Leandri E, Fermand-Brule S, Dubreuil-Lemaire ML, Hill C. Analgesic effect of auricular acupuncture for cancer pain: a randomized, blinded, controlled trial. J Clin Oncol. 2003;21(22):4120–6.
5. Lee H, Schmidt K, Ernst E. Acupuncture for the relief of cancer-related pain – a systematic review. Eur J Pain. 2005;9(4):437–44.
6. Filshie J, Hester J. Guideline for providing acupuncture treatment for cancer patients – a peer-reviewed sample policy document. Acupunct Med. 2006;24:172–82.
7. Chaitow L. The acupuncture treatment of pain. Rochester: Healing Arts Press; 1990.
8. Ronald M, Stillwell DM, Fox EJ. Trigger points and acupuncture points for pain: correlations and implications. Pain. 1977;3(1):3–23.
9. Redfearn T. Surrounding the dragon. Acupunct Med. 1992;10(2):73–4.
10. Stannard C, Booth S. Churchill's pocketbook of pain. 2nd ed. Churchill Livingstone; 2004.
11. Walsh DM. TENS clinical applications and related theory. Edinburgh: Churchill Livingstone; 1997.
12. Johnson MI. Transcutaneous electrical nerve stimulation (TENS). In: Watson T, editor. Electrotherapy, evidence based practice. 11th ed. Edinburgh: Churchill Livingstone; 2008. p. 253–96.
13. Ma YT, Sluka KA. Reduction in inflammation-induced sensitization of dorsal horn neurons by transcutaneous electrical nerve stimulation in anaesthetized rats. Exp Brain Res. 2001;137:94–102.
14. Robb K, Oxberry SG, Bennet MI, Johnson MI, Simpson KH, Searle RD. A Cochrane systematic review of transcutaneous electrical nerve stimulation for cancer pain. J Pain Symptom Manage. 2009;137(1):746–53.
15. Goreszeniuk T, Kothari S. Chapter 31. Subcutaneous targeted stimulation. In: Krames E, editor. Neuromodulation. Oxford: Elsevier. 2009. p. 418.
16. Goreszeniuk T, Kothari S. Targeted external area stimulation. Reg Anesth Pain Med. 2004; 29(4 Suppl 5):98.
17. Kothari S, Goreszeniuk T. External neuromodulation as a diagnostic and therapeutic procedure. Eur J Pain. 2006;10 Suppl 1:S158.
18. Gauchi CA. Manual of RF techniques. 2nd ed. Amsterdam: Flivopress; 2008.
19. Berger P. Electrical pain modulation for the chronic pain patient. S Afr J Anaesthesiol Analg. 1999;5:14–9.
20. Odendaal CL. APS therapy – a new way of treating chronic backache – a pilot study. S Afr J Anaesthesiol Analg. 1999;5:26–9.
21. British National Formulary 60; Sept 2010.
22. Noto C et al. NGX-4010, a high concentration capsaicin dermal patch for lasting relief of peripheral neuropathic pain. Curr Opin Investig Drugs. 2009;10(7):702–10.
23. Backonja M, Wallace MS, Blonsky ER, Cutler BJ, Malan Jr P, Rauck R, et al. NGX-4010, a high-concentration capsaicin patch, for the treatment of postherpetic neuralgia: a randomised, double-blind study.NGX-4010 C116 study group. Lancet Neurol. 2008;7(12):1106–12. Epub 2008 Oct 30. Erratum in: Lancet Neurol. 2009;8(1):31.
24. Simpson DM, Brown S, Tobias J. Controlled trial of high-concentration capsaicin patch for treatment

of painful HIV neuropathy.; NGX-4010 C107 study group. Neurology. 2008;70(24):2305–13.

25. BOTOX 100U UK Summary of product characteristic, Allergan Ltd: http://www.medicines.org.uk/emc/medicine/112, llast updated on the eMC: 21/12/2012.

26. Greene CS, Goddard G, Macaluso GM, Mauro G. Topical review: placebo responses and therapeutic responses. How are they related? Journal of Orofacial Pain. 2009;23(2):93–107.

27. Benedetti F, Amanzio M. The neurobiology of placebo analgesia: from endogenous opioids

to cholecystokinin. Prog Neurobiol. 1997;52: 109–25.

28. Di Blasi Z, Harkness E, Ernst E, Georgiou A, Kleijnen J. Influence of context effects on health outcomes: a systematic review. Lancet. 2001;357:757–62.

29. Kaptchuk TJ. The placebo effect in alternative medicine: can the performance of a healing ritual have clinical significance? Ann Intern Med. 2002;136: 817–25.

30. Brody H. The placebo response. Recent research and implications for family medicine. Family practice. 2000;49(7):649–54.

New Drugs in Management of Pain in Cancer

Marie Fallon

Abstract

Cancer-related pain can be difficult to treat in some cases, and clinicians need to be knowledgeable about new developments in analgesics and interventional approaches to pain management [1]. There have been few genuinely new drugs for the management of pain in the last decade; however, there have been new formulations and exploration of the optimum use of old drugs.

Keywords

Advances • Pain assessment • Somatosensory markers • Prediction of response • Descending noxious inhibitory control • New drugs • Interventional analgesia

The gabapentinoids, the various fentanyl formulations for breakthrough pain, and tapentadol, a novel, centrally acting analgesic with both mu opioid receptor agonist and noradrenaline reuptake inhibition activity (minimal serotonin reuptake inhibition), are new, along with ziconotide, the first in a new class of non-opioid intrathecal (IT) drugs. Cannabinoids are at advanced stages of development for cancer-related pain, and topical capsaicin patch is licensed for peripheral neuropathic pain.

Single-agent analgesics are frequently ineffective and analgesic rotation of combinations is prescribed with little evidence of additive or synergistic benefits [2]. Multiple adjuvant analgesics are frequently used with opioids without strong evidence as to their effectiveness [3–6].

Evidence for benefits in neuropathic pain is often based on disease-oriented trials, but recent research is starting to focus on pathophysiological mechanisms of action of analgesics [7, 8]. A developing hypothesis is that the underlying neurobiology of the pain is the driving factor of an analgesic response rather than the pain aetiology [9]. This forms the basis of using somatosensory characteristics as predictors of an individual's analgesic response. The realisation that we have to explore reliable ways of predicting a likely clinical response to analgesia is a key advance. While this will involve much time-consuming clinical and translational research

M. Fallon, MBChB, MD, FRCP
University of Edinburgh, Western General Hospital, Edinburgh, UK

Department of Palliative Medicine,
Edinburgh Cancer Research Centre,
Crewe Road South, Edinburgh EH5 3AP, UK
e-mail: marie.fallon@ed.ac.uk

M. Hanna, Z. Zylicz (eds.), *Cancer Pain*,
DOI 10.1007/978-0-85729-230-8_12, © Springer-Verlag London 2013

and there will be no quick answers, linking neurobiology of pain rather than pain diagnosis to treatment is a critical advance. This is of particular importance in relation to choice of adjuvant analgesics in cancer pain, when time is often limited and can run out before optimum pain relief is established.

Assessment

The clinical benefits of analgesics can be difficult to evaluate. Confounders such as baseline pain variability, emotional state, and associated disease-related symptoms bias outcomes [10]. Placebo responses are substantial, over-inflating analgesic response in single-arm studies and diminishing anticipated benefits in randomised studies. Frequently, individuals with cancer pain have several pains, one of which responds better to an analgesic than the other(s).

In some setting assessment of neurobiology of pain is already part of routine practice.

Descending Inhibitory Control and Antidepressants

Experimental pain models involve acute skin, nasal, and dental mucosa pain; muscle pain; diffuse noxious inhibitory control (DNIC); and hyperalgesia/central sensitisation. Pain intensity, location, frequency, and duration are controlled in these models to limit confounders and better explore analgesic responses to pain mechanisms. These models are valuable tools for characterising analgesic actions beyond pharmacodynamic information derived from receptor or channel interactions [11]. Using these models, Staahl and colleagues [12] recently reported a systematic review of non-opioid analgesic responses in human experimental pain. Aspirin improved acute pain, was ineffective in ischemic muscle pain but, interestingly, improved hyperalgesia and central sensitisation. Ibuprofen had the same spectrum of activity, including reduction of mechanical hyperalgesia. In contrast, N-methyl D-aspartate (NMDA) receptor antagonists did not reduce acute pain but did reduce muscle pain and secondary hyperalgesia. Gabapentin did not enhance DNIC,

whereas lamotrigine did but did not relieve cutaneous hyperalgesia. Tricyclic antidepressants reduced acute pain and visceral pain but did not enhance DNIC [13–15]. While there are clear limitations to such models, such information can be useful in developing further evaluation of analgesics.

Elucidation of descending inhibitory control by Anthony Dickenson has been illuminating from aspects of understanding how analgesia attenuates pain signalling centrally but also how the traditional palliative care concept of "Total Pain" is represented by this wiring in the brain and spinal cord (Fig. 12.1).

The ability of a descending noradrenergic mechanism to protect from pain puts pathways from the brain to the spinal cord once again at the forefront of pain modulation. The ideas of descending inhibitions and facilitations in different pain states have expanded since the seminal studies of Basbaum and Fields [16]. There is now evidence for gain of facilitation and/or loss of inhibition in preclinical pain models [17], and in patients, comparable anatomical regions have been implicated in both descending inhibition (placebo analgesia) [18] and facilitation (patients with high osteoarthritis pain) [19]. Indeed, Diffuse Noxious Inhibitory Controls has been reported to be deficient in a number of pain states and may also be predictive of subsequent pain problems [20–22].

Opioids and Adjuvant Analgesics

Several recent studies have demonstrated benefits from combinations of opioids and adjuvant analgesics, which produce superior pain control compared to single analgesics even though the maximum tolerable doses of both drugs are less in combination. Effective combinations include oxycodone plus pregabalin [23], morphine plus gabapentin [24], and nortriptyline plus gabapentin [25]. The mechanisms behind the added benefits are not known but presumably are due to complementary receptor interactions that diminish pain or reduce opioid analgesic tolerance. It is speculated that gabapentin and pregabalin block calcium channels that are upregulated by opioids [26]. Gabapentin required activated $5HT_3$ (serotonin) receptors for analgesia [27, 28].

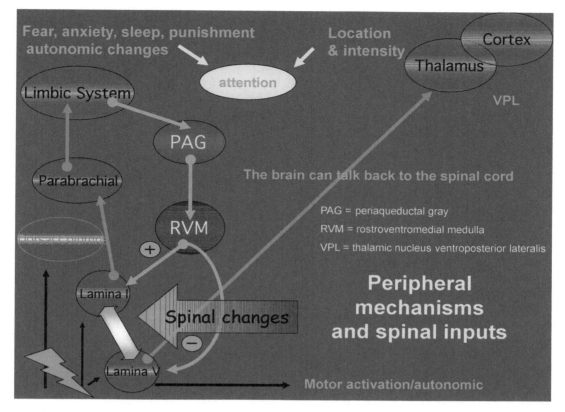

Fig. 12.1 Peripheral mechanisms and spinal inputs (Reproduced by kind permission of Prof A Dickenson)

The choice of antidepressants for chronic pain is clinically important [29]. Tricyclic antidepressants have greater evidence for benefit in acquired pain processing disorders (neuropathic pain, headaches, low back pain, fibromyalgia, and irritable bowel syndrome), while newly developed selective serotonin and norepinephrine reuptake inhibitors have less supportive evidence. Selective serotonin reuptake inhibitors are generally ineffective. Overall adrenergic (alpha-2-adrenergic) receptor activation is more important to antidepressant analgesic activity than activation of serotonin receptors.

There is good evidence that alpha-2-adrenoceptors mediate inhibitory descending brain stem control over dorsal horn nociceptive traffic and that the serotonin 5HT$_3$ receptor facilitates dorsal horn nociceptive processing [30]. Pain processing disorders such as fibromyalgia and irritable bowel syndrome are putatively the result of endogenous central monoamine imbal-ances, which cause the brain stem nociceptive modulator to malfunction. This may be the reason why antidepressants that selectively reduce serotonin reuptake are less effective adjuvant analgesics and why norepinephrine is the important monoamine when dampening pain processing [30].

Cannabinoids

Interest in cannabinoids as an analgesic has been long-standing; however, recently we have seen progress in a clinical development program focusing on the therapeutic use in cancer pain. Recent studies reported that the combination of tetrahydrocannabinol (THC) and cannabidiol was more effective in relieving cancer pain than THC alone [13–15]. Combinations may improve pain and/or diminish side effects, thus extending the THC therapeutic index.

Cannabinoids are undergoing further investigation as potential adjuvant analgesics in cancer pain. *Cannabis sativa* L. contains 60 or more cannabinoids, the most abundant of which are delta-9-tetrahydrocannabinol (THC) and cannabidiol (CBD). Both of these have a pharmacology which suggests they may be useful in the relief of pain. The endogenous cannabinoids (anandamide, 2-arachidonoyl glycerol [2-AG]) act primarily via specific cannabinoid receptors: CB_1 receptors are predominantly distributed in the CNS; CB_2 receptors are located in both the CNS and extensively in the periphery (especially the immune system). THC is a partial CB_1 and CB_2 receptor agonist and its principal pharmacological effects include analgesia, muscle relaxation, anti-emesis, appetite stimulation, and psychoactivity. CBD has analgesic and anti-inflammatory effects in its own right and has been shown to reduce the anxiogenic and psychoactive effects of THC

Several animal studies in both acute and chronic pain models suggest analgesic synergy between cannabinoids and opioids. The mechanism of such synergy is unclear but may involve cross talk between the cannabinoid and opioid receptor. Cannabinoid and opioid receptors co-localise in brain and spinal cord areas relevant to descending pain pathways, and cannabinoids provoke the release of endogenous opioid precursors. Furthermore, studies have also shown that cannabinoids are able to reduce tolerance to opioids in acute pain settings. These studies provide a rationale for the development of cannabinoid drugs for analgesic purposes. Studies of these compounds to date suggest that they may be able to enhance the analgesic efficacy of opioids, but the investigations are short-term and in small samples.

Nabiximols (Sativex®, GW Pharma Ltd, UK) is a standardised extract of *Cannabis sativa L,* which contains THC+CBD at a fixed ratio. Delivered as an oromucosal spray, each 100 μl delivers 2.7 mg of THC and 2.5 mg of CBD. Nabiximols has been shown to have analgesic efficacy in neuropathic pain and spasticity in MS [15]. Studies are in progress to confirm efficacy as an add-on therapy in opioid-treated cancer patients and to clarify the doses that are most likely to be safe and effective. This work is at advanced stages.

Capsaicin

Topical capsaicin creams have been used for post herpetic neuralgia and other peripheral neuropathic pain for decades. The mechanism of action of capsaicin involves primarily a reversible defunctionalisation of cutaneous nociceptors that have been shown to be hyperactive in painful peripheral neuropathies. This hyperactivity has been shown to be associated with decreased epidermal nerve fibre density [31–35] and a reduction of TRPV1 immunoreactivity [36, 37]. Data also suggest a positive correlation between the extent of epidermal nerve fibre loss and the severity of pain [38–42]. Although capsaicin most likely exerts its effect through TRPV1 receptors expressed on cutaneous nociceptors, TRPV1 receptors have also been reported to be expressed in keratinocytes and other epithelial and mesenchymal cell types. It is possible that despite a loss of TRPV1-expressing epidermal nerve fibres in peripheral neuropathies, TRPV1 expression in keratinocytes and other epidermal and dermal cells persists [43], although the physiological relevance of TRPV1 in these cells remains unclear [44].

In summary, a new treatment with a single 60-min topical application of a capsaicin 8 % patch provided a significant reduction in pain that was maintained for up to 3 months in patients with peripheral herpetic neuralgia and was generally well tolerated [45]. In the clinic we can see significant pain during patch application associated with a transient worsening of pain for 1–2 days. This should be anticipated and management planned in the event of this occurring. Exploration of which patients with cancer-related pain may respond to topical capsaicin 8 % patch is being studied.

Bone Pain

Animal models for cancer-induced bone pain (CIBP) have been very helpful in the formulation of clinical research which may lead directly to new treatments.

The results of the clinical randomised controlled trial of pregabalin as an adjuvant for CIBP are imminent. Ibandronate has shown promise in the RCT of palliative radiotherapy *versus* ibandronate (personal communication with P. Hoskins, results presented at ECCO 2012). The emergence of a monoclonal antibody to Rank-L (denosumab) certainly shows promise as an easier to administer method of delaying symptomatic bone disease; however, the data on cancer bone pain per se require further study.

Breakthrough Pain

One of the key challenges in pain, and in particular bone pain, is the concept of breakthrough pain.

The characteristics of this breakthrough pain are shown in Table 12.1. The results of a breakthrough pain questionnaire are shown in Table 12.1. Forty-one patients (75 % of all patients in the sample with CIBP) had breakthrough pain.

The median (IQR) number of episodes of breakthrough pain over 24 h was 4 [2–8]. The median severity of the breakthrough pain episodes was 8 (based on a 0–10 NRS). The speed of onset (time from being first aware of pain to pain reaching its peak) was less than 5 min in 33 (79 %) patients. Thirty-two patients (78 %) had breakthrough pain of less than 30 min duration. Eighteen patients (44 %) had pain which was unpredictable (including those patients who had onset of pain in less than 10 s). Twenty patients (48 %) had breakthrough pain which was rapid onset (less than 5 min) and of short duration (less than 15 min) [46].

New Formulations for the Management of Breakthrough Pain

True breakthrough pain can be challenging to manage. With growing recognition of the prevalence and potential negative consequences of breakthrough pain, a short-acting drug is usually offered as needed during regular opioid treatment. Recently, a variety of rapid-onset transmucosal fentanyl formulations have become available with the intention of addressing the

Table 12.1 Breakthrough pain (BTP) characteristics ($n=41$)

	Median	IQR
Number of BTP episodes in 24 h	4	2–8
Severity of BTP episodes (0–10 NRS)	8	4–9
	n	%
Speed of onset of BTP		
Unpredictable	5	12
<10 s	13	32
10 s–5 min	15	37
6–30 min	6	15
31–60 min	1	2
Unable to quantify	1	2
Duration of BTP		
<1 min	6	15
1–15 min	15	37
16–30 min	11	27
31–60 min	2	5
60–120 min	5	12
>120 min	2	5
Rapid onset (5 min) and short duration (<15 min)	20	49

mismatch between the time course of a typical breakthrough pain and the time to action of an oral drug (see Table 12.1). Available fentanyl formulations include an oral transmucosal lozenge, an effervescent buccal tablet, a buccal patch, a sublingual tablet, and nasal sprays. There are other products in development which use other routes or other lipophilic drugs. Clearly, the success of more rapid onset of opioid analgesia (10– 15 min) will depend on the profile of the patient's breakthrough pain. Pain with a very rapid onset, early peak, and fast resolution (<10 min) will be the pain which is irrelevant to these new fentanyl formulations. The clear message is that for some patients, even fast-acting novel opioid formulations will not be helpful.

Interventional Analgesia

Pain flares for patients with spinal analgesia also present a challenge. Rarely do spinal opioids completely relieve such pain, but this may be due to patient selection. In general, individuals considered for spinal analgesia are highly opioid-tolerant, and as a result, systemic opioid doses for transient flares of pain are less likely to be effective or are required in high doses, leading to toxicity. Mercadante and colleagues [47] reported the use of either spinal bolus levobupivacaine or sublingual ketamine for breakthrough pain episodes. Individuals in the study were treated by spinal analgesia (local anaesthetics, clonidine, and morphine) and experienced unacceptable side effects and/or little pain relief from systemic morphine (mean dose 36 mg) for pain flares. Spinal bolus levobupivacaine (mean dose 1.5 mg/0.6 ml) through a side port or sublingual ketamine (25 mg) reduced pain severity by 50 % within 5 min of administration. Leg weakness was seen in 10 % of episodes treated with spinal levobupivacaine. There is very little published evidence on how to manage pain flares on spinal opioids, and this research paradigm described by Mercadante could be useful for other studies.

Steroids

Steroids have been used in cancer pain for decades and we know dexamethasone reduces pain in several clinical scenarios. Perioperative studies have demonstrated the analgesic benefits of dexamethasone [48–52].

A study which involved ten individuals with intractable lower hemibody cancer pain was conducted. Weekly intrathecal betamethasone (2 mg) produced analgesia quickly (within 30 min). Half of the individuals had pain relief lasting 7 days [49]. Repeat intrathecal injections at 7-day intervals may be clinically problematic unless an intrathecal catheter is in place. Analgesic tolerance to intrathecal dexamethasone was not determined in this study. Persistent responses with repeated injections would be an important outcome. However, in those with a short time to live (1–2 weeks), this may be a reasonable option in lieu of spinal analgesia if the latter is not possible.

The mechanism by which dexamethasone improves analgesia is not well understood. Morphine increases central nervous system glutamate levels, and dexamethasone increases glutamate transporter expression, which increases glutamate clearance from synaptic clefts [53–55].

Hence, dexamethasone appears acutely to reduce morphine analgesic tolerance or blunt counter-opioid responses. It would be of interest to know if cerebrospinal fluid glutamate levels are reduced by dexamethasone in morphine-tolerant individuals. Further research with dexamethasone would be very useful.

Ziconotide

Ziconotide is the first in a new class of non-opioid intrathecal (IT) drugs that produces potent antinociceptive effects. Isolated from the venom of the marine snail *Conus magus*, this agent is a synthetic version of the omega-conotoxin MVIIA [8]. For two decades, it has been well known that ziconotide selectively and reversibly blocks the *N*-type voltage-sensitive calcium channels, thus decreasing neurotransmission from primary nociceptive afferents [56–60]. Ziconotide has been approved for use in managing severe, chronic pain in patients who are intolerant or refractory to other treatments [61–64]. The safety and efficacy of ziconotide were evaluated in 3 double-blind, placebo-controlled clinical trials [65–67]. These studies showed that ziconotide was associated with a statistically significant reduction in visual analogue scale of pain intensity (VASPI) scores from baseline in patients with both malignant and nonmalignant pain, but a high incidence of adverse events (AEs), such as dizziness and nystagmus, was observed. A small starting dose and a slow-titration regimen resulted in a lower incidence of serious AEs [67].

Ziconotide can be also used in combination with other IT drugs [65, 68–70], and clinical trial results suggest that it has an additive or synergistic analgesic effect with opioids, with minimal risk for dependency and tolerance development [59, 60, 71, 72]. Disadvantages of the drug include a variable therapeutic window and numerous known adverse events [72–75]. Recently two studies demonstrated the efficacy of IT combination of morphine and ziconotide in reducing pain that was inadequately controlled by only one of these two drugs in patients with chronic nonmalignant pain [76, 77]. There do not seem to be any studies investigating the efficacy of an IT combination of morphine and ziconotide in patients with severe cancer pain refractory to high doses of systemic opioid therapy apart from the study described below in some detail [78].

The aim of the ziconotide study was to assess the safety and efficacy of intrathecal (IT) combination of ziconotide and morphine in malignant pain refractory to high doses of oral opioids. Patients with malignant pain refractory to high oral opioids doses with a mean visual analogue scale of pain intensity (VASPI) score of 70 mm were enrolled, and an IT combination therapy was administered: Ziconotide was started at a dose of 2.4 mcg/day, followed by increases of 1.2 mcg/day at intervals of at least 7 days, and an initial IT daily dose of morphine was calculated based on its oral daily dose. Percentage change in VASPI scores from baseline was calculated at 2 days, at 7 days, and weekly until the first 28 days. The mean percentage change of VASPI score from baseline was used for efficacy assessment. Safety was monitored based on adverse events and routine laboratory values. Twenty patients were enrolled, with a mean daily VASPI score at rest of 90 ± 7. All had a disseminated cancer with bone metastases involving the spine. The percentage changes in VASPI mean scores from baseline to 2 days, 7 days, and 28 days were 39 ± 13 % (95 % confidence interval [CI] $=13.61–64.49$, $P<.001$), 51 ± 12 % (95 % CI $= 27.56–74.56$, $P<.001$), and 62 ± 13 % (95 % CI $= 36.03–87.89$ %, $P<.001$), respectively. Four patients experienced mild adverse events related to the study drugs. In this study, an IT combination of low doses of ziconotide and morphine was reported as allowing safe and rapid control of oral opioid-refractory malignant pain.

Ziconotide may be a drug to be considered for severe cancer pain that is unresponsive to systemic opioids and appropriate adjuvants.

Tapentadol

Several mechanisms can be proposed to explain an apparent synergistic analgesic action between μ-opioid and α2-adrenergic receptor agonists.

Combining both effects in a single molecule eliminates the potential for drug-drug interactions inherent in multiple drug therapy. Tapentadol is the first approved centrally acting analgesic having both μ-opioid receptor agonist and noradrenaline (norepinephrine) reuptake inhibition activity with minimal serotonin reuptake inhibition. This dual mode of action may make tapentadol particularly useful in the treatment of neuropathic pain. Having limited protein binding, no active metabolites, and no significant microsomal enzyme induction or inhibition, tapentadol has a limited potential for drug-drug interactions. Clinical trial evidence in acute and chronic non-cancer pain and neuropathic pain seems to support an opioid-sparing effect that reduces some of the typical opioid-related adverse effects. Specifically, the reduction in treatment-emergent gastrointestinal adverse effects for tapentadol compared with equianalgesic pure μ-opioid receptor agonists resulted in improved tolerability and adherence to therapy for both the immediate and extended release formulations of tapentadol [79, 80].

Tapentadol represents one of the very few new molecules for analgesia made commercially available in recent years. As a new agent, relatively few data have been published regarding its use to date. The following summarises the data available on efficacy, safety, and tolerability data for both tapentadol immediate release (IR) and tapentadol extended release (ER) formulations.

Tapentadol binds to the μ-opioid receptor selectively, with a>10-fold affinity [81, 82]. Despite μ-opioid binding that is nearly 50 times lower than morphine, the analgesic potency of tapentadol was only two to three times lower than morphine when tested in multiple preclinical pain models [82]. The inhibition of noradrenaline reuptake by tapentadol was similar to that for venlafaxine in a synaptosomal monoamine reuptake assay in the rat. Clearly, the overall analgesic effect is greater than the sum of the expected analgesia provided exclusively by noradrenaline reuptake inhibition and direct μ-receptor agonist effects. While alternative explanations also exist, it may be that the non-opioid-mediated complementary mechanism for analgesia, i.e., potent noradrenaline reuptake inhibition with minimal serotonin effects, accounts for this additive or possibly synergistic effect.

The relative contribution from noradrenaline reuptake inhibition versus opioid analgesia varies with the pain model tested [83]. This is consistent with the hypothesis that this dual action may be particularly beneficial in neuropathic pain states. This notion has some preclinical support in that tapentadol, but not morphine, inhibited thermal hyperalgesia in a rodent model for diabetic neuropathic pain [84]. In addition, a recent study in another rodent model for neuropathic pain (spinal nerve ligation) suggests that the primary site of action of tapentadol is the spinal cord and that the analgesia it induces depends solely on opioid and noradrenaline reuptake mechanisms [85]. This study also provides evidence consistent with a shift from a normal state with predominant opioid inhibitory mechanisms to a noradrenaline inhibitory predominance in neuropathic pain states. Consequently, an agent with strong noradrenaline reuptake inhibition, such as tapentadol, might be particularly appropriate for use in clinical neuropathic pain states.

Synergistic effects between two drugs are often demonstrated using isobolographic analyses. However, proving dual synergistic mechanisms in a single agent requires modification of this approach. In two recent sets of experiments, the dual synergistic opioid and noradrenaline effects of tapentadol were demonstrated in preclinical models of both acute pain and chronic neuropathic pain [83, 86]. In the first set of experiments, dose–response curves developed in the presence of tapentadol with the opioid-blocking agent naloxone were compared with those developed with tapentadol in combination with the α2-adrenergic receptor antagonist yohimbine [83]. Analogous brain receptor occupancy studies were then performed in the acute pain rodent model. Modified isobolographic analyses were sequentially constructed using tapentadol in the presence of naloxone and yohimbine [86]. Supra-additive effects were reported in both studies. Taken together, these studies present compelling evidence for true synergism between the dual mech-

anisms of action of tapentadol in both acute and neuropathic preclinical pain models.

While rapidly absorbed, the oral bioavailability of tapentadol under fasting conditions is only 32 % due to an extensive first-pass effect [81, 87]. Only 20 % of the drug is bound to plasma protein. Its half-life of 4.9 h permits achievement [20] of steady-state concentrations at 25–30 h when tapentadol is administered orally every 6 h [81, 82]. Extensive metabolism, primarily by the uridine diphosphate-glucuronosyltransferase (UGT) enzymes UGT1A9 and UGT2B7, results in renal elimination of inactive glucuronide or sulfate conjugates, with tapentadol-0-glucuronide being the major metabolite [81, 88]. Tapentadol follows first-order elimination kinetics over a wide range of conditions. Moderate hepatic dysfunction, however, warrants dose reduction [87, 89]. Tapentadol is not recommended and should not be given to patients with severe hepatic dysfunction.

Tapentadol neither significantly inhibits nor induces any clinically important CYP enzymes [88]. It does not require metabolism for its activity and has no active metabolites [90]. Having low protein binding, displacement reactions are unlikely. Overall, tapentadol has a low potential for pharmacokinetic drug-drug interactions. Drug interaction studies examining paracetamol, naproxen, or aspirin (acetylsalicylic acid) administered with tapentadol revealed no significant changes in serum tapentadol concentration [91]. Data also suggest there are no drug-drug interactions between tapentadol and omeprazole, metoclopramide, and probenecid [92–94].

As a noradrenaline reuptake inhibitor, tapentadol is contraindicated in patients receiving monoamine oxidase inhibitors (MAOIs) within the previous 14 days. Despite minimal serotonergic effect, theoretically a serotonin syndrome might be precipitated by concomitant use with serotonin noradrenaline reuptake inhibitor (SNRI), selective serotonin reuptake inhibitor (SSRI), TCA, MAOI or serotonin 5-HTIB/ID receptor agonist (triptan) medications [87].

Duloxetine

Duloxetine is a selective noradrenalin reuptake inhibitor. Use of duloxetine in cancer-related neuropathic pain has increased, although evidence is lacking. A randomised, placebo-controlled phase III trial to determine whether duloxetine reduced painful chemotherapy-induced peripheral neuropathy (CIPN) was reported at the American Society of Clinical Oncology (ASCO) in 2012. The secondary study endpoint was treatment-related adverse effects. The authors concluded that duloxetine 60 mg daily was an efficacious and well-tolerated intervention for the treatment of taxane or platinum-related painful CIPN [95]. This work is clearly of interest as such neuropathies are notoriously difficult to treat.

Opioids

Finally, one of the main advances in cancer pain has been the acceptance that for some patients, morphine may not be the opioid of choice and that the armamentarium of opioid analgesics should be considered in all patients as clinically indicated [96].

Conclusion

There have been advances which can be drawn on for cancer pain management, but work is required which explores some of the unique aspects of cancer pain which are related to tumour factors.

References

1. Brennan F, Carr D, Cousins M. Pain management, a fundamental human right. Anesth Analg. 2007;105:205–21.
2. Breivik H, Cherny N, Collett B, et al. Cancer-related pain: a pan-European survey of prevalence, treatment and patient attitudes. Ann Oncol. 2009;20:1420–33.
3. Apolone G, Corli A, Caraceni A, et al. Pattern and quality of care of cancer pain management. Results from the cancer pain outcome research study group. Br J Cancer. 2009;100:1566–74.
4. Mantyh P. Cancer pain and its impact on diagnosis, survival and quality of life. Nat Rev Neurosci. 2006;7:797.
5. Christo P, Maxloomdoost D. Cancer pain and analgesia. Ann NY Acad Sci. 1008;1138:278–98.
6. Hanks GW, de Conno F, Cherny N, et al. Morphine and alternative opioids in cancer pain: the EAPC recommendations. Br J Cancer. 2001;84:587–93.
7. Pappagallo M, Oaklander A, Quatrano-Piacentin A, et al. Heterogenous patterns of sensory dysfunction in postherpetic neuralgia suggest multiple pathophysiologic mechanisms. Anaesthesiol. 2000;92:691–8.
8. Attal N, Fermanian C, Fermanian J, et al. Neuropathic pain: are there distinct subtypes depending on the aetiology or anatomical lesion? Pain. 2008;138:343–53.
9. Baron R, Tolle TR, Gockel U, Brosz M, Freynhagen R. A cross-sectional cohort survey in 2100 patients with painful diabetic neuropathy and postherpetic neuralgia: differences in demographic data and sensory symptoms. Pain. 2009;146:34–40.
10. Drewes A, Gregersen H, Arendt-Nielsen L. Experimental pain in gastroenterology: a reappraisal of human studies. Scand J Gastroenterol. 2003;38:115–30.
11. Arendt-Nielsen L, Curatolo M, Drewes A. Human experimental pain models in drug development; translational pain research. Curr Opin Investig Drugs. 2007;8:41–53.
12. Staahl C, Estrup Olesen A, Andresen T, et al. Assessing efficacy of non-opioid analgesics in experimental pain models in healthy volunteers – an updated review. Br J Clin Pharmacol. 2009;68:322–41.
13. Johnson JR, Burnell-Nugent M, Lossignol D, et al. Multicenter, double-blind, randomized, placebo-controlled, parallel group study of the efficacy, safety and tolerability of the THC:CBD extract and THC extract in patients with intractable cancer-related pain. J Pain Symptom Manage. 2010;39:167–79.
14. Johnson J, Lossignol D, Burnell-Nugent M, Fallon M. An open-label extension study to investigate the long-term safety and tolerability of THC/CBD spray and THC spray in patient with cancer-related pain. J Pain Symptom Manage. 2012; [Epub, 7 Nov 2012].
15. Portenoy R, Ganae-Motan E, Yanagihara R, Shimkus B, Shaiova L, Allende S, et al. Nabiximols for Opioid-treated cancer patients with poorly-controlled chronic pain: a randomized placebo-controlled, graded-dose trial. J Pain. 2012. doi:10.1016/j.jpain.2012.01.003.
16. Basbaum AI, Fields HL. Endogenous pain control mechanisms: review and hypothesis. Ann Neurol. 1978;4:451–62.
17. Bannister K, Bee LA, Dickenson AH. Preclinical and early clinical investigations related to monoaminergic pain modulation. Neurotherapeutics. 2009;6:703–12.
18. Eippert F, Bingel U, Schoell ED, Yacubian J, Klinger R, Lorenz J, et al. Activation of the opioidergic descending pain control system underlies placebo analgesia. Neuron. 2009;63:533–43.
19. Gwilym SE, Keltner JR, Warnaby CE, Carr AJ, Chizh B, Chessell I, et al. Psychophysical and functional imaging evidence supporting the presence of central

sensitization in a cohort of osteoarthritis patients. Arthritis Rheum. 2009;61:1226–34.

20. van Wijk G, Veldhuijzen DS. Perspective on diffuse noxious inhibitory controls as a model of endogenous pain modulation in clinical pain syndromes. J Pain. 2010;11:408–19.

21. Dickensen AH. Descending controls: insurance against pain? Pain. 2011;152:2677–8.

22. De Felice M, Sanoja R, Wang R, et al. Engagement of descending inhibition from the rostral ventromedial medulla protects against chronic neuropathic pain. Pain. 2011;152:2701–9.

23. Gatti A, Sabato A, Occhioni R, et al. Controlled-release oxycodone and pregabalin in the treatment of neuropathic pain: results of a multicenter Italian study. Eur Neurol. 2009;61:129–37.

24. Gilron A, Bailey J, Dongsheng T, et al. Morphine, gabapentin or their combination for neuropathic pain. N Engl J Med. 2005;352:1324–34.

25. Gilron I, Bailey J. Nortriptyline and gabapentin, alone and in combination for neuropathic pain: a double-blind, randomized controlled crossover trial. Lancet. 2009;374:1252–61.

26. Shibasaki M, Kurokawa K, Ohkuma S. Role of alpha2/delta subunit in the development of morphine-induced rewarding effect and behavioural sensitization. Neuroscience. 2009;163:731–4.

27. D'Mello R, Dickensen AH. Spinal cord mechanisms of pain. Br J Anaesth. 2008;101:8–16.

28. Suzuki R, Rygh L, Dickensen A. Bad news from the brain; descending 5-HT pathways that control spinal pain processing. Trends Pharmacol Sci. 2004;25:613–7.

29. Verdu B, Decosterd I, Buclin T, et al. antidepressants for the treatment of chronic pain. Drugs. 2008;68:2611–32.

30. Bannister K, Bee LA, Dickensen AH. Preclinical and early clinical investigations related to monoaminergic pain modulation. Neurotherapeutics. 2009;6:703–12.

31. Rowbotham MC, Petersen KL. Zoster-associated pain and neural dysfunction. Pain. 2001;93:1–5.

32. Bley KR. Recent developments in transient receptor potential vanilloid receptor 1 agonist-based therapies. Expert Opin Investig Drugs. 2004;13:1445–56.

33. Kennedy WR, Wendelschafer-Crabb G, Johnson T. Quantitation of epidermal nerves in diabetic neuropathy. Neurology. 1996;47:1042–8.

34. Oaklander AL, Romans K, Horasek S, et al. Unilateral postherpetic neuralgia is associated with bilateral sensory neuron damage. Ann Neurol. 1998;44:789–95.

35. Polydefkis M, Yiannoutsos CT, Cohen BA, et al. Reduced intraepidermal nerve fiber density in HIV-associated sensory neuropathy. Neurology. 2002;58:115–9.

36. Facer P, Casula MA, Smith GD, et al. Differential expression of the capsaicin receptor TRPV1 and related novel receptors TRPV3, TRPV4 and TRPM8 in normal human tissues and changes in traumatic and diabetic neuropathy. BMC Neurol. 2007;7:11.

37. Lauria G, Morbin M, Lombardi R, et al. Expression of capsaicin receptor immunoreactivity in human peripheral nervous system and in painful neuropathies. J Peripher Nerv Syst. 2006;11:262–71.

38. Bodó E, Kovács I, Telek A, et al. Vanilloid receptor-1 (VR1) is widely expressed on various epithelial and mesenchymal cell types of human skin. J Invest Dermatol. 2004;123:410–3.

39. Denda M, Fuziwara S, Inoue K, et al. Immunoreactivity of VR1 on epidermal keratinocyte of human skin. Biochem Biophys Res Commun. 2001;285:1250–2.

40. Inoue K, Koizumi S, Fuziwara S, et al. Functional vanilloid receptors in cultured normal human epidermal keratinocytes. Biochem Biophys Res Commun. 2002;291:124–9.

41. Southall MD, Li T, Gharibova LS, et al. Activation of epidermal vanilloid receptor-1 induces release of proinflammatory mediators in human keratinocytes. J Pharmacol Exp Ther. 2003;304:217–22.

42. Ständer S, Moormann C, Schumacher M, et al. Expression of vanilloid receptor subtype 1 in cutaneous sensory nerve fibers, mast cells, and epithelial cells of appendage structures. Exp Dermatol. 2004;13:129–39.

43. Wilder-Smith EP, Ong W-Y, Guo Y, Chow AW-L. Epidermal transient receptor potential vanilloid 1 in idiopathic small nerve fibre disease, diabetic neuropathy and healthy human subjects. Histopathology. 2007;51:674–80.

44. Pecze L, Szabó K, Széll M, et al. Human keratinocytes are vanilloid resistant. PLoS One. 2008;3:e3419.

45. Iriving GA, Backonja MM, Dunteman E, et al. A multicenter, randomized, double-blind, controlled study of NGX-4010, a high-concentration capsaicin patch, for the treatment of postherpetic neuralgia. Pain Med. 2011;12:99–109.

46. Laird B, Walley J, Murray G, et al. Characterization of cancer-induced bone pain: an exploratory study. Support Care Cancer. 2011;19:1393–401.

47. Mercadante S, Arcuri E, Ferrera P, Villari P, Mangione S. Alternative treatments of breakthrough pain in patients receiving spinal analgesics for cancer pain. J Pain Symptom Manage. 2005;30:5.

48. Kardash K, Sarrazin F, Tessler M, Velly AM. Single dose dexamethasone reduces dynamic pain after total hip arthroplasty. Anesth Analg. 2008;106:1253–7.

49. Taguchi H, Oishi K, Sakamoto S, Shingu K. Intrathecal betamethasone for cancer pain in the lower half of the body: a study of its analgesic efficacy and safety. Br J Anaesth. 2007;3:385–9.

50. Thangaswamy CR, Rewari V, Trikha A, Dehran M, Chandralekha. Dexamethasone before total laparoscopic hysterectomy: a randomized controlled dose response study. J Anesth. 2010;24:24–30.

51. Jokela RM, Ahonen JV, Tallgren MK, Marjakangas PC, Korttila KT. The effective analgesic dose of dexamethasone after laparoscopic hysterectomy. Anesth Analg. 2009;109:607–15.

52. Mathiesen O, Rasmussen ML, Dierking G, Lech K, Hilsted KL, Fomsgaard JS, et al. Pregabalin and dexamethasone in combination with paracetamol for postoperative pain control after abdominal hysterectomy. A randomized clinical trial. Acta Anaesthesiol Scand. 2009;53:227–35.

53. Wen ZH, Wu GH, Chang YC, Wang JJ, Wong CS. Dexamethasone modulates the development of

morphine tolerance and expression of glutamate transporters in rats. Neuroscience. 2005;133:807–17.

54. Wen ZH, Chang YC, Cherng CH, Wang JJ, Tao PL, Wong CS. Increasing of intrathecal CSF excitatory amino acids concentration following morphine challenge in morphine-tolerant rats. Brain Res. 2004;995:253–9.

55. Zschocke J, Bayatti N, Clement AM, Witan H, Figiel M, Engele J, et al. Differential promotion of glutamate transporter expression and function by glucocorticoid in astrocytes from various brain regions. J Biol Chem. 2005;280:34924–32.

56. Bowersox SS, Luther R. Pharmacotherapeutic potential of omega-conotoxin MVIIA (SNX-111), an N-type neuronal calcium channel blocker found in the venom of Conus magus. Toxicon. 1998;36:1651–8.

57. Molinski TF, Dalisay DS, Lievens SL, Saludes JP. Drug development from marine natural products. Nat Rev Drug Discov. 2009;8:69–85.

58. Schmidtko A, Lötsch J, Freynhagen R, Geisslinger G. Ziconotide for treatment of severe chronic pain. Lancet. 2010;375:1569–77.

59. Wang Y-X, Bowersox SS. Analgesic properties of ziconotide, a selective blocker of N-type neuronal calcium channels. CNS Drug Rev. 2000;6:1–20.

60. Wang YX, Bezprozvannaya S, Bowersox SS, et al. Peripheral versus central potencies of Ntype voltage-sensitive calcium channel blockers. Naunyn Schmiedebergs Arch Pharmacol. 1998;357:159–68.

61. Prialt prescribing information. 2008. Available from: http://www.prialt.com/Images/product_information.pdf. Accessed 3 Jan 2010.

62. Rauck RL, Wallace MS, Burton AW, Kapural L, North JM. Intrathecal ziconotide for neurophatic pain: a review. Pain Pract. 2009;9:327–37.

63. Smith HS, Deer TR. Safety and efficacy of intrathecal ziconotide in the management of severe chronic pain. Ther Clin Risk Manage. 2009;5:521–34.

64. Williams JA, Day M, Heavner JE. Ziconotide: an update and review. Expert Opin Pharmacother. 2008;9:1575–83.

65. Rauck RL, Wallace MS, Leong MS, et al. Ziconotide 301 study group. A randomized, double-blind, placebo-controlled study of intrathecal ziconotide in adults with severe chronic pain. J Pain Symptom Manage. 2006;31:393–406.

66. Staats PS, Yearwood T, Charapata SG, et al. Intrathecal ziconotide in the treatment of refractory pain in patients with cancer or AIDS: a randomized controlled trial. JAMA. 2004;291:63–70.

67. Wallace MS, Charapata SG, Fisher R, et al. The Ziconotide nonmalignant pain study 96–002 group. Intrathecal ziconotide in the treatment of chronic nonmalignant pain: a randomized, double blind, placebo-controlled clinical trial. Neuromodulation. 2006;9: 75–86.

68. Madaris L. Ziconotide: a non-opioid alternative for chronic neuropathic pain, a case report. SCI Nurs. 2008;25:19–23.

69. Saulino M. Successful reduction of neuropathic pain associated with spinal cord injury via a combination of intrathecal hydromorphone and ziconotide: a case report. Spinal Cord. 2007;45:749–52.

70. Saulino M, Burton AW, Danyo DA, et al. Intrathecal ziconotide and baclofen provide pain relief in seven patients with neuropathic pain and spasticity: case reports. Eur J Phys Rehabil Med. 2009;45:61–7.

71. Wallace MS, Rauck RL, Deer T. Ziconotide combination intrathecal therapy: rationale and evidence. Clin J Pain. 2010;26:635–44.

72. Wallace MS, Kosek PS, Staats P, et al. Phase II, open-label, multicenter study of combined intrathecal morphine and ziconotide: addition of ziconotide in patients receiving intrathecal morphine for severe chronic pain. Pain Med. 2008;9:271–81.

73. Deer T, Krames ES, Hassenbusch SJ, et al. Polyanalgesic consensus conference 2007: recommendations for the management of pain by intrathecal (intraspinal) drug delivery: report of an interdisciplinary expert panel. Neuromodulation. 2007;10:300–28.

74. Ellis D, Dissanayake S, McGuire D, et al. The ELAN Study 95–002 group. Continuous intrathecal infusion of ziconotide for treatment of chronic malignant and nonmalignant pain over 12 months: a prospective, open-label study. Neuromodulation. 2008;1:40–9.

75. Ver Donck A, Collins R, Rauck RL, et al. An open-label, multicenter study of the safety and efficacy of intrathecal ziconotide for severe chronic pain when delivered via an external pump. Neuromodulation. 2008;11:103–10.

76. Wallace MS, Rauck R, Fisher R, et al. Ziconotide 98–022 Study group. Intrathecal ziconotide for severe chronic pain: safety and tolerability results of an open-label, long-term trial. Anesth Anal. 2008; 106:628–37.

77. Webster LR, Keri LF, Charapata S, et al. Open-label, multicenter study of combined intrathecal morphine and ziconotide: addition of morphine in patients receiving ziconotide for severe chronic pain. Pain Med. 2008;9:282–90.

78. Alicino I, Giglio M, Manca F, et al. Intrathecal combination of ziconotide and morphine for refractory cancer pain: a rapidly acting and effective choice. Pain. 2012;153:245–9.

79. Hatrick CT, Rozek RJ. Tapentadol in pain management: a μ-opioid receptor agonist and noradrenaline reuptake inhibitor. CNS Drugs. 2011;25(5):359–70.

80. Riemsma R, Forbes C, Harker J, et al. Systematic review of tapentadol in chronic severe pain. Curr Med Res Opin. 2011;27(10):1907–30.

81. Tzschentke TM, De Vry J, Terlinden R, et al. Tapentadol hydrochloride: analgesic mu-opioid receptor agonist noradrenaline reuptake inhibitor. Drugs Future. 2006;31(12):1053–61.

82. Tzschentke TM, Christoph T, Kögel B, et al. (−)-(1 R,2R)-3-(3-dimethylamino-1-ethyl-2-methyl-propyl)-phenol hydrochloride (tapentadol HCl): a novel mu-opioid receptor agonist norepinephrine reuptake inhibitor with broad-spectrum analgesic properties. J Pharmacol Exp Ther. 2007;323(1):265–76.

83. Schröder W, Vry JD, Tzschentke TM, et al. Differential contribution of opioid and noradrenergic mechanisms of tapentadol in rat models of nociceptive and neuropathic pain. Eur J Pain. 2010;14(8):814–21.

84. Christoph T, De Vry J, Tzschentke TM. Tapentadol, but not morphine, selectively inhibits disease-related thermal hyperalgesia in a mouse model of diabetic neuropathic pain. Neurosci Lett. 2010;470(2):91–4.

85. Bee LA, Bannister K, Rahman W, et al. Mu-opioid and noradrenergic a(2)-adrenoceptor contributions to the effects of tapentadol on spinal electrophysiological measures of nociception in nerve-injured rats. Pain. 2011;152(1):131–9.

86. Schroder W, Tzschentke TM, Terlinden R, et al. Synergistic interaction between the two mechanisms of action of tapentadol in analgesia. J Pharmacol Exp Ther. 2011;337(1):312–20. doi:10.1124/jpet.110.175042

87. Nucynta™ (tapentadol hydrochloride immediate-release oral tablets) [US prescribing information; online]. 2011. Available from URL: http://www.labeldataplus.com/detail.php?c=22871. Accessed 12 Jan 2011.

88. Kneip C, Terlinden R, Beier H, et al. Investigations into drug-drug interaction potential of tapentadol in human liver microsomes and fresh human hepatocytes. Drug Metab Lett. 2008;2:67–75.

89. Xu XS, Smit JW, Lin R, et al. Population pharmacokinetics of tapentadol immediate release (IR) in healthy subjects and patients with moderate or severe pain. Clin Pharmacokinet. 2010;49(10):671–82.

90. Terlinden R, Kogel BY, Englberger W, et al. In vitro and in vivo characterization of tapentadol metabolites. Methods Find Exp Clin Pharmacol. 2010;32(1):31–8.

91. Smit JW, Oh C, Rengelshausen J, et al. Effects of acetaminophen, naproxen, and acetylsalicylic acid on tapentadol pharmacokinetics: results of two randomized, open-label, crossover, drug-drug interaction studies. Pharmacotherapy. 2010;30(1):25–34.

92. Mangold B, Oh C, Jaeger D, et al. The pharmacokinetics of tapentadol are not affected by omeprazole: results of a 2-way crossover drug-interaction study in healthy subjects [abstract no. PI 126]. Pain Pract. 2007;1(7 Suppl):55.

93. Smit J, Oh C, Mangold B, et al. Effects of Metoclopramide on tapentadol pharmacokinetics: results of an open-label, cross-over, drug-drug interaction study [abstract no. 62]. J Clin Pharmacol. 2009;49:1104.

94. Smit J, Oh C, Lannie C, et al. Effects of probenecid on tapentadol immediate release pharmacokinetics: results of an open-label, crossover, drug-drug interaction study [abstract no. 61]. J Clin Pharmacol. 2009;49:1104.

95. Lavoie Smith E, Pang H, Cirrincione C, et al. A Phase III double-blind trial of duloxetine to treat painful chemotherapy-induced peripheral neuropathy (CIPN). J Clin Orthod. 2012;30 Suppl 18:CRA9013.

96. Caraceni A, Hanks G, Kaasa S, Bennett M, Brunelli C, Cherny N, et al. Use of opioid analgesics in the treatment of cancer pain: the 2011 EAPC recommendations. Lancet Oncol. 2012;13:e58–8.

Neuropathic Component of Pain in Cancer

13

Jung Hun Kang and Eduardo Bruera

Abstract

The prevalence of neuropathic pain in cancer patients is increasing as more patients are exposed to neurotoxic chemotherapies including taxane and platinum agents. Up to 40 % of cancer patients may experience neuropathic pain during the course of the disease.

The neuropathic cancer pain generally originates from tumour-related and treatment-related causes. Various mechanisms such as mechanical or chemical destruction of neurons, distortion of the surrounding nerve environment, and central sensitisation are involved in the development of neuropathic cancer pain. No single symptom or sign could confirm neuropathic pain, but diagnosis only can be established by a combination of unique symptoms, physical examinations, and appropriate tests. Opioids are recommended as first-line agents for the treatment of neuropathic cancer pain. Antidepressants and anticonvulsants have beneficial effects as adjuvants.

Keywords

Neuropathic pain • Peripheral neuropathies • Cancer • Central sensitisation • Opioids • Pharmaceutical adjuvants

J.H. Kang, MD
Division of Oncology,
Department of Internal Medicine,
Gyeongsang National University Hospital,
Chilam-dong 90, Faculty Building. No 404,
Jinju, Gyeongnam 660-702, South Korea
e-mail: newatp@gnu.ac.kr

E. Bruera, MD (✉)
Department of Palliative Care and Rehabilitation Medicine,
University of Texas M.D. Anderson Cancer Center,
1400 Pressler St, Pickens Academic Tower,
FCT 5. 6090, Houston,
TX 77030, USA
e-mail: ebruera@mdanderson.org

Introduction

Chronic cancer pain is usually categorised into three classes: nociceptive pain, neuropathic pain, and coexisting nociceptive and neuropathic pain [1]. Neuropathic pain is a common symptom in cancer patients and can be manifested as either pure neuropathic pain or a mixed component pain [2].

The management of neuropathic pain is often a challenging issue for physicians, and it is often difficult to control satisfactorily. Poorly controlled neuropathic pain may not only weaken

M. Hanna, Z. Zylicz (eds.), *Cancer Pain*,
DOI 10.1007/978-0-85729-230-8_13, © Springer-Verlag London 2013

patients' physical and psychological ability to struggle through cancer but can also affect patient outcomes due to delayed treatment, dose reductions, and discontinuations of cancer therapy.

The definition of neuropathic pain has changed over time. The International Association for the Study of Pain (IASP) originally defined neuropathic pain as "pain initiated or caused by a primary lesion or dysfunction in the nervous system" [3]. Although this definition has been useful in distinguishing some characteristics of neuropathic and nociceptive pain, it cannot easily differentiate neuropathic dysfunction from normal plasticity of the nociceptive system [4]. In addition, the pain that originates from mechanical compression of nerves may develop through normal activation of nociceptors. To cover this imperfection, IASP revised the definition to "Pain arising as a direct consequence of a lesion or disease affecting the somatosensory system" [5], and IASP recently refined the definition again to "pain caused by a lesion or disease of the somatosensory nervous system" [6]. This revised definition means that the presence of a symptom hinting at neuropathic pain, such as touch-evoked pain alone, does not justify the use of the term neuropathic pain.

The frequency of neuropathic pain is increasing as more cancer patients are exposed to neurotoxic chemotherapies for adjuvant purposes and as more patients enter the palliative setting. Because neuropathic pain is one of the well-known factors for poor pain control [7], all clinicians should be well acquainted with neuropathic pain. This chapter will focus on the characteristics and management of neuropathic pain.

Epidemiology

Most epidemiologic studies of cancer pain do not classify pain according to pain pathophysiology, and there is a significant limit to the information available about the incidence of neuropathic pain in the cancer pain population. Despite recent accumulation of evidences from a development in the definition and grading of neuropathic pain [8], our understanding about the prevalence of neuropathic pain is far from complete. Furthermore, most prevalence studies of neuropathic pain in cancer have been uncontrolled, physician-based, or simple retrospective surveys involving a single medical centre.

At least 15–20 % of patients develop neuropathic pain during the course of cancer, and the proportion of patients with neuropathic pain is presumed to increase to almost a third in advanced stages of the cancer [9]. IASP reported in a prospective, international survey that up to 40 % of 1,095 cancer patients with cancer pain and receiving opioid medication had pain involving neuropathic mechanisms [10]. However, only 8 % of these cancer pain patients with neuropathic characteristics had pure neuropathic pain; the others in the survey had mixed neuropathic pain. The incidence of neuropathic pain from direct tumour involvement to the nervous system was 28 %, and cancer treatment-related pain was 10 %.

In research analysing cancer pain characterisation, 746 consecutive patients referred to palliative care consultation services were screened for cancer pain. Of 619 patients with cancer pain, 17 % had pain from neuropathic mechanisms with or without nociceptive origin [11]. Another retrospective study also found a similar prevalence rate of 12 % for neuropathic pain in cancer [12].

Recently a large prospective study investigated the prevalence of neuropathic pain in 8,615 cancer patients [13]. In this population, 6 % of patients were identified as having neuropathic pain with moderate and severe intensity; 55 % of patients with confirmed neuropathic pain also had a nociceptive pain component.

Neuropathic pain syndrome is common in patients receiving chemotherapy. The incidence of chemotherapy-induced neuropathic pain (CINP) depends on the cumulative dose, type of agent, and preexisting nerve damage such as diabetic neuropathy. The incidence of peripheral neuropathy ranges from 30 to 50 % for patients receiving common neurotoxic anticancer drugs [14–16], and about 90 % of patients receiving oxaliplatin experience acute neuropathic pain [17].

Neuropathic pain conditions may persist in cancer-free survivors and significantly diminish the quality of life. Of 240 breast cancer survivors who had undergone chemotherapy, 18 % continued to experience neuropathic pain [18].

Aetiology

There are several causes of neuropathic pain in cancer patients. Nerve damage occurring through various mechanisms can result in neuropathic pain. The origin of neuropathic pain can be divided into tumour-related and treatment-related causes (Table 13.1), and pain arising from these factors may occur simultaneously or subsequently. In a prospective survey, pain origin was tumour related in 69 % of these patients and treatment related in 43 % [13].

Tumour-related neuropathic pain can develop from direct compression of the peripheral nerve or from infiltration by the growing cancer, and cancer involvement of the brain or spinal cord may also induce neuropathic pain. The peripheral nerve damaged by cancer invasion or compression generates its own signals despite there being no real problem in the innervating tissue. The false signal is transmitted through the lateral spinothalamic tract and perceived as uncomfortable pain. Patients usually describe such pain as a burning, shooting, or electrical sensation or as a deep ache. This symptom is commonly observed in oncologic patients with involvement of nerve plexuses (brachial, lumbar, sacral) or of individual nerves by the metastasised or primary cancer.

Neuropathic pain from a central origin is associated with central nervous system tumours, stroke, or radiation sequela. It is less frequently observed than peripheral neuropathic pain in cancer patients. Central neuropathic pain tends to be more resistant to pharmacologic treatment than peripheral neuropathic pain.

Neuropathic pain may also result from treatment-related causes such as chemotherapy, radiotherapy, surgery, or postprocedural pain [19, 20]. Chemotherapeutic agents, such as oxaliplatin, cisplatin, paclitaxel, docetaxel, vincristine,

Table 13.1 Common causes of neuropathic pain in cancer patients

Cancer related
Brachial, cervical, or sacral plexus neuropathies by cancer compression
Cranial neuropathy
Radiculopathy from vertebral body and leptomeningeal metastases
Paraneoplastic neuropathy
Treatment related
Postsurgical neuropathic pain
Postmastectomy syndrome
Post-thoracotomy syndrome
Post-radical neck dissection syndrome
Phantom limb pain
Complex regional pain syndrome
Radiation-induced neuropathic pain
Radiation myelopathy
Chemotherapy-induced neuropathy
Cisplatin
Oxaliplatin
Paclitaxel
Docetaxel
Vincristine
Thalidomide
Bortezomib
Other
Postherpetic neuropathy
Chronic alcoholism
Nutritional deficiency

bortezomib, and thalidomide, have been extensively reported to induce peripheral neuropathy [21]. The incidence and severity of chemotherapy-induced neuropathic pain are usually dose dependent or related to concomitant administration of neurotoxic agents and coexisting neuropathy such as diabetic neuropathy. When paclitaxel/cisplatin combination chemotherapy was administered, neuropathic pain of more than moderate intensity developed in 60 % of patients [22, 23].

Pathophysiology

Most of our current knowledge regarding the pathophysiology of neuropathic pain originated from experimental data. Although the mechanisms of cancer-related neuropathic pain are not fully understood, the mechanisms and neural pathways are essentially like those for noncancer patients [24]. Accumulated data indicate that several mechanisms are involved in neuropathic pain.

Neuropathic pain can result from mechanical destruction of neurons, chemical injury to neuronal cells, distortion of the surrounding nerve environment such as loss of blood supply leading to nerve ischemia, exposure to an inflammatory microenvironment, or central alteration of pain modulation. The subsequent responses after nerve injury in the structure and function of the nerve conduction system are totally different from that of nonneuronal damage. This phenomenon, called neuroplasticity, is essential to the understanding of neuropathic pain in cancer. Injuries to the nerve tissues lead to key pathophysiologic changes in neuropathic pain (see Fig. 13.1): peripheral sensitisation, spontaneous nerve activity, and central sensitisation.

Peripheral Sensitisation and Spontaneous Nerve Activity

Noxious pain sense is transmitted through afferent unmyelinated C-fibres and thinly myelinated (Aδ−) neurons. These nociceptors are usually activated at high thresholds under normal conditions (see Fig. 13.1a). However, if the peripheral nerve is injured by cancer invasion or various chemotherapeutic agents, these neurons are abnormally sensitised. After peripheral nerve injury, chemical mediators can be subsequently released abnormally by the degenerating distal neurons, as in Wallerian degeneration or signals produced by descending inhibitory neurons [25, 26]. Chemical mediators such as nerve growth factor are released in the vicinity of intact nerve fibres that house diverse ion channels and receptors such as the sodium channel, calcium channel, transient receptor potential V1 (TRPV1), and adrenoreceptor [27]. These chemical mediators expedite increased expression and redistribution of the sodium channel or other receptors not only at the site of the nerve lesion but also at the intact neurons (see Fig. 13.1b). Because these ion channels and receptors are key elements for generating action potential, changes in the number of ion channels or receptors on peripheral nerves would follow spontaneous activation in both injured and intact nerves through these mechanisms [28–31].

TRPV1 is a receptor protein that is located on the peripheral nerve endings and activated by noxious heat under normal physiologic conditions. When a neuron is harmed, TRPV1 is upregulated on injured C-fibres [32, 33]. These changes in TRPV1 expression might lead to spontaneous nerve activation at normal body temperature (heat hyperalgesia). The TRPM8 channel, which is a critical sensor for cold, is activated in the 8–28 °C range and is expressed on the small diameter of the dorsal root ganglion (DRG) [34]. A similar phenomenon of abnormal

→

Fig. 13.1 Pathophysiologic mechanism of peripheral and central sensitisation. (**a**) Normal afferent pathways and their connections in the spinal cord dorsal horn. Red line represents nociceptive C-fibres which form synapse at upper laminae with spinothalamic projection neuron (*yellow neuron*), while non-nociceptive myelinated A-fibres (*blue line*) project to the deeper laminae. Glial cell (*grey line*) in spinal cord facilitates synaptic transmission, whereas GABAergic interneurons (*green line*) normally exert inhibitory action on the afferent neuron. (**b**) Peripheral changes of afferent neurons after a partial nerve lesion. Axons 1 and 3 depict damaged or degenerated axons. Axon 2 and 4 show intact and connected to the peripheral tissues. Peripheral sensitisation develops through various mechanisms; release of products such as nerve growth factor from nearby degenerated nerves fibre (axon 1) leading to expression of channels and receptors on intact nerve (axon 2), increased expression of sodium channel (axon 3). (**c**) Central sensitisation. Autonomous activities in C-nociceptors lead to spinal cord hyperexcitability (*star in yellow neuron*) which causes signal input from mechanoreceptive A-fibres for light touch (*blue line*) to be perceived as pain (allodynia). Inhibitory neural systems (*green neurons*) are also impaired after nerve lesions. (**d**) Chemokines from injured peripheral nerve activates spinal cord glial cells (*grey cell*). Activated microglia further enhance excitability in wide dynamic range neurons by releasing cytokines and growth factors such as tumour necrosis factor α and bone-derived nerve factor (Courtesy of Baron R. Lancet Neurol. from the Elsevier Science Publishers)

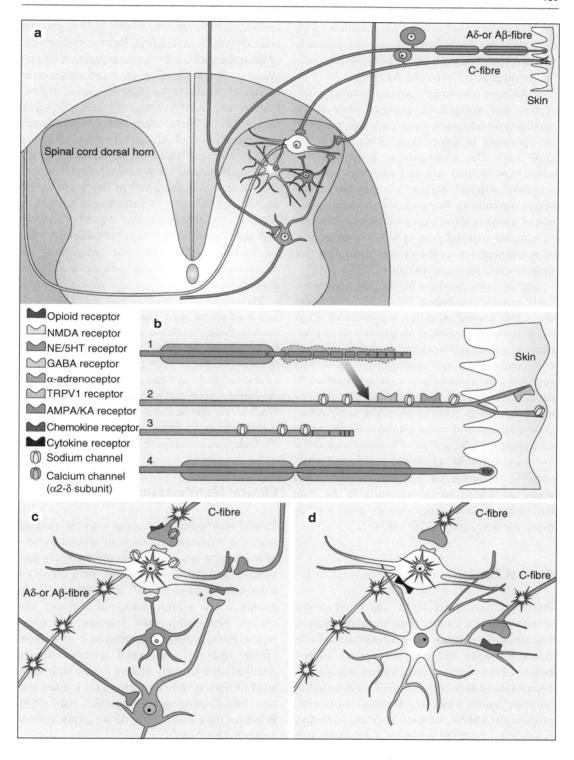

TRPM8 upregulation is observed in patients with cold allodynia [35]. Acid-sensing ion channels (ASICs) have been suggested as being responsible for mechanical hyperalgesia [36].

Pathologic adrenergic coupling between nociceptors and sympathetic postganglionic fibres may increase adrenoceptors on afferent nerves or the sprouting of sympathetic fibres within the DRG [27]. The expression of functional α1-adrenoceptors and α2-adrenoceptors on the peripheral afferent nerves is augmented when nerves are injured. In patients who had amputation of a limb or those with postherpetic neuralgia or complex regional pain syndrome, application of norepinephrine to the symptomatic area can trigger severe spontaneous pain [37, 38].

The exact mechanisms for the development of CINP are not established. However, it is evident that CINP caused by different anticancer drugs has a similarity to clinical manifestations of symmetrical glove-and-stocking sensation and predominantly sensory neuropathy. This fact suggests that common pathways are involved in the development of neuropathic pain. Neurotoxic anticancer drugs such as platinum compounds, taxane agents, and vinca alkaloid usually target either one or multiple sites of microtubules, distal axon, and DRG [39–43]. Loss of epidermal innervations, activation of Langerhans cells, and abnormal activity of mitochondria in the axon have been recently suggested as other mechanisms for developing CINP [44, 45].

Central Sensitisation

Protracted nociceptive inputs can cause central sensitisation. Patients become more sensitive to pain through this mechanism. Glutamate and substance P, the fast transmitter of primary afferent neurons, bind to several receptors on postsynaptic neurons in the dorsal horn of spinal cord, including inotropic amino-3-hydroxy-5-methyl-4-isoxazole propionate (AMPA), kainate (KA), and N-methyl-D-aspartate (NMDA) receptors. Glutamate, substance P, and prostaglandin are key mediators for neuronal excitation, whereas inhibitory mediators for suppressing conduction of pain signals are opioids, norepinephrine, serotonin, and gamma-aminobutyric acid (GABA). Relentless discharge of neurotransmitters from overexpression on presynaptic afferent nerves might cause activation of sodium channels [46] or phosphorylation of these NMDA and AMPA receptors on postsynaptic nerves [47]. These alternations subsequently induce activation of Aβ- and Aδ-neuronal fibres, which are low-threshold mechanoreceptors, resulting in normally non-noxious stimuli such as soft touch being perceived as severe pain (see Fig. 13.1c) [27, 48]. In particular, activation of NMDA receptor is an essential step in both peripheral and central sensitisation [49]. Based on this mechanism, NMDA receptor antagonists are occasionally applied to neuropathic pain in cancer patients [50, 51].

Peripheral nerve injuries may also cause activation of spinal cord non-neural glial cells. The excited glial cells release various cytokines, which further enhance excitability in the spinal sensory neurons (see Fig. 13.1d). Imbalance between pain inhibition and facilitation could contribute to developing neuropathic pain. Loss of inhibitory GABAergic interneurons, which normally play a potent role in inhibition of pain transmission to the thalamus, could cause neuropathic pain [52].

Clinical Manifestation

Painful neuropathy may occur anytime, ranging from the immediate moment to several months after injury to any afferent nerves that carry pain signals, and once neuropathic pain develops from either cancer-related or treatment-related causes, it has a high chance of evolving into chronic neuropathic pain. Patients with nerve injury have several characteristic symptoms (Table 13.2) [6]. Abnormal sensation in the involved area virtually always exists, with some level of sensory deficit nearby. This is a key feature in diagnosing neuropathic pain [53]. However, the clinical terms do not imply a mechanism for neuropathic pain.

Peripheral sensory nerve injury and regeneration play a key role in the development of neuropathic pain, which is characterised by partial or

Table 13.2 Common symptoms and signs suggestive of neuropathic pain

Terms	Definition
Allodynia	Pain due to a stimulus that does not normally provoke pain
Hyperalgesia	Increased pain from a stimulus that normally provokes pain. For pain evoked by stimuli that usually are not painful, the term allodynia is preferred, whereas hyperalgesia is more appropriately used for cases with an increased response at a normal threshold or at an increased threshold
Paresthesia	An abnormal sensation, whether spontaneous or evoked
Dysesthesia	An unpleasant abnormal sensation, whether spontaneous or evoked. Paresthesia is used to describe an abnormal sensation that is not unpleasant, whereas dysesthesia is preferentially used for an abnormally unpleasant sensation
Causalgia	A syndrome of sustained burning pain, allodynia, and hyperpathia after a traumatic nerve lesion, often combined with vasomotor and sudomotor dysfunction and later trophic changes
Hyperpathia	A painful syndrome characterised by an abnormally painful reaction to a stimulus, especially a repetitive stimulus, as well as an increased threshold. It may occur with allodynia, hyperesthesia, hyperalgesia, or dysesthesia
Hypoesthesia	Decreased sensitivity to stimulation, excluding the special senses
Hypoalgesia	Diminished pain in response to a normally painful stimulus

complete sensory loss in the painful area and stimulus-independent or abnormally exaggerated pain (allodynia, hyperalgesia, hyperpathia) [5, 54]. Injuries to the sensory afferent transmission result in loss of sensory input to the peripheral nerve endings. Consequently, patients feel less pain than under normal conditions. The regeneration and changes in the injured nerves and intact nerves in the vicinity cause secondary hypersensitivity or stimulus-independent pain [55].

The quality of the neuropathic pain is quite diverse: patients describe their symptoms as "pins and needles," "electric shooting," "fireworks," "walking on broken glass or ice," "painful numbness," "cold," "wet," "hot," and "burning." Some patients experience deep aching pains occurring anywhere in the dermatomal region innervated by the damaged neural structure, and others experience abnormal sensations, including spontaneous or evoked paresthesias, allodynia, and hyperalgesia. However, patients cannot readily distinguish between true neuropathic pain and other neuropathic distressing symptoms such as tingling, pressure, and burning [56].

Patients with neuropathic pain may or may not develop motor and/or autonomic dysfunction in the distribution of the involved nerve. Signs of sympathetic hyperactivity with excessive sweating, skin temperature, and colour change may occur simultaneously with neuropathic pain. Symptoms may differ with the cause and location of the lesion.

Cancer-Related Neuropathic Pain

Cancer-Related Plexus Neuropathy

Plexopathy is a form of peripheral neuropathy from lesions that affect a network of nerves, blood vessels, and lymph vessels, a so-called plexus [57]. Common plexus neuropathies include cervical, brachial, and lumbosacral plexopathies. Neurologic manifestations of neoplastic and radiation-induced plexopathies are characterised initially by severe, unrelenting pain followed by development of weakness and focal sensory disturbances [58]. Imaging workups such as magnetic resonance imaging (MRI), computed tomography (CT), and/or positron emission tomography (PET) scanning should be considered in cancer patients with symptoms compatible with plexus neuropathy. Although there is no strong evidence of superiority, MRI with its superior soft tissue discrimination and multi-planar imaging capabilities tends to be adopted for the workup [59, 60].

Cervical plexopathies are usually due to head and neck cancer or lymph node metastasis. When the cervical plexus is invaded by cancer, patients may complain of pre- and postauricular anterior neck pain. In addition, pain may radiate to lateral aspect of the face, head, and shoulder. Pain may be aggravated by head movement or swallowing, and ipsilateral Horner's syndrome or hemidiaphragmatic paralysis could be associated with pain.

Brachial plexopathies occur in breast cancer patients from axillary lymph node metastasis or postoperative radiation, in patients with lymphoma, and in patients with apical lung cancer (so-called Pancoast's tumour). Pain usually precedes muscle weakness and sensory abnormality by several months [61]. Lower plexus (C7–T1) infiltration with tumour leads to pain in the elbow, medial forearm, and fourth or fifth fingers. Cancer involvement of the upper plexus is less common than in the lower plexus. Pain may localise to the elbow or medial forearm. When the upper plexus (C5 and C6) is involved, characteristic pain develops in the shoulder girdle in the lateral arm and hand.

Lumbosacral plexopathies that affect the function of the lumbar, sacral, and coccygeal nerves are conditions in the lumbosacral plexus, which constitutes the neurovascular supply to the pelvis and lower limbs. Lumbosacral plexopathies are commonly associated with lymphoma, colorectal cancer, cervical cancer, or sarcoma. When cancer patients present with pain in the lumbosacral dermatome and dysfunction in a leg, lumbosacral plexopathy should be included in the differential diagnosis [62]. As in other plexus neuropathies, almost all patients experience typical pain that precedes neurologic signs. The qualities of pain include aching, stabbing, and pressure-like characteristics. Paresthesia, numbness, and weakness commonly develop weeks to months after pain initiation. Pain may be localised in the buttocks and perineum or posterolateral thigh if the lower lumbosacral plexus is involved. Other autonomic symptoms include bladder or bowel dysfunction, leg edema, and sacral area allodynia. Sensory change or motor weakness may be observed in the L5 and L1 dermatomes and positive results on the straight-leg-raising test. Other findings include bladder or bowel dysfunction and leg edema [63].

The main differential diagnosis is between cancer-induced lumbosacral plexopathy and radiation-induced plexopathy, which is often a difficult determination [58]. Radiation-induced lumbosacral plexopathy is a rare complication, occurring in 0.3–1.3 % of patients treated with radiation, and it develops several months to years after completion of radiotherapy [64]. Patients with radiation-induced lumbosacral plexopathy present with progressive motor weakness of innervated lesion. Pain is not the predominant symptom and progressive motor weakness precede the pain in the L5–S1 innervating area in radiation-induced plexopathy, whereas cancer-induced lumbosacral plexopathy has opposite symptoms [63]. Additionally, radiation-induced plexopathy may present with bilateral symptoms and signs.

Radiculopathy from Leptomeningeal Metastases or the Vertebral Body

With cancers disseminated over the leptomeninges, clinical manifestations are diverse depending on the involved sites. Focal or multifocal neurologic symptoms or signs may be present at any level of the neuraxis. Thus, patients typically present with multifocal symptoms. Patients commonly have generalised headache and radicular pain in the upper and lower limbs, lower back, and neck. On physical examination, lower motor neuron weakness is the most common sign in the majority of patients, with accompanying reflex loss and dermatomal sensory loss often seen [65]. Concurrent seizures, gait disturbance, diplopia, and mental changes such as lethargy, confusion, or loss of memory also occur frequently.

Involvement of metastatic cancer to vertebral bodies with extradural compression of the spinal cord or its nerve roots is most common in lung cancer, breast cancer, multiple myeloma, and prostate cancer [66]. Paraspinal or retroperitoneal lymph node enlargement may compress nerves from the spinal cord in 5–10 % of patients with lymphoma [67], and any nerve compressing lesions could cause radicular pain. The local pain is usually the earliest sign of the spinal cord compression and may precede radicular pain and motor weaknesses by weeks. Radicular pain from the nerve compression or irritation in the vertebral bodies is likely to be localised to the distribution of the nerves involved and to be constant in duration. Sensory changes occur later, with numbness and anaesthesia distal to the level of involvement [68]. Autonomic and sphincter dysfunction also can develop in the later stage. Coughing, sneezing, and Valsalva maneuvers often exacerbate this radicular pain [69]. The characteristic sign of electric-like pain, so-called Lhermitte's sign, which is induced by forward flexion of the head, can be observed in cervical and thoracic epidural spinal cord compression. The pain is usually worse at night, whereas the opposite pattern is observed with degenerative disease. Interestingly, radicular pain does not necessarily correlate with the dermatomal distribution of the disease location [70].

When lesions damage the cauda equina, patients typically present with marked neurologic disability. The symptoms are dominated by bilateral lower extremity weakness (L3–S1) and sphincter weakness as well as saddle paresthesia (S2–4).

Cranial Nerve Neuropathy

Twelve pairs of nerves, the cranial nerves, come directly from the brain, and pain in the head and neck is mediated through these nerves. When cancers metastasise to the skull base or leptomeninges and affect cranial nerve(s), the injured nerves can produce cranial neuropathic pain. Because skull bone metastasis is common in patients with prostate or lung cancer, cranial neuropathies are most commonly observed in such patients. Direct invasion from head and neck cancer may also cause cranial nerve neuralgias. Pain from cranial nerve neuropathy is often accompanied by other neurologic symptoms such as ptosis, swallowing difficulties, and facial numbness [71]. All cancer patients with symptoms compatible with cranial neuralgia should be scrutinised for the underlying tumour.

Glossopharyngeal neuralgia is characterised by severe transient stabbing pains in the ear, tongue base, tonsillar regions, or angle of the jaw that is innervated by the glossopharyngeal

nerve [72]. Pain is commonly induced by swallowing, talking, or coughing. Syncope may occur simultaneously with glossopharyngeal neuralgia [73].

Trigeminal neuralgia is a unilateral disorder characterised by brief electric shock-like pain that is characterised by abrupt onset and termination. Leptomeningeal metastases or cancer involving the middle or posterior fossa can induce trigeminal neuralgia.

Paraneoplastic Neuropathy

Neuropathic pain can occur rarely by a remote effect of the cancer and not due to the direct spread of cancer. Paraneoplastic neuropathy (PNN) is most commonly associated with small cell lung cancer [74, 75]. Lymphoma also affects the peripheral nervous system and may occasionally cause neuropathic pain [76]. Symptoms precede the diagnosis of the causative cancer in 50 to 80 % of patients with PNN [77].

The mechanism responsible is considered to be injury to the sensory neuronal cell bodies in the DRG by autoantibodies. Cancer can stimulate the immune system to mediate production of antibodies against intracellular antigens of neurons.

Patients can present with sensory ataxia or mechanical hyperalgesia, either symmetrically or in a multifocal area in the extremities, trunk, and face. The diverse symptoms in PNN may be best explained by differences in the sensory nerves involved. In contrast to small nerve fibres for pain conduction damaged in painful cases of PNN, loss of large sensory neurons in the DRG was observed in the ataxic forms of PNN [78]. The course is typically independent of cancer prognosis. PNN rarely improves with treatment of the cancer [79].

Treatment-Related Neuropathic Pain

Neuropathic pain may also come from treatment such as surgery, radiotherapy, and chemotherapy. The common presentations after surgery are postmastectomy pain with breast cancer, post-thoracotomy pain, pain after post-radical neck dissection, and phantom limb pain after amputation. Peripheral nerve injuries are a common cause of persistent postoperative pain. Chemotherapeutic agents including platinum, taxane, and vinca alkaloid are also frequent causes.

Postmastectomy Pain Syndrome

Chronic pain is not uncommon after surgical resection of breast cancer. The prevalence of postmastectomy pain syndrome (PMPS) has been reported to be 24–68 % in patients with breast cancer [80–82]. In a national-wide study in Denmark of patients who received surgery 1–3 years before and/or adjuvant therapy for breast cancer, about half of the patients with PMPS still had moderate or severe pain, and 20 % of patients revisited the clinic because of the pain [82].

The mechanisms of PMPS are believed to be damage to the intercostal nerves in the axilla and/or formation of neuromas [83]. Pain is often localised to the axilla, medial upper arm, and/or anterior chest wall of the operated side and is described as "burning" or "shooting" pain induced by pressure. Dissection of axillary lymph node may increase the development of PMPS [81].

Post-thoracotomy Pain Syndrome

Retrospective studies have reported that about 12–26 % of patients have had chronic pain of more than moderate intensity after thoracotomy [84–87]. Intercostal nerve damage has been suggested as a main cause of post-thoracotomy pain syndrome (PTPS), and studies have found that 35–83 % of such patients had a neuropathic component to their pain, including stabbing sensations, burning pains, and dysesthesia [85, 86]. In some patients, post-thoracotomy pain may originate from a taut muscular band within the scapular area [88].

It is currently not possible to predict which patients are vulnerable to developing PTPS. Most studies of PTPS have been retrospectively designed and have been too inconsistent and heterogeneous to draw conclusive risk factors [89].

Post-radical Neck Dissection Pain

Radical neck dissection (RND) is a key procedure in the surgical treatment of head and neck cancer (HNC). However, cervical nerve damage after RND can result in chronic shoulder and neck pain, and hence chronic pain after surgical operation for HNC is not uncommon [90, 91]. Dysesthesia, intermittent shock-like pain, or lancinating pain may develop. Nociceptive pain may also develop from musculoskeletal imbalance and subsequent changes in the shoulder.

Persistently increasing pain in HNC patients who underwent RND may signify cancer recurrence or soft tissue infection. CT or MRI scanning workups are warranted to exclude cancer relapse.

Phantom Limb Pain

Patients may perceive pain in the distal part of an amputated limb as if it were still attached to the body. Pain in the limb that is no longer present, so-called phantom limb pain (PLP), is commonly confused with pain in the residual limb. Pain commonly persists after the injured tissue has healed. In addition, PLP frequently resembles the pain felt in the limb before amputation.

From recent reports, PLP occurs at rates of 47–69 % in amputees [92, 93]. Patients describe a wide range of pain characteristics such as "burning," "tingling," "lancinating electrical shock," "throbbing," and a "cramping" sense.

Although numerous theories have been proposed, the mechanism of PLP development is not fully understood. Both central and peripheral mechanisms are believed to be involved in PLP. The most common theory in the development of PLP is central reorganisation. After extremities are amputated, the somatosensory cortical areas for extremities are occupied by neighboring representational zones, and a remapping of the location of amputated limb into the mouth and chin areas occurs [94]. Patients may experience PLP by stimulation of the mouth or face.

The peripheral nerve system could also be involved in PLP. When extremities are amputated, many severed nerve endings commonly form neuromas at the distal portion of the residual limb. These abnormally produced neuromas evoke an aberrant action potential that can lead to pain with neurologic characteristics [95]. Phantom pain is not limited to limb amputation but also occurs with surgical resection of many other organs, such as the breast, rectum, penis, and bladder [96–100].

Complex Regional Pain Syndrome

Complex regional pain syndrome (CRPS) is a chronic painful condition in which the pain intensity is disproportionate to the inciting event. The concept of CRPS was introduced by IASP to replace the conditions previously known as reflex sympathetic dystrophy (corresponding to CRPS type I) and causalgia (corresponding to CRPS type II) [101]. The definition was modified to "an array of painful conditions that are characterised by a continuing regional pain that is seemingly disproportionate in time or degree to the usual course of any known trauma or other lesion" [102].

Common clinical characteristics of CRPS include sensory disturbance with neuropathic pain features, sudomotor, vasomotor, and motor disturbance. Diagnosis is based on clinical criteria, and no gold standard has been established. IASP proposed diagnostic criteria for CRPS that include at least one symptom in three and one sign in two out of four categories [102]:

1. *Sensory*: Hyperesthesia (to pinprick) and/or allodynia (to light touch and/or temperature sensation and/or deep somatic pressure and/or joint movement)
2. *Vasomotor*: Temperature asymmetry (≥1 °C) and/or asymmetric skin colour change

3. *Sudomotor*: Edema and/or asymmetric sweating
4. *Motor/trophic*: Motor dysfunction (weakness, tremor, dystonia) and/or changes in nail, hair, skin

Diagnosis can be made with a sensitivity of 0.76 and a specificity of 0.81. Cancer patients are at risk of CRPS from surgery or direct cancer invasion. Considering that 20 % of patients with CRPS have a history of surgery in the affected area, the actual incidence of CRPS in postoperative cancer patients may be underestimated [103]. Information about CRPS-associated plexopathy is not unknown but only rarely reported [104].

The mechanism is poorly understood, although CRPS is presumed to be a systemic disease with both peripheral and central nervous system involvement. Several pathways are thought to be involved in CRPS development [105], and no single mechanism can explain its development satisfactorily. The clinical course is quite variable.

Radiation-Induced Neuropathic Pain

Cancer patients who have undergone radiation therapy may have neuropathic pain as a sequela after a latency period. Radiation-induced neuropathy (RNP) is presumed to be mediated by injuries to myelinated nerve fibres and blood vessels, and several factors including total radiation dose are contributing factors for its occurrence. Both higher doses per fraction and greater total radiation dose are likely to increase the incidence of RNP [106]. According to a retrospective report, the risk of RNP was less than 0.5 % in patients who received a total dose of 45–50 Gy in 1.8–2 Gy daily fractions [107]. The complication rate for RNP increased to up to 5 % in patients who received a radiation dose of 57–61 Gy.

In contrast to early pain that occurs within weeks after spinal cord irradiation and is often reversible, delayed RNP typically occurs after several months to years [108, 109]. Slowly progressing symptoms, a latency period, and the absence of a space-occupying mass suggest RNP.

Chemotherapy-Induced Neuropathic Pain

Many essential anticancer drugs commonly cause serious neuropathic pain. These chemotherapeutic agents include platinum agents, taxanes, vinca alkaloids, thalidomide, and bortezomib. Such pain not only interferes with daily activities for a lengthy period in cancer survivors [110] but also may cause a reduction or discontinuation of planned anticancer treatment [111]. Nonetheless, this unavoidable side effect is often underestimated by healthcare providers and is seen as the cost of eradicating cancer. There is a substantial discrepancy in the perception of chemotherapy-induced peripheral neuropathy (CIPN) between patients and physicians [112]. CIPN is frequently considered one of the most distressing side effects of cancer treatment by patients and their family members.

The incidence of CIPN depends on cumulative dose, type of chemotherapeutic agent, and preexisting neuropathy such as diabetic or alcoholic neuropathy. It usually involves peripheral sensory nerves, and the symptoms or signs of CIPN depend on which nerves are damaged. Distal deep tendon reflexes (e.g., Achilles or brachioradialis) of the affected extremities can be lost completely. Physical examination often reveals impairment of touch sense, two-point discrimination, temperature, and vibration in the involved area.

There are several common clinical manifestations in CIPN, as follows:

1. Pain is characterised by continuous distal symmetric painful paresthesia, such as a "shooting," "stabbing," "burning," or "tingling" sense in the feet and/or hands, as well as the so-called "glove-and-stocking" sensation. The intensity of CIPN may be increased by contact.
2. Although manifestations of CIPN may include motor, autonomic, and sensory neuropathy, CIPN is predominantly sensory neuropathy. Motor or autonomic functions are usually saved.
3. Symptoms have temporal relationship in the onset of CIPN and can develop during or after

stopping of the chemotherapy, so-called coasting.
4. Signs and symptoms in neurosensory dysfunction are present concurrently. Patients can have numbness or just less ability to sense pressure, touch, heat, or cold. They often have trouble in using their fingers to pick up things. They may have problems in balance and often trip or stumble while walking

Platinum Agents (Cisplatin, Carboplatin, Oxaliplatin)

All platinum anticancer drugs can cause dose-dependent, cumulative CIPN. The platinum drugs also share the coast phenomenon, which is a worsening of the severity of symptoms for weeks or months after quitting chemotherapy. CIPN associated with platinum agents is usually considered to originate from injury to neuronal cells in the DRG (neuronopathy) that leads to anterograde axonal degeneration related to development of axonopathy [113, 114]. Pathologic evaluation reveals loss of large fibres with secondary damage to the myelin sheath. Consequently, marked reduction in the conduction velocities and amplitude of sensory nerve potentials are observed. Predictive factors for CIPN with the use of platinum agents include dose, schedule of administration, and the combination of agents. CIPN starts as sensory neuropathy such as paresthesias and a tingling sense in a stocking-glove wearing zone, progressing to decreased or absent reflexes in the affected extremities. Because patients may have permanent sensory disturbances after DRG damage [16], great care should be taken to minimise CIPN.

Cisplatin-induced neuropathy appeared after cumulative doses of more than 300 mg/m^2, with tingling to painful paresthesia, loss of distal tendon reflex, and reduced vibration sense [115]. The incidence of CIPN increased to 50–90 % in patients who had received a cumulative dose of 500 mg/m^2 [116]. Cisplatin-induced neuropathy may develop up to 3 months after last administration of cisplatin and can progress in intensity. About 30 % of patients still have symptoms years after therapy [17, 24].

Carboplatin-induced sensory neuropathy is clinically indistinguishable from that of cisplatin. Although carboplatin is generally considered to be less neurotoxic [17, 116], some studies comparing the clinical effect and toxicity have indicated that the incidence and severity of neuropathic pain is not less than with cisplatin [117, 118].

Persistent sensory neuropathy remains the key dose-limiting adverse effect in treatment using oxaliplatin. Oxaliplatin shares features of cumulative toxicity with other platinum anticancer agents. It was reported that up to 20 % of patients developed severe neurotoxicity at 750–850 mg/m^2 [119]. Oxaliplatin-induced nerve damage commonly does not resolve at long-term follow-up, with symptoms of moderate foot numbness and tingling neuropathic pain in 22 % of patients [120]. In recent small prospective studies, up to 79 % of patients had chronic residual neuropathy, primarily numbness in the extremities [121, 122].

Compared with other platinum agents, oxaliplatin has a distinct acute neurotoxicity with a rapid onset of hours to days following treatment. Up to 90 % of patients experience painful numbness when drinking a cold beverage or upon exposure to cold temperature. Rather than structural damage, the suggested mechanism is ion channel dysfunction: the release of oxalates from oxaliplatin chelates calcium with an effect on sodium channels in the axonal membrane and synapses [123, 124]. Disrupted sodium channels subsequently increase sensory nerve excitability.

Taxanes (Paclitaxel, Docetaxel)

Taxane compounds stabilise GDP-bound tubulin in the microtubules and subsequently interfere with cellular microtubule dynamics. When patients are exposed to taxanes, marked microtubule aggregation is observed in large myelinated axons [114]. Accordingly, taxane administration interrupts axonal transport. Paclitaxel and docetaxel are two main anticancer agents that cause CIPN. Although there are differences between the two chemotherapeutic agents in the incidence of side effects and in predisposing conditions, it is impossible to distinguish between their clinical side effects [24]. Docetaxel tends to induce

neuropathy less often than does paclitaxel (11 % vs. 30 %) [125].

Neurotoxicity from taxanes seems to be influenced both by infusion time and cumulative dose, compared with only the dose for platinum agents. Weekly administration of taxanes has been previously shown to be a contributing factor for increasing the incidence of neurotoxicity. However, recent studies have raised questions about this association with neurotoxicity incidence. Two randomised phase III trials that considered the neurotoxicity incidence of weekly paclitaxel compared with administration every 3 weeks reported inconsistent results [126, 127]. Another randomised phase III trials of docetaxel also showed conflicting data concerning the incidence of neuropathy, depending on the schedule [128–130].

The duration of infusion may be a factor in the incidence of neuropathy. One study reported that grade 3 neurosensory toxicity was experienced by 13 % of patients with a 3-h infusion of paclitaxel compared with 7 % for the 24-h infusion group [131].

Patients who experienced acute myalgia or arthralgia within a few days after paclitaxel administration are more likely to have chronic sensory neuropathy and more likely to have numbness or a tingling sense rather than a shooting or burning sense [132]. Combined taxane and platinum agents is a popular regimen in the clinical field, and thus dose-limiting neurotoxicity is quite common [133].

Although various experimental agents have been tried to protect against neuropathic pain, most results are empirical or from a small non-randomised trial [134]. Thus, the evidence for routine use of such medications with taxanes is scarce.

Vinca Alkaloid (Vincristine, Vinblastine, Vinorelbine, Vindesine)

In contrast to taxane compounds, which exert their anticancer effect through aggregating microtubules in the cell, vinca alkaloids destabilise tubulin and thereby prevent the formation of microtubules. Because microtubules are a key element in axonal transport, these alterations in neuronal cells by vinca alkaloids disturb normal signal transduction by impulse. Thirty to forty percent of patients who receive vinca alkaloids were estimated to experience sensory neuropathy [17, 135]. The peak incidence occurs after 2–3 weeks, and most patients recover between 1 and 3 months after quitting the drug. However, peripheral neuropathy may persist in some patients [24]. CIPN by vincristine is usually similar to symptoms caused by other agents, with symmetrical glove-stocking area neuropathic pain. However, motor symptoms and autonomic function may be impaired, with difficulties in the dorsiflexion and wrist extension, postural hypotension, urogenital dysfunction, and paralytic ileus [15, 136]. Foot drop may cause gait disturbance. Vincristine-induced neuropathy seems to increase significantly in cases of a cumulative dose of more than 20 mg/m^2 [24, 136]. Other vinca alkaloids such as vinblastine, vinorelbine, and vindesine have similar toxicity, but the severity and prevalence are reportedly less than for vincristine [24].

Thalidomide

Thalidomide is an immunomodulatory agent used primarily for treating multiple myeloma. The exact mechanism of its neuropathic side effects is unknown. A recent report suggested that polymorphisms in genes mediating gene repair and neuroinflammation may increase the risk of thalidomide-induced neuropathy [137]. Incidence rates are 15–70 % and vary with duration of chemotherapy and cumulative dose [138]. The usual symptoms are a painful tingling sense and numbness. Motor function is usually preserved.

Bortezomib

Bortezomib is a proteasome-inhibiting agent used for multiple myeloma. CIPN caused by bortezomib is common, occurring in 23–37 % of patients [139, 140]. The mechanism of bortezomib-induced neuropathy is not well established. Onset is quite variable but frequently occurs within 3 months of administration. In general, symptoms present are the common features of CIPN, including allodynia, burning dysesthesia complicated by numbness, and symmetric glove-and-stocking sensation. Bortezomib-related neuropathic pain can be managed according to dose

modification guidelines [141], and up to 71 % of patients improve after dose reduction or stopping [142]. Recovery may take longer in patients with grade 3 or greater neurotoxicity compared with grade 1 or 2 neurotoxicity [143].

Other Causes of Neuropathic Pain

Postherpetic Neuralgia

Postherpetic neuralgia (PHN) is a common and painful complication of herpes zoster. Herpes zoster results from reactivation of the varicella zoster virus that hibernates in DRG neurons after chicken pox infection in childhood and may reactivate, for unclear reasons. PHN can follow recovery of herpes zoster infection at an incidence of 10–20 % of patients [144]. One study reported that 12 % of patients with herpes zoster infection had PHN at 3 months, and PHN persisted at least 6 months in 5 % of patients [145].

PHN can present with diverse manifestations of pain including burning, aching, shooting, or lancinating pain. Patients may experience allodynia or hyperalgesia with decreased touch sense in the involved dermatome. Some patients cannot tolerate even air conditioning or cloth contact. Such allodynia or hyperalgesia comes from formation of new connections between non-nociceptive large diameter afferent nerves and central pain transmission neurons. Early use of antiviral agents can reduce both acute pain and the risk of PHN [146]. However, these medications are not helpful after the development of PHN.

Assessment

No single symptom or sign suffices to confirm neuropathic pain. Diagnosis can be established by combinations of characteristic symptoms, bedside examinations, and diagnostic tests for confirming neurologic lesions [147]. Even thorough clinical examination can never prove any pain to be neuropathic pain; it can only provide supporting evidence for alterations in the somatosensory conduction system [148]. The European

Federation of Neurological Societies (EFNS) suggested three steps, as below, when assessing neuropathic pain [149]:

1. A clinical history will be taken to ascertain whether patients have symptoms compatible with neuropathic pain or relevant lesions in the painful area. Patients usually present with burning, lancinating, itchy, stinging, stabbing, or shooting qualities with unusual tingling, crawling, or electrical sensations [150]. Pain is distributed in a distinct neuroanatomically plausible area.

2. Physical examination will determine the presence of reduced and exaggerated sensory signs (Table 13.2). Abnormal sensory findings would match neuroanatomically with a localised lesion for neuropathic pain [151]. Thus, the neurologic examination is directed to find possible abnormalities correlated to the lesion and the anatomic level of sensory abnormalities. Clinical examination includes mapping of sensory abnormalities, touch, pinprick, pressure, cold, heat, vibration, and temporal summation. The sensory deficit is usually to noxious and thermal stimuli [152].

3. Neuroimaging tests or skin biopsy could be performed to confirm specific underlying neurologic disease or sensory lesion within the pain distribution.

Definite neuropathic pain is diagnosed in patients with positive findings for all three of the above steps, probable neuropathic pain for patients with step 1 plus either step 2 or 3, and possible neuropathic pain for patients with step 1 without step 2 or 3 [5]. Conventional electrophysiological techniques such as nerve conduction studies or somatosensory evoked potential can assess only the function of the myelinated peripheral axonal systems or lemniscal system, not affection of nerves for somatosensory conduction. Thus, these tests are not usually necessary for making the diagnosis.

Although several screening tools for neuropathic pain have been developed [153–156], a standard method has not been established. These screening tools may help detect undiagnosed neuropathic pain in cancer patients [157]. Specific screening tools for neuropathic pain are discussed in greater detail elsewhere in this textbook (Chap. 8).

The pain intensity can be evaluated with the same methods used for nociceptive pain. However, pain intensity should be described separately, if the pain has a mixed pain component (e.g., dull aching and concurrent lancinating pain) [151]. The scale includes a descriptive method ("mild," "moderate," "severe"), numeric ratings, visual analogues, and colour and graphical representation.

Treatment

Neuropathic pain is hard to control, and its management in cancer patients is a challenging issue. Patients with neuropathic pain tend to have a higher average pain intensity and lower quality of life [158, 159].

Although numerous randomised trials have been conducted and various medications have been developed, results for most treatments for pain are disappointing, and less than 50 % of patients achieve satisfactory pain relief [160]. Several studies have indicated that patients may have persistent neuropathic pain with more than moderate intensity even after medication [161]. Furthermore, lack of head-to-head comparison trials, diverse disease conditions, and inconsistent study designs make the choice of specific medications difficult for physicians. To evaluate the effectiveness of drugs for neuropathic pain and to avoid confusion, the concept of numbers needed-to-treat (NNT) is commonly used. NNT is the number of patients that need to be treated with a certain medication to obtain a benefit in one patient compared with a control in a clinical trial and is the opposite definition of absolute risk reduction [162]. The ideal NNT is 1. If NNT is 1 for a certain medication, every patient can improve with treatment, and no one improves with the control. The higher the NNT, the less effective is the treatment. In general, effective medications for treating neuropathic pain have NNTs between 2 and 6, which means up to six patients must be treated for one additional patient to experience meaningful pain improvement [160].

Despite several guidelines for neuropathic pain having been introduced and updated repeatedly based on randomised controlled trials [148, 163, 164], most trials have investigated patients with noncancer neuropathic pain. Thus, there could be a problem for application directly to cancer patients. For example, opioids are not recommended as first-line medications in noncancer neuropathic pain owing to concerns over their long-term safety. However, opioids are unique medications that could provide immediate pain relief in neuropathic patients. Sequelae such as addiction and immunologic changes from the long-term use of opioids are less problematic in patients with advanced cancer. For these reasons, opioids are recommended as first-line medications in neuropathic cancer pain [165]. Of the diverse opioid analgesics, methadone plays an important role in treatment owing to its peculiar mechanism of action. In contrast to their use for nociceptive pain, nonsteroidal anti-inflammatory drugs (NSAIDs) are not effective, and their role in controlling neuropathic pain is limited [166, 167].

The non-opioid medications, so-called adjuvant analgesics, have to be combined with opioid analgesics for uncontrolled neuropathic cancer pain. Steroids also should be considered in cases of pain from nerve compression [168]. The adjuvant pharmacologic agents for neuropathic pain include antidepressants, anticonvulsants, and topical agents (Table 13.3). The evidence for the use of adjuvants for neuropathic cancer pain was derived from randomised controlled trials for chronic noncancer neuropathic pain, because there are few randomised controlled or comparative trials concerning cohorts with neuropathic cancer pain.

Pharmacologic Treatment of Neuropathic Cancer Pain

Opioids

Opioids are a mainstay for the treatment of neuropathic cancer pain. To optimise opioid use before trials of other adjuvant drugs, opioids should be titrated and adverse events (such as constipation, nausea, and itching) should be managed properly [169]. Opioids are often avoided by clinicians and patients for first-line treatment of neuropathic cancer pain. This reluctance is usually attributed to a misunderstanding of the responsiveness of neuropathic pain to opioids and to fear of addiction. Although neuropathic cancer pain may require higher opioid doses than for nociceptive pain [170, 171], the mechanisms of neuropathic pain do not provide inherent resistance to opioids. Pain relief may be achieved by opioids alone, rotation to other opioids, or combination with other drugs [171, 172]. When the opioid alone is found to be not effective or when side effects of opioids are not tolerable, the addition of adjuvants is appropriate [165, 168]. Specific opioids for neuropathic pain are discussed in depth in another part (Chap. 9) of this book.

Antidepressants

Antidepressants have well-established beneficial effects on neuropathic pain, and their analgesic effects are independent of their antidepressant effects. However, antidepressants might be preferred to anticonvulsants in the management of neuropathic cancer pain in patients with depression. Antidepressants for neuropathic pain can be categorised as tricyclic antidepressants (TCAs) and selective serotonin noradrenaline reuptake inhibitors (SNRIs). Selective serotonin reuptake inhibitors (SSRIs) have limited analgesic effects in the management of neuropathic pain [163, 173, 174].

Numerous randomised controlled trials have confirmed the efficacy of TCAs for the various types of neuropathic pain. TCAs have analgesic effects through multiple modes of action. They can inhibit reuptake of serotonin and noradrenaline from presynaptic terminals and subsequently potentiate endogenous pain-suppressing pathways down from the brainstem. They also block voltage-gate sodium channels and other cholinergic and histaminergic channels. Several kinds of TCAs (amitriptyline, imipramine, nortriptyline, and desipramine) are available.

Table 13.3 Adjuvant analgesics for neuropathic cancer pain (Courtesy of Baron R. Lancet Neurol. from the Elsevier Science Publishers)

Drug/category	Mechanism of action	Titration	Starting dose/maximal dose (mg)	Major adverse events
Antidepressants				
Tricyclic antidepressants				
Amitriptyline	Inhibition reuptake of serotonin, noradrenaline from presynaptic terminals, and cholinergic Na+ channel blocking	Increase by 25 mg daily every 3–5 days if tolerated	10–25/150	Anticholinergic side effects such as sedation, dry mouth, constipation, urinary retention, sweating. Cardiac conduction disturbances
Imipramine			25–50/300	
Nortriptyline			10–25/150	
Desipramine			10–25/150	
SNRIs				
Duloxetine	Inhibition both serotonin and norepinephrine reuptake	Increase by 60 mg daily as tolerated	20–30/120	Nausea, hepatic and renal dysfunction
Venlafaxine		Increase by 37.5–75 mg each week	50–75/225	Nausea, withdrawal syndrome with abrupt discontinuation
Dopamine and norepinephrine receptor inhibitor				
Bupropion	Inhibition of neuronal noradrenaline reuptake and a weak inhibitor of dopamine reuptake at presynaptic level		100–150/450	Lower seizure threshold, contraindicated in patients with history of seizures
Anticonvulsants				
Gabapentin	Inhibit $\alpha_2\delta$ subunit of calcium channels in presynaptic sites and subsequently decrease release of glutamate, norepinephrine, substance P	Increase by 100–300 mg three times daily every 1–7days	100–300/3,600	Sedation, dizziness, peripheral edema
Pregabalin		Increase by 50 mg three times or 75 mg twice daily	150/300	
Topical agents				
5 % Lidocaine	Blocking of sodium channels		1–3 Patch/3 patches	Local erythema, rash

Studies comparing drugs within the same class reported similar efficacies for neuropathic pain [175]. The NNT for TCAs in multiple randomised controlled trials is reported as 3.6 (95 % CI 3–4.5) [176].

TCAs should be started at low doses (10–25 mg), administered at night, and the dose increased every 3–5 days. The tertiary amines (amitriptyline, imipramine) may be more efficacious, but anticholinergic adverse effects such as sedation, dryness of mouth, and urinary retention are more likely to occur with amitriptyline and imipramine than with secondary amines (desipramine, nortriptyline) [165]. For this reason, secondary amines are advocated as first-line medication in

the certain guideline [177]. The risk of sedation and confusion may be present in the initial phase of treatment and particularly in elderly patients. TCAs especially may present a safety problem in high dosages in elderly patients and no superior analgesic efficacy over gabapentin [178]. TCAs may also cause cardiac conduction problems in 5 % of patients [163]. Therefore, the ECG should be checked before starting TCAs as medication, and TCAs are contraindicated in patients with heart failure and cardiac conduction blocks. Sudden cardiac death was reported to increase in the patients receiving more than 100 mg daily [179]. On the basis of these data, the Neuropathic Pain Special Interest Group (NeuPSIG) guidelines recommend using TCAs at less than 100 mg/day with caution in patients with cardiac disease, whenever possible [160].

The effectiveness of two SNRIs, duloxetine and venlafaxine, in neuropathic pain was established through multiple randomised controlled trials [180, 181]. Venlafaxine has an NNT of 3.1 (95 % CI 2.2–5.1) in a meta-analysis [176].

The SNRIs are generally well tolerated, and adverse events tend to diminish after discontinuation of medication. Nausea is the most common adverse event with SNRIs, with other adverse events including somnolence, dry mouth, constipation, reduced appetite, dizziness, and hyperhidrosis. Elevations of hepatic enzymes, blood pressure, and plasma glucose can rarely occur. Duloxetine is contraindicated in patients with hepatic dysfunction. Withdrawal syndrome was observed in patients receiving venlafaxine. Therefore, venlafaxine should be cautiously tapered. Venlafaxine withdrawal syndrome may resemble a stroke or psychiatric symptoms [182].

Duloxetine can be started at the dose of 20–30 mg daily to avoid nausea and increased to a range of 60–120 mg daily after a 1-week run-in period at lower doses. There is no clear superior benefit of a dose of 120 mg daily over a lower dose. Venlafaxine should be started at a low dose (37.5 mg) and can be increased by 75 mg weekly to a higher dosage (up to 225 mg) than for duloxetine. It generally requires 2–4 weeks to titrate to effectiveness.

Bupropion is a nontricyclic antidepressant that specifically inhibits neuronal noradrenaline reuptake and weakly blocks dopamine reuptake at the presynaptic level. It does not affect other ion channels, muscarinic, or histaminergic receptors. Thus, it tends to be better tolerated than other TCAs [183]. However, the data to support its use for managing neuropathic pain are not sufficient [184, 185]. Bupropion can intensify seizure activity and should be not used in patients with a history of seizures or abrupt alcohol abuse. Duloxetine and bupropion may expedite the metabolism of tamoxifen and careful note should be taken. Doses are 100–150 mg daily initially and can be increased to 450 mg daily. The recommendations of bupropion for the management of neuropathic

cancer pain are not consistent within the existing guidelines [165, 168].

Selective serotonin reuptake inhibitors have limited evidence for their usefulness for neuropathic pain [55, 176].

Anticonvulsants

Anticonvulsants have equal preference with antidepressants as medications for neuropathic cancer pain. Of the anticonvulsants, calcium channel $\alpha_2\delta$ blocking agents (gabapentin, pregabalin) are the most established agents for treating neuropathic pain. Gabapentin and pregabalin are structural analogues of GABA. However, these agents do not affect GABAergic receptors in the neuron but bind to the $\alpha_2\delta$ subunit of calcium channels in presynaptic neuron terminals. Consequently, calcium influx into the neuronal cells is reduced to decrease the release of neurotransmitters. The action mechanism of gabapentin and pregabalin contributes to side effects in the central nervous system, where calcium channels are widely distributed [55].

Both gabapentin and pregabalin have equal effectiveness, few drug interactions, and good tolerability in neuropathic pain. However, pregabalin has a more favourable pharmacokinetic profile than gabapentin, with more rapid titration. Gabapentin is administered three times daily and should be initiated at low doses (100–300 mg) with gradual titration. It can be increased by 300 mg every 1–7 days up to 3,600 mg. Pregabalin can be administered at 150 mg daily initially and increased by 150 mg every 3–7 days up to 600 mg daily. Titration time is shorter than gabapentin. The oral bioavailability of pregabalin is better than that of gabapentin. Pregabalin also has an anxiolytic effect and can be considered as a first-line medication in neuropathic cancer pain patients with anxiety disorder [186]. It can be started at 75–150 mg daily. The NNT of calcium channel $\alpha_2\delta$ blocking anticonvulsants in the management of neuropathic pain is 4.1 (95 % CI 3.6–4.8) [187].

In head-to-head comparison trials, TCAs and calcium channel $\alpha_2\delta$ binding anticonvulsants had similar efficacy [188, 189]. However, TCA had a less favourable safety profile at high doses and in elderly patients [178].

Several studies have confirmed the benefit of a combination of calcium channel $\alpha_2\delta$ binding anticonvulsants with either strong opioids or antidepressants and have supported the rationale of adding another agent, when monotherapy does not have a sufficient analgesic effect [178, 188, 190]. Thus, when cancer patients have partially controlled neuropathic pain with strong opioids, the NCCN guideline recommends antidepressants, anticonvulsants, or both [165].

Older anticonvulsants, such as phenytoin and carbamazepine, have less favourable toxicity profiles than gabapentin and lack supporting evidence for their use in neuropathic pain.

Topical Agents

Topical lidocaine blocks sodium channels on the ectopic peripheral afferent nerve fibres. When patients receive topical applications of lidocaine, reduced ectopic discharges on sensory afferent fibres are believed to be the pain-relieving mechanism. The positive data about topical lidocaine have usually come from studies of postherpetic neuralgia, and lidocaine is approved by the US Food and Drug Administration for use in the management of neuropathic pain.

Placebo-controlled studies have shown that 5 % lidocaine plasters are as effective as pregabalin for neuropathic pain relief with little adverse events in PHN [191–194]. The most common side effects are local irritation without systemic reaction. Lidocaine plaster also could be considered for add-on treatment in patients with a partial response to monotherapy [192]. Topical 5 % lidocaine in patients with localised peripheral neuropathic pain had an NNT of 4.4 (95 % CI 2.5–17) [195]. On the basis of these data, NCCN guidelines recommend lidocaine patches applied to the site of pain in combination with an opioid, antidepressant, and/or anticonvulsant. Up to four patches daily for no more than 12 h within a 24-h period can be applied.

Other Pharmacological Agents

Tramadol is a unique opioid that not only stimulates mu-opioid receptors but also inhibits reuptake of serotonin and norepinephrine at the synapse. However, the binding affinity is relatively weaker than strong opioids to the mu-receptor and lower efficiency in the blocking of serotonin reuptake than SSRIs or SNRIs. Tramadol has relatively rapid analgesic effects in neuropathic pain with an NNT of 3.8 (95 % CI 2.8–6.3) [196]. A small randomised trial documented the beneficial effect of tramadol for neuropathic cancer pain [197]. The adverse events are nausea, constipation, vomiting, dry mouth, and sedation. Tramadol should be used with caution in patients with a history of seizure or depression. It may lower the seizure threshold or cause fatal serotonin syndrome when combined with SNRIs or especially SSRIs. Tramadol should be initiated at a low dose in elderly patients (50 mg once or twice daily) and can be increased gradually up to 400 mg daily. Dose reduction is needed in patients with renal or hepatic dysfunction.

The NMDA receptor plays a key role in central pain sensitisation. Activation of NMDA receptors results in the opening of calcium channels in postsynaptic neurons and consequently causes neuronal hyperexcitability. Given the important roles in neuropathic pain, the NMDA receptor might be fascinating target for controlling neuropathic pain. Common NMDA receptor antagonists include amantadine, ketamine, dextromethorphan, memantine, and riluzole. The effect of NMDA receptor antagonists has been extensively investigated [198]. Despite a large number of studies, the clinical trials have reported mixed results, and there is limited evidence to support wide application of NMDA antagonists in neuropathic pain. Ketamine appears to have the best effectiveness among these agents, but the incidence of adverse events is high [169].

Cannabinoids have potent analgesic effects through stimulating cannabinoid receptors (CBR). Activated CBRs inhibit calcium channels and subsequently reduce the release of neurotransmitters in the neuron terminals. CBR and mu-receptor have been shown to colonise on the same neurons. They also share similar biological effects including strong pain relief, addictive properties, and adverse events of hypothermia, sedation, and hypotension [199]. However, clinical data are not sufficient to warrant the wide use of cannabinoids in neuropathic pain [200–202].

References

1. Baron R. Mechanisms of disease: neuropathic pain – a clinical perspective. Nat Clin Pract Neurol. 2006; 2(2):95–106.
2. Stromgren AS, Groenvold M, Petersen MA, et al. Pain characteristics and treatment outcome for advanced cancer patients during the first week of specialized palliative care. J Pain Symptom Manage. 2004;27(2): 104–13.
3. Merskey H, Bogduk N. Classification of chronic pain: descriptions of chronic pain syndromes and definitions of pain terms. 2nd ed. Seattle: IASP Press; 1994.
4. Max MB. Clarifying the definition of neuropathic pain. Pain. 2002;96(3):406–7; author reply 407–8.
5. Treede RD, Jensen TS, Campbell JN, et al. Neuropathic pain: redefinition and a grading system for clinical and research purposes. Neurology. 2008;70(18):1630–5.
6. International Association for the Study of Pain | IASP taxonomy. 2011. http://www.iasp-pain.org/ AM/Template.cfm?Section=Pain_Defi…isplay. cfm&ContentID=1728. Accessed 20 June 2011.
7. Bruera E, Lawlor P. Cancer pain management. Acta Anaesthesiol Scand. 1997;41(1 Pt 2):146–53.
8. Ochoa JL. Neuropathic pain: redefinition and a grading system for clinical and research purposes. Neurology. 2009;72(14):1282–3.
9. Argyra E. Neuropathic pain in cancer patients. Prevalence and assessment. In: 3rd international congress on neuropathic pain, Athens; 2010.
10. Caraceni A, Portenoy RK. An international survey of cancer pain characteristics and syndromes IASP Task Force on Cancer Pain. International Association for the Study of Pain. Pain. 1999;82(3):263–74.
11. Fainsinger RL, Nekolaichuk CL, Lawlor PG, Neumann CM, Hanson J, Vigano A. A multicenter study of the revised Edmonton Staging System for classifying cancer pain in advanced cancer patients. J Pain Symptom Manage. 2005;29(3):224–37.
12. Bhatnagar S, Mishra S, Roshni S, Gogia V, Khanna S. Neuropathic pain in cancer patients – prevalence and management in a tertiary care anesthesia-run referral clinic based in urban India. J Palliat Med. 2010;13(7): 819–24.
13. Garcia de Paredes ML, del Moral Gonzalez F, Martinez del Prado P, et al. First evidence of oncologic neuropathic pain prevalence after screening 8615 cancer patients. Results of the on study. Ann Oncol. 2011;22(4):924–30.
14. Velasco R, Bruna J. Chemotherapy-induced peripheral neuropathy: an unresolved issue. Neurologia. 2010;25(2):116–31.
15. Quasthoff S, Hartung HP. Chemotherapy-induced peripheral neuropathy. J Neurol. 2002;249(1):9–17.
16. Windebank AJ, Grisold W. Chemotherapy-induced neuropathy. J Peripher Nerv Syst. 2008;13(1):27–46.
17. Farquhar-Smith P. Chemotherapy-induced neuropathic pain. Curr Opin Support Palliat Care. 2011;5(1): 1–7.
18. Reyes-Gibby CC, Morrow PK, Buzdar A, Shete S. Chemotherapy-induced peripheral neuropathy as a predictor of neuropathic pain in breast cancer patients previously treated with paclitaxel. J Pain. 2009;10(11): 1146–50.
19. Urch CE, Dickenson AH. Neuropathic pain in cancer. Eur J Cancer. 2008;44(8):1091–6.
20. Cleeland CS, Bennett GJ, Dantzer R, et al. Are the symptoms of cancer and cancer treatment due to a shared biologic mechanism? A cytokine-immunologic model of cancer symptoms. Cancer. 2003;97(11): 2919–25.
21. Cavaletti G, Marmiroli P. Chemotherapy-induced peripheral neurotoxicity. Nat Rev Neurol. 2010;6(12):657–66.
22. Argyriou AA, Polychronopoulos P, Koutras A, et al. Peripheral neuropathy induced by administration of cisplatin – and paclitaxel-based chemotherapy. Could it be predicted? Support Care Cancer. 2005;13(8):647–51.
23. Cavaletti G, Bogliun G, Marzorati L, et al. Early predictors of peripheral neurotoxicity in cisplatin and paclitaxel combination chemotherapy. Ann Oncol. 2004;15(9):1439–42.
24. Hausheer FH, Schilsky RL, Bain S, Berghorn EJ, Lieberman F. Diagnosis, management, and evaluation of chemotherapy-induced peripheral neuropathy. Semin Oncol. 2006;33(1):15–49.
25. Charo IF, Ransohoff RM. The many roles of chemokines and chemokine receptors in inflammation. N Engl J Med. 2006;354(6):610–21.
26. White FA, Jung H, Miller RJ. Chemokines and the pathophysiology of neuropathic pain. Proc Natl Acad Sci U S A. 2007;104(51):20151–8.
27. Baron R, Binder A, Wasner G. Neuropathic pain: diagnosis, pathophysiological mechanisms, and treatment. Lancet Neurol. 2010;9(8):807–19.
28. Lai J, Hunter JC, Porreca F. The role of voltage-gated sodium channels in neuropathic pain. Curr Opin Neurobiol. 2003;13(3):291–7.
29. Black JA, Nikolajsen L, Kroner K, Jensen TS, Waxman SG. Multiple sodium channel isoforms and mitogen-activated protein kinases are present in painful human neuromas. Ann Neurol. 2008;64(6): 644–53.
30. Siqueira SR, Alves B, Malpartida HM, Teixeira MJ, Siqueira JT. Abnormal expression of voltage-gated sodium channels Nav1.7, Nav1.3 and Nav1.8 in trigeminal neuralgia. Neuroscience. 2009;164(2): 573–7.
31. Cummins TR, Sheets PL, Waxman SG. The roles of sodium channels in nociception: implications for mechanisms of pain. Pain. 2007;131(3):243–57.

32. Ma W, Zhang Y, Bantel C, Eisenach JC. Medium and large injured dorsal root ganglion cells increase TRPV-1, accompanied by increased alpha2C-adrenoceptor co-expression and functional inhibition by clonidine. Pain. 2005;113(3):386–94.

33. Hong S, Wiley JW. Early painful diabetic neuropathy is associated with differential changes in the expression and function of vanilloid receptor 1. J Biol Chem. 2005;280(1):618–27.

34. McKemy DD, Neuhausser WM, Julius D. Identification of a cold receptor reveals a general role for TRP channels in thermosensation. Nature. 2002; 416(6876):52–8.

35. Serra J, Sola R, Quiles C, et al. C-nociceptors sensitized to cold in a patient with small-fiber neuropathy and cold allodynia. Pain. 2009;147(1–3):46–53.

36. Price MP, McIlwrath SL, Xie J, et al. The DRASIC cation channel contributes to the detection of cutaneous touch and acid stimuli in mice. Neuron. 2001; 32(6):1071–83.

37. Baron R, Schattschneider J, Binder A, Siebrecht D, Wasner G. Relation between sympathetic vasoconstrictor activity and pain and hyperalgesia in complex regional pain syndromes: a case–control study. Lancet. 2002;359(9318):1655–60.

38. Ali Z, Raja SN, Wesselmann U, Fuchs PN, Meyer RA, Campbell JN. Intradermal injection of norepinephrine evokes pain in patients with sympathetically maintained pain. Pain. 2000;88(2):161–8.

39. Cavaletti G, Cavalletti E, Oggioni N, et al. Distribution of paclitaxel within the nervous system of the rat after repeated intravenous administration. Neurotoxicology. 2000;21(3):389–93.

40. Screnci D, McKeage MJ, Galettis P, Hambley TW, Palmer BD, Baguley BC. Relationships between hydrophobicity, reactivity, accumulation and peripheral nerve toxicity of a series of platinum drugs. Br J Cancer. 2000;82(4):966–72.

41. Cavaletti G, Fabbrica D, Minoia C, Frattola L, Tredici G. Carboplatin toxic effects on the peripheral nervous system of the rat. Ann Oncol. 1998;9(4):443–7.

42. Topp KS, Tanner KD, Levine JD. Damage to the cytoskeleton of large diameter sensory neurons and myelinated axons in vincristine-induced painful peripheral neuropathy in the rat. J Comp Neurol. 2000;424(4):563–76.

43. Cavaletti G, Gilardini A, Canta A, et al. Bortezomib-induced peripheral neurotoxicity: a neurophysiological and pathological study in the rat. Exp Neurol. 2007;204(1):317–25.

44. Siau C, Xiao W, Bennett GJ. Paclitaxel- and vincristine-evoked painful peripheral neuropathies: loss of epidermal innervation and activation of Langerhans cells. Exp Neurol. 2006;201(2):507–14.

45. Bennett GJ. Pathophysiology and animal models of cancer-related painful peripheral neuropathy. Oncologist. 2010;15 Suppl 2:9–12.

46. Ultenius C, Linderoth B, Meyerson BA, Wallin J. Spinal NMDA receptor phosphorylation correlates with the presence of neuropathic signs following peripheral nerve injury in the rat. Neurosci Lett. 2006;399(1–2):85–90.

47. Hains BC, Saab CY, Klein JP, Craner MJ, Waxman SG. Altered sodium channel expression in second-order spinal sensory neurons contributes to pain after peripheral nerve injury. J Neurosci. 2004;24(20): 4832–9.

48. Luo ZD, Chaplan SR, Higuera ES, et al. Upregulation of dorsal root ganglion (alpha)2(delta) calcium channel subunit and its correlation with allodynia in spinal nerve-injured rats. J Neurosci. 2001;21(6): 1868–75.

49. Woolf CJ, Thompson SW. The induction and maintenance of central sensitization is dependent on N-methyl-D-aspartic acid receptor activation; implications for the treatment of post-injury pain hypersensitivity states. Pain. 1991;44(3):293–9.

50. Pud D, Eisenberg E, Spitzer A, Adler R, Fried G, Yarnitsky D. The NMDA receptor antagonist amantadine reduces surgical neuropathic pain in cancer patients: a double blind, randomized, placebo controlled trial. Pain. 1998;75(2–3):349–54.

51. Okon T. Ketamine: an introduction for the pain and palliative medicine physician. Pain Physician. 2007; 10(3):493–500.

52. Moore KA, Kohno T, Karchewski LA, Scholz J, Baba H, Woolf CJ. Partial peripheral nerve injury promotes a selective loss of GABAergic inhibition in the superficial dorsal horn of the spinal cord. J Neurosci. 2002;22(15):6724–31.

53. Hansson P. Neuropathic pain: clinical characteristics and diagnostic workup. Eur J Pain. 2002;6(Suppl A):47–50.

54. Jensen TS, Gottrup H, Sindrup SH, Bach FW. The clinical picture of neuropathic pain. Eur J Pharmacol. 2001;429(1–3):1–11.

55. Jensen TS, Madsen CS, Finnerup NB. Pharmacology and treatment of neuropathic pains. Curr Opin Neurol. 2009;22(5):467–74.

56. Cassileth BR, Keefe FJ. Integrative and behavioral approaches to the treatment of cancer-related neuropathic pain. Oncologist. 2010;15 Suppl 2: 19–23.

57. Dictionary of cancer terms. http://www.cancer.gov/dictionary. Accessed 26 May 2011.

58. Jaeckle KA. Neurologic manifestations of neoplastic and radiation-induced plexopathies. Semin Neurol. 2010;30(3):254–62.

59. van Es HW. MRI of the brachial plexus. Eur Radiol. 2001;11(2):325–36.

60. Taylor BV, Kimmel DW, Krecke KN, Cascino TL. Magnetic resonance imaging in cancer-related lumbosacral plexopathy. Mayo Clin Proc. 1997;72(9): 823–9.

61. Kori SH. Diagnosis and management of brachial plexus lesions in cancer patients. Oncology (Williston Park). 1995;9(8):756–60; discussion 765.

62. Jaeckle KA, Young DF, Foley KM. The natural history of lumbosacral plexopathy in cancer. Neurology. 1985;35(1):8–15.

63. Hanks G, Cherny NI, Christakis NA, Fallon M, Kaasa S, Portenoy RK, editors. Oxford textbook of palliative medicine. 4th ed. New York: Oxford University Press; 2009.

64. Georgiou A, Grigsby PW, Perez CA. Radiation induced lumbosacral plexopathy in gynecologic tumors: clinical findings and dosimetric analysis. Int J Radiat Oncol Biol Phys. 1993;26(3):479–82.

65. DeAngelis LM. Current diagnosis and treatment of leptomeningeal metastasis. J Neurooncol. 1998; 38(2–3):245–52.

66. Schiff D. Spinal cord compression. Neurol Clin. 2003;21(1):67–86, viii.

67. Bach F, Larsen BH, Rohde K, et al. Metastatic spinal cord compression. Occurrence, symptoms, clinical presentations and prognosis in 398 patients with spinal cord compression. Acta Neurochir (Wien). 1990;107(1–2):37–43.

68. Coleman RE. Clinical features of metastatic bone disease and risk of skeletal morbidity. Clin Cancer Res. 2006;12(20 Pt 2):6243s–9.

69. Penas-Prado M, Loghin ME. Spinal cord compression in cancer patients: review of diagnosis and treatment. Curr Oncol Rep. 2008;10(1):78–85.

70. Murphy DR, Hurwitz EL, Gerrard JK, Clary R. Pain patterns and descriptions in patients with radicular pain: does the pain necessarily follow a specific dermatome? Chiropr Osteopath. 2009;17:9.

71. McDermott RS, Anderson PR, Greenberg RE, Milestone BN, Hudes GR. Cranial nerve deficits in patients with metastatic prostate carcinoma: clinical features and treatment outcomes. Cancer. 2004;101(7): 1639–43.

72. Headache Classification Subcommittee of the International Headache Society. The international classification of headache disorders: 2nd edition. Cephalalgia. 2004;24 Suppl 1:9–160.

73. Metheetrairut C, Brown DH. Glossopharyngeal neuralgia and syncope secondary to neck malignancy. J Otolaryngol. 1993;22(1):18–20.

74. Graus F, Keime-Guibert F, Rene R, et al. Anti-Hu-associated paraneoplastic encephalomyelitis: analysis of 200 patients. Brain. 2001;124(Pt 6):1138–48.

75. Sillevis Smitt P, Grefkens J, de Leeuw B, et al. Survival and outcome in 73 anti-Hu positive patients with paraneoplastic encephalomyelitis/sensory neuronopathy. J Neurol. 2002;249(6):745–53.

76. Kelly JJ, Karcher DS. Lymphoma and peripheral neuropathy: a clinical review. Muscle Nerve. 2005;31(3): 301–13.

77. Graus F, Dalmau J. Paraneoplastic neurological syndromes: diagnosis and treatment. Curr Opin Neurol. 2007;20(6):732–7.

78. Oki Y, Koike H, Iijima M, et al. Ataxic vs painful form of paraneoplastic neuropathy. Neurology. 2007;69(6):564–72.

79. Braik T, Evans AT, Telfer M, McDunn S. Paraneoplastic neurological syndromes: unusual presentations of cancer. A practical review. Am J Med Sci. 2010;340(4): 301–8.

80. Peintinger F, Reitsamer R, Stranzl H, Ralph G. Comparison of quality of life and arm complaints after axillary lymph node dissection vs sentinel lymph node biopsy in breast cancer patients. Br J Cancer. 2003;89(4):648–52.

81. Vilholm OJ, Cold S, Rasmussen L, Sindrup SH. The postmastectomy pain syndrome: an epidemiological study on the prevalence of chronic pain after surgery for breast cancer. Br J Cancer. 2008;99(4):604–10.

82. Gartner R, Jensen MB, Nielsen J, Ewertz M, Kroman N, Kehlet H. Prevalence of and factors associated with persistent pain following breast cancer surgery. JAMA. 2009;302(18):1985–92.

83. Jung BF, Ahrendt GM, Oaklander AL, Dworkin RH. Neuropathic pain following breast cancer surgery: proposed classification and research update. Pain. 2003;104(1–2):1–13.

84. Pluijms WA, Steegers MA, Verhagen AF, Scheffer GJ, Wilder-Smith OH. Chronic post-thoracotomy pain: a retrospective study. Acta Anaesthesiol Scand. 2006;50(7):804–8.

85. Steegers MA, Snik DM, Verhagen AF, van der Drift MA, Wilder-Smith OH. Only half of the chronic pain after thoracic surgery shows a neuropathic component. J Pain. 2008;9(10):955–61.

86. Maguire MF, Ravenscroft A, Beggs D, Duffy JP. A questionnaire study investigating the prevalence of the neuropathic component of chronic pain after thoracic surgery. Eur J Cardiothorac Surg. 2006;29(5): 800–5.

87. Tiippana E, Nilsson E, Kalso E. Post-thoracotomy pain after thoracic epidural analgesia: a prospective follow-up study. Acta Anaesthesiol Scand. 2003;47(4): 433–8.

88. Hamada H, Moriwaki K, Shiroyama K, Tanaka H, Kawamoto M, Yuge O. Myofascial pain in patients with postthoracotomy pain syndrome. Reg Anesth Pain Med. 2000;25(3):302–5.

89. Wildgaard K, Ravn J, Kehlet H. Chronic post-thoracotomy pain: a critical review of pathogenic mechanisms and strategies for prevention. Eur J Cardiothorac Surg. 2009;36(1):170–80.

90. Talmi YP, Horowitz Z, Pfeffer MR, et al. Pain in the neck after neck dissection. Otolaryngol Head Neck Surg. 2000;123(3):302–6.

91. Dijkstra PU, van Wilgen PC, Buijs RP, et al. Incidence of shoulder pain after neck dissection: a clinical explorative study for risk factors. Head Neck. 2001;23(11):947–53.

92. Probstner D, Thuler LC, Ishikawa NM, Alvarenga RM. Phantom limb phenomena in cancer amputees. Pain Pract. 2010;10(3):249–56.

93. Byrne KP. Survey of phantom limb pain, phantom sensation and stump pain in Cambodian and New Zealand amputees. Pain Med. 2011;12(5):794–8.

94. Ramchandran K, Hauser J. Phantom limb pain #212. J Palliat Med. 2010;13(10):1285–6.

95. Weeks SR, Anderson-Barnes VC, Tsao JW. Phantom limb pain: theories and therapies. Neurologist. 2010;16(5):277–86.

96. Hansen DM, Kehlet H, Gartner R. Phantom breast sensations are frequent after mastectomy. Dan Med Bull. 2011;58(4):A4259.

97. Rothemund Y, Grusser SM, Liebeskind U, Schlag PM, Flor H. Phantom phenomena in mastectomized patients and their relation to chronic and acute pre-mastectomy pain. Pain. 2004;107(1–2):140–6.

98. Ovesen P, Kroner K, Ornsholt J, Bach K. Phantom-related phenomena after rectal amputation: prevalence and clinical characteristics. Pain. 1991; 44(3):289–91.

99. Biley FC. Phantom bladder sensations: a new concern for stoma care workers. Br J Nurs. 2001;10(19): 1290–6.

100. Fisher CM. Phantom erection after amputation of penis. Case description and review of the relevant literature on phantoms. Can J Neurol Sci. 1999; 26(1):53–6.

101. Stanton-Hicks M, Janig W, Hassenbusch S, Haddox JD, Boas R, Wilson P. Reflex sympathetic dystrophy: changing concepts and taxonomy. Pain. 1995;63(1):127–33.

102. Harden RN, Bruehl S, Stanton-Hicks M, Wilson PR. Proposed new diagnostic criteria for complex regional pain syndrome. Pain Med. 2007;8(4):326–31.

103. Reuben SS. Preventing the development of complex regional pain syndrome after surgery. Anesthesiology. 2004;101(5):1215–24.

104. Gallo AC, Codispoti VT. Complex regional pain syndrome type II associated with lumbosacral plexopathy: a case report. Pain Med. 2010;11(12):1834–6.

105. Bennett MI, editor. Neuropathic pain. 2nd ed. New York: Oxford University Press; 2010.

106. Johansson S, Svensson H, Denekamp J. Dose response and latency for radiation-induced fibrosis, edema, and neuropathy in breast cancer patients. Int J Radiat Oncol Biol Phys. 2002;52(5):1207–19.

107. Marcus Jr RB, Million RR. The incidence of myelitis after irradiation of the cervical spinal cord. Int J Radiat Oncol Biol Phys. 1990;19(1):3–8.

108. Gibbs IC, Patil C, Gerszten PC, Adler Jr JR, Burton SA. Delayed radiation-induced myelopathy after spinal radiosurgery. Neurosurgery. 2009;64(2 Suppl):A67–72.

109. Lin Z, Wu VW, Ju W, Yamada Y, Chen L. Radiation-induced changes in peripheral nerve by stereotactic radiosurgery: a study on the sciatic nerve of rabbit. J Neurooncol. 2011;102(2):179–85.

110. Hershman DL, Weimer LH, Wang A, et al. Association between patient reported outcomes and quantitative sensory tests for measuring long-term neurotoxicity in breast cancer survivors treated with adjuvant paclitaxel chemotherapy. Breast Cancer Res Treat. 2011;125(3):767–74.

111. Tofthagen C, Overcash J, Kip K. Falls in persons with chemotherapy-induced peripheral neuropathy. Support Care Cancer. 2012;20(3):583–9.

112. Shimozuma K, Ohashi Y, Takeuchi A, et al. Feasibility and validity of the Patient Neurotoxicity Questionnaire during taxane chemotherapy in a phase III randomized trial in patients with breast cancer: N-SAS BC 02. Support Care Cancer. 2009; 17(12):1483–91.

113. Meijer C, de Vries EG, Marmiroli P, Tredici G, Frattola L, Cavaletti G. Cisplatin-induced DNA-platination in experimental dorsal root ganglia neuronopathy. Neurotoxicology. 1999;20(6):883–7.

114. Park SB, Krishnan AV, Lin CS, Goldstein D, Friedlander M, Kiernan MC. Mechanisms underlying chemotherapy-induced neurotoxicity and the potential for neuroprotective strategies. Curr Med Chem. 2008;15(29):3081–94.

115. Krarup-Hansen A, Helweg-Larsen S, Schmalbruch H, Rorth M, Krarup C. Neuronal involvement in cisplatin neuropathy: prospective clinical and neurophysiological studies. Brain. 2007;130(Pt 4):1076–88.

116. Screnci D, McKeage MJ. Platinum neurotoxicity: clinical profiles, experimental models and neuroprotective approaches. J Inorg Biochem. 1999;77(1–2): 105–10.

117. Ozols RF, Bundy BN, Greer BE, et al. Phase III trial of carboplatin and paclitaxel compared with cisplatin and paclitaxel in patients with optimally resected stage III ovarian cancer: a Gynecologic Oncology Group study. J Clin Oncol. 2003;21(17):3194–200.

118. Rosell R, Gatzemeier U, Betticher DC, et al. Phase III randomised trial comparing paclitaxel/carboplatin with paclitaxel/cisplatin in patients with advanced non-small-cell lung cancer: a cooperative multinational trial. Ann Oncol. 2002;13(10):1539–49.

119. de Gramont A, Figer A, Seymour M, et al. Leucovorin and fluorouracil with or without oxaliplatin as first-line treatment in advanced colorectal cancer. J Clin Oncol. 2000;18(16):2938–47.

120. Land SR, Kopec JA, Cecchini RS, et al. Neurotoxicity from oxaliplatin combined with weekly bolus fluorouracil and leucovorin as surgical adjuvant chemotherapy for stage II and III colon cancer: NSABP C-07. J Clin Oncol. 2007;25(16):2205–11.

121. Park SB, Lin CS, Krishnan AV, Goldstein D, Friedlander ML, Kiernan MC. Long-term neuropathy after oxaliplatin treatment: challenging the dictum of reversibility. Oncologist. 2011;16(5):708–16.

122. Baek KK, Lee J, Park SH, et al. Oxaliplatin-induced chronic peripheral neurotoxicity: a prospective analysis in patients with colorectal cancer. Cancer Res Treat. 2010;42(4):185–90.

123. Gamelin E, Gamelin L, Bossi L, Quasthoff S. Clinical aspects and molecular basis of oxaliplatin neurotoxicity: current management and development of preventive measures. Semin Oncol. 2002;29(5 Suppl 15):21–33.

124. Krishnan AV, Goldstein D, Friedlander M, Kiernan MC. Oxaliplatin and axonal Na+ channel function in vivo. Clin Cancer Res. 2006;12(15):4481–4.

125. Vasey PA, Jayson GC, Gordon A, et al. Phase III randomized trial of docetaxel-carboplatin versus paclitaxel-carboplatin as first-line chemotherapy for ovarian carcinoma. J Natl Cancer Inst. 2004;96(22): 1682–91.

126. Seidman AD, Berry D, Cirrincione C, et al. Randomized phase III trial of weekly compared with every-3-weeks paclitaxel for metastatic breast cancer, with trastuzumab for all HER-2 overexpressors and random assignment to trastuzumab or not in HER-2 nonoverexpressors: final results of Cancer and Leukemia Group B protocol 9840. J Clin Oncol. 2008;26(10):1642–9.

127. Belani CP, Ramalingam S, Perry MC, et al. Randomized, phase III study of weekly paclitaxel in combination with carboplatin versus standard every-3-weeks administration of carboplatin and paclitaxel for patients with previously untreated advanced non-small-cell lung cancer. J Clin Oncol. 2008;26(3):468–73.

128. Stemmler HJ, Harbeck N, Groll de Rivera I, et al. Prospective multicenter randomized phase III study of weekly versus standard docetaxel plus doxorubicin (D4) for first-line treatment of metastatic breast cancer. Oncology. 2010;79(3–4):204–10.

129. Stemmler HJ, Harbeck N, Groll de Rivera I, et al. Prospective multicenter randomized phase III study of weekly versus standard docetaxel (D2) for first-line treatment of metastatic breast cancer. Oncology. 2010;79(3–4):197–203.

130. Camps C, Massuti B, Jimenez A, et al. Randomized phase III study of 3-weekly versus weekly docetaxel in pretreated advanced non-small-cell lung cancer: a Spanish Lung Cancer Group trial. Ann Oncol. 2006;17(3):467–72.

131. Smith RE, Brown AM, Mamounas EP, et al. Randomized trial of 3-hour versus 24-hour infusion of high-dose paclitaxel in patients with metastatic or locally advanced breast cancer: National Surgical Adjuvant Breast and Bowel Project Protocol B-26. J Clin Oncol. 1999;17(11):3403–11.

132. Loprinzi CL, Reeves BN, Dakhil SR, et al. Natural history of paclitaxel-associated acute pain syndrome: prospective cohort study NCCTG N08C1. J Clin Oncol. 2011;29(11):1472–8.

133. Verstappen CC, Postma TJ, Hoekman K, Heimans JJ. Peripheral neuropathy due to therapy with paclitaxel, gemcitabine, and cisplatin in patients with advanced ovarian cancer. J Neurooncol. 2003;63(2):201–5.

134. Wickham R. Chemotherapy-induced peripheral neuropathy: a review and implications for oncology nursing practice. Clin J Oncol Nurs. 2007;11(3):361–76.

135. Swain SM, Arezzo JC. Neuropathy associated with microtubule inhibitors: diagnosis, incidence, and management. Clin Adv Hematol Oncol. 2008;6(6):455–67.

136. Hartman A, van den Bos C, Stijnen T, Pieters R. Decrease in motor performance in children with cancer is independent of the cumulative dose of vincristine. Cancer. 2006;106(6):1395–401.

137. Johnson DC, Corthals SL, Walker BA, et al. Genetic factors underlying the risk of thalidomide-related neuropathy in patients with multiple myeloma. J Clin Oncol. 2011;29(7):797–804.

138. Mileshkin L, Prince HM. The troublesome toxicity of peripheral neuropathy with thalidomide. Leuk Lymphoma. 2006;47(11):2276–9.

139. Richardson PG, Briemberg H, Jagannath S, et al. Frequency, characteristics, and reversibility of peripheral neuropathy during treatment of advanced multiple myeloma with bortezomib. J Clin Oncol. 2006;24(19):3113–20.

140. Richardson PG, Sonneveld P, Schuster MW, et al. Bortezomib or high-dose dexamethasone for relapsed multiple myeloma. N Engl J Med. 2005;352(24):2487–98.

141. Richardson PG, Sonneveld P, Schuster MW, et al. Reversibility of symptomatic peripheral neuropathy with bortezomib in the phase III APEX trial in relapsed multiple myeloma: impact of a dose-modification guideline. Br J Haematol. 2009;144(6):895–903.

142. Cavaletti G, Jakubowiak AJ. Peripheral neuropathy during bortezomib treatment of multiple myeloma: a review of recent studies. Leuk Lymphoma. 2010;51(7):1178–87.

143. Badros A, Goloubeva O, Dalal JS, et al. Neurotoxicity of bortezomib therapy in multiple myeloma: a single-center experience and review of the literature. Cancer. 2007;110(5):1042–9.

144. Johnson RW, Wasner G, Saddier P, Baron R. Postherpetic neuralgia: epidemiology, pathophysiology and management. Expert Rev Neurother. 2007;7(11):1581–95.

145. Oxman MN, Levin MJ, Johnson GR, et al. A vaccine to prevent herpes zoster and postherpetic neuralgia in older adults. N Engl J Med. 2005;352(22):2271–84.

146. Johnson RW, Whitton TL. Management of herpes zoster (shingles) and postherpetic neuralgia. Expert Opin Pharmacother. 2004;5(3):551–9.

147. Rasmussen PV, Sindrup SH, Jensen TS, Bach FW. Symptoms and signs in patients with suspected neuropathic pain. Pain. 2004;110(1–2):461–9.

148. Haanpaa M, Attal N, Backonja M, et al. NeuPSIG guidelines on neuropathic pain assessment. Pain. 2011;152(1):14–27.

149. Cruccu G, Sommer C, Anand P, et al. EFNS guidelines on neuropathic pain assessment: revised 2009. Eur J Neurol. 2010;17(8):1010–8.

150. Dobratz MC. Word choices of advanced cancer patients: frequency of nociceptive and neuropathic pain. Am J Hosp Palliat Care. 2008–2009;25(6):469–75.

151. Haanpaa ML, Backonja MM, Bennett MI, et al. Assessment of neuropathic pain in primary care. Am J Med. 2009;122(10 Suppl):S13–21.

152. Baron R, Tolle TR. Assessment and diagnosis of neuropathic pain. Curr Opin Support Palliat Care. 2008;2(1):1–8.

153. Bennett M. The LANSS Pain Scale: the Leeds assessment of neuropathic symptoms and signs. Pain. 2001;92(1–2):147–57.

154. Portenoy R. Development and testing of a neuropathic pain screening questionnaire: ID Pain. Curr Med Res Opin. 2006;22(8):1555–65.

155. Bouhassira D, Attal N, Fermanian J, et al. Development and validation of the Neuropathic Pain Symptom Inventory. Pain. 2004;108(3):248–57.

156. Bastyr 3rd EJ, Price KL, Bril V. Development and validity testing of the neuropathy total symptom

score-6: questionnaire for the study of sensory symptoms of diabetic peripheral neuropathy. Clin Ther. 2005;27(8):1278–94.

157. Reyes-Gibby C, Morrow PK, Bennett MI, Jensen MP, Shete S. Neuropathic pain in breast cancer survivors: using the ID pain as a screening tool. J Pain Symptom Manage. 2010;39(5):882–9.

158. Torrance N, Smith BH, Watson MC, Bennett MI. Medication and treatment use in primary care patients with chronic pain of predominantly neuropathic origin. Fam Pract. 2007;24(5):481–5.

159. Smith BH, Torrance N, Bennett MI, Lee AJ. Health and quality of life associated with chronic pain of predominantly neuropathic origin in the community. Clin J Pain. 2007;23(2):143–9.

160. O'Connor AB, Dworkin RH. Treatment of neuropathic pain: an overview of recent guidelines. Am J Med. 2009;122(10 Suppl):S22–32.

161. O'Connor AB. Neuropathic pain: quality-of-life impact, costs and cost effectiveness of therapy. Pharmacoeconomics. 2009;27(2):95–112.

162. Cook RJ, Sackett DL. The number needed to treat: a clinically useful measure of treatment effect. BMJ. 1995;310(6977):452–4.

163. Attal N, Cruccu G, Baron R, et al. EFNS guidelines on the pharmacological treatment of neuropathic pain: 2010 revision. Eur J Neurol. 2010;17(9): e1113–88.

164. Moulin DE, Clark AJ, Gilron I, et al. Pharmacological management of chronic neuropathic pain – consensus statement and guidelines from the Canadian Pain Society. Pain Res Manag. 2007;12(1):13–21.

165. NCCN Clinical Practical Guidelines for Cancer Pain. http://www.nccn.org/professionals/physician_gls/f_guidelines.asp. Accessed 22 June 2011.

166. Morlion B. Pharmacotherapy of low back pain: targeting nociceptive and neuropathic pain components. Curr Med Res Opin. 2011;27(1):11–33.

167. Gallagher RM. Management of neuropathic pain: translating mechanistic advances and evidence-based research into clinical practice. Clin J Pain. 2006;22(1 Suppl):S2–8.

168. Jost L, Roila F. Management of cancer pain: ESMO Clinical Practice Guidelines. Ann Oncol. 2010;21 Suppl 5:v257–60.

169. For neuropathic pain, optimize opioids. J Support Oncol. 2006;4(2):95–6.

170. Mercadante S, Portenoy RK. Opioid poorly-responsive cancer pain. Part 1: clinical considerations. J Pain Symptom Manage. 2001;21(2):144–50.

171. Mercadante S, Gebbia V, David F, et al. Tools for identifying cancer pain of predominantly neuropathic origin and opioid responsiveness in cancer patients. J Pain. 2009;10(6):594–600.

172. Mercadante S, Bruera E. Opioid switching: a systematic and critical review. Cancer Treat Rev. 2006;32(4):304–15.

173. Hawley P. Nontricyclic antidepressants for neuropathic pain #187. J Palliat Med. 2009;12(5):476–7.

174. Otto M, Bach FW, Jensen TS, Brosen K, Sindrup SH. Escitalopram in painful polyneuropathy: a randomized, placebo-controlled, cross-over trial. Pain. 2008;139(2):275–83.

175. Finnerup NB, Sindrup SH, Jensen TS. The evidence for pharmacological treatment of neuropathic pain. Pain. 2010;150(3):573–81.

176. Saarto T, Wiffen PJ. Antidepressants for neuropathic pain: a Cochrane review. J Neurol Neurosurg Psychiatry. 2010;81(12):1372–3.

177. Dworkin RH, O'Connor AB, Backonja M, et al. Pharmacologic management of neuropathic pain: evidence-based recommendations. Pain. 2007;132(3): 237–51.

178. Gilron I, Bailey JM, Tu D, Holden RR, Jackson AC, Houlden RL. Nortriptyline and gabapentin, alone and in combination for neuropathic pain: a double-blind, randomised controlled crossover trial. Lancet. 2009;374(9697):1252–61.

179. Ray WA, Meredith S, Thapa PB, Hall K, Murray KT. Cyclic antidepressants and the risk of sudden cardiac death. Clin Pharmacol Ther. 2004;75(3):234–41.

180. Sindrup SH, Bach FW, Madsen C, Gram LF, Jensen TS. Venlafaxine versus imipramine in painful polyneuropathy: a randomized, controlled trial. Neurology. 2003;60(8):1284–9.

181. Goldstein DJ, Lu Y, Detke MJ, Lee TC, Iyengar S. Duloxetine vs. placebo in patients with painful diabetic neuropathy. Pain. 2005;116(1–2):109–18.

182. Taylor D, Stewart S, Connolly A. Antidepressant withdrawal symptoms-telephone calls to a national medication helpline. J Affect Disord. 2006;95(1–3) :129–33.

183. Dhillon S, Yang LP, Curran MP. Bupropion: a review of its use in the management of major depressive disorder. Drugs. 2008;68(5):653–89.

184. Semenchuk MR, Sherman S, Davis B. Double-blind, randomized trial of bupropion SR for the treatment of neuropathic pain. Neurology. 2001;57(9): 1583–8.

185. Semenchuk MR, Davis B. Efficacy of sustained-release bupropion in neuropathic pain: an open-label study. Clin J Pain. 2000;16(1):6–11.

186. Frampton JE, Foster RH. Pregabalin: in the treatment of generalised anxiety disorder. CNS Drugs. 2006;20(8):685–93; discussion 694–5.

187. Finnerup NB, Otto M, McQuay HJ, Jensen TS, Sindrup SH. Algorithm for neuropathic pain treatment: an evidence based proposal. Pain. 2005;118(3):289–305.

188. Chandra K, Shafiq N, Pandhi P, Gupta S, Malhotra S. Gabapentin versus nortriptyline in post-herpetic neuralgia patients: a randomized, double-blind clinical trial–the GONIP Trial. Int J Clin Pharmacol Ther. 2006;44(8):358–63.

189. Bansal D, Bhansali A, Hota D, Chakrabarti A, Dutta P. Amitriptyline vs. pregabalin in painful diabetic neuropathy: a randomized double blind clinical trial. Diabet Med. 2009;26(10):1019–26.

190. Hanna M, O'Brien C, Wilson MC. Prolonged-release oxycodone enhances the effects of existing

gabapentin therapy in painful diabetic neuropathy patients. Eur J Pain. 2008;12(6):804–13.

191. Baron R, Mayoral V, Leijon G, Binder A, Steigerwald I, Serpell M. Efficacy and safety of 5 % lidocaine (lignocaine) medicated plaster in comparison with pregabalin in patients with postherpetic neuralgia and diabetic polyneuropathy: interim analysis from an open-label, two-stage adaptive, randomized, controlled trial. Clin Drug Investig. 2009;29(4): 231–41.

192. Baron R, Mayoral V, Leijon G, Binder A, Steigerwald I, Serpell M. Efficacy and safety of combination therapy with 5 % lidocaine medicated plaster and pregabalin in post-herpetic neuralgia and diabetic polyneuropathy. Curr Med Res Opin. 2009;25(7): 1677–87.

193. Baron R, Mayoral V, Leijon G, Binder A, Steigerwald I, Serpell M. 5 % lidocaine medicated plaster versus pregabalin in post-herpetic neuralgia and diabetic polyneuropathy: an open-label, non-inferiority two-stage RCT study. Curr Med Res Opin. 2009;25(7): 1663–76.

194. Rehm S, Binder A, Baron R. Post-herpetic neuralgia: 5 % lidocaine medicated plaster, pregabalin, or a combination of both? A randomized, open, clinical effectiveness study. Curr Med Res Opin. 2010; 26(7):1607–19.

195. Wolff RF, Bala MM, Westwood M, Kessels AG, Kleijnen J. 5 % lidocaine-medicated plaster vs other relevant interventions and placebo for post-herpetic

neuralgia (PHN): a systematic review. Acta Neurol Scand. 2011;123(5):295–309.

196. Hollingshead J, Duhmke RM, Cornblath DR. Tramadol for neuropathic pain. Cochrane Database Syst Rev. 2006;(3):CD003726.

197. Arbaiza D, Vidal O. Tramadol in the treatment of neuropathic cancer pain: a double-blind, placebo-controlled study. Clin Drug Investig. 2007;27(1): 75–83.

198. Collins S, Sigtermans MJ, Dahan A, Zuurmond WW, Perez RS. NMDA receptor antagonists for the treatment of neuropathic pain. Pain Med. 2010; 11(11):1726–42.

199. Bushlin I, Rozenfeld R, Devi LA. Cannabinoid-opioid interactions during neuropathic pain and analgesia. Curr Opin Pharmacol. 2010;10(1):80–6.

200. Karst M, Salim K, Burstein S, Conrad I, Hoy L, Schneider U. Analgesic effect of the synthetic cannabinoid CT-3 on chronic neuropathic pain: a randomized controlled trial. JAMA. 2003;290(13): 1757–62.

201. Berman JS, Symonds C, Birch R. Efficacy of two cannabis based medicinal extracts for relief of central neuropathic pain from brachial plexus avulsion: results of a randomised controlled trial. Pain. 2004;112(3):299–306.

202. Rog DJ, Nurmikko TJ, Friede T, Young CA. Randomized, controlled trial of cannabis-based medicine in central pain in multiple sclerosis. Neurology. 2005;65(6):812–9.

Noncancer-Related Pain in Daily Practice

14

Zbigniew (Ben) Zylicz

Abstract

Noncancer-related pain could be experienced by many cancer patients. Many treatments as well as degenerative disorders only distantly related to cancer (e.g. cachexia) may result in persistent, difficult-to-treat pain. Prevalence of this type of pain can be growing as cancer patients tend to live longer with their disease and many of them can be cured, sometimes at the cost of persistent noncancer-related pain. In this chapter, I shall discuss in more details pain that originates from nerve compression due to the atrophy of supporting tissues. This atrophy can be spontaneous as in cachexia, or it may be induced by the frequent and chronic use of corticosteroids, mainly dexamethasone. Another pain problem frequently encountered by patients suffering or cured from cancer is osteoporosis induced by either steroids or opioids. Skin can also get atrophic and is prone to damages, which can be painful and may heal poorly. Specific treatment of noncancer-related pain might help in keeping the opioid and other analgesics doses as low as possible and contribute to better overall pain control and better mobility of the patients.

Keywords

Localised pain • Noncancer-related pain • Skin pain • Nerve compression pain • Osteoporosis

Introduction

Noncancer-related pain is seldom discussed in the texts concerning the treatment of pain in patients with cancer. However, because patients suffering from or surviving cancer are living longer, the noncancer-related pain is increasing and should be taken into account. In this chapter, we will concentrate on pains that are not specific to cancer but may either be preexisting or occur in patients deteriorating physically towards the end of their lives. We shall exclude here pains due to the treatment of cancer, as these have been discussed elsewhere (see Chap. 7). Noncancer-related pain can

Z. Zylicz, MD, PhD
Department of Research and Education,
Hildegard Hospiz, St. Alban Ring 151,
Basel 4020, Switzerland
e-mail: ben.zylicz@hildegard-hospiz.ch

M. Hanna, Z. Zylicz (eds.), *Cancer Pain*,
DOI 10.1007/978-0-85729-230-8_14, © Springer-Verlag London 2013

contribute significantly to the total pain experienced by patients with cancer and cancer survivors (see Chap. 15).

One of the common elements of many non-cancer-related pains is the fact that they are mostly related to the loss of tissue integrity and normal function. Deterioration of tissue elasticity causes compression and/or ischemia of nerves and pain-sensitive tissues. Another common characteristic is relative insensitivity to opioids, which has not been studied systematically.

The lack of a specific diagnosis and the classification of these pains generally as "cancer pains" simply because they occur in patients with cancer, now or in the past, may result in treatment with increasing doses of opioids, excessive toxicity, and, finally, treatment failure. A specific diagnosis may lead to more precise and less toxic treatment.

Pains which will be discussed here are as follows: compression (mono)neuropathies; pain due to muscle wasting and muscle overuse; skin pain due to wounds, scars, and bedsores; and pain due to osteoarthritis, osteoporosis, bone remodelling, and fractures. An important role in the origin of these pains is credited to the widespread use of corticosteroids, especially dexamethasone, towards the end of life, which will be discussed separately.

Compression (Mono)neuropathies

Compression (mono)neuropathies (CMN), sometimes called entrapment neuropathies, are characterised by spontaneous and/or paroxysmal pain felt in the cutaneous or deep distribution of an involved sensory or mixed nerve or corresponding to the anatomical course of the nerve trunk or its branches [1]. Pain may spread into the distribution of other nerves of the same limb and even to corresponding nerves on the opposite side, which suggests central facilitation of pain [2]. The pain due to CMN is more severe with movement and at those points where nerves can become compressed passing through narrow fibro-osseous tunnels or around bony prominences [3]. These areas can be extremely sensitive to palpation, sometimes initiating a pain cascade similar to those seen in trigeminal neuralgia [4]. Spontaneous symptoms

are described as unusual tactile and thermal sensations associated with numbness, tingling, pins and needles, burning, shooting, and electric shock-like sensations.

The paroxysmal pain caused by CMN may be responsible for many so-called "breakthrough" pains encountered in patients with advanced cancer (see Chap. 9) and needs specific diagnosis and treatment. There are no epidemiological studies supporting this notion. Neuropathies affecting only motor nerves may cause painful muscle cramps, which are often seen in motor neuron disease.

Nothing specific is known about the epidemiology of CMN, especially in patients with cancer. Clinical descriptions of CMN have been known for many decades but tend to be forgotten in academic teaching, possibly because the changes are below the radar of modern imaging techniques. Rediscovering these phenomena may lead to improvement in pain control in patients with cancer.

Neuropathic pain (see Chap. 13) can be divided into two different categories. The first is nerve compression or nerve trunk pain [1]. This neurogenic pain has been attributed to increased activity in, as well as abnormal processing of non-nociceptive input from, the nervi nervorum [5]. With time, there may be a progressive loss of small and myelinated nerve fibres [5]. It is unclear how important local inflammation is in this process. Nerves subjected to stress, by either toxicity or pressure, will respond with distal edema [6–8]. Distal edema may cause entrapment of a nerve in a distant anatomically narrow space [3]. In this situation, the stressor may act proximally (e.g., compression of the nerve root due to vertebral fracture), but the pain will be experienced distally in a typical place. Another situation will occur when the nerve is compressed directly in a narrow space, for example, by nerve traction. Here, local inflammation may play an important role.

The other type of neuropathic pain is dysesthetic [1]. Here, there is no inflammation in the damaged nerve, but the pain depends on axonal damage, ectopic axonal discharges, and central sensitisation. This type of pain is discussed extensively in Chap. 13.

In the first type of neuropathic pain, there will be skin hyperalgesia, while in the second, hyperalgesia may be accompanied by allodynia. Relieving the pressure (decompression) on the nerve will result in recovery, while recovery may be problematic or impossible in dysesthetic type of pain. Long-standing pressure may evolve from reversible nerve trunk pain to irreversible dysesthetic pain. Both syndromes may show decreased sensitivity to opioids [9]. We do not know exactly whether nerve compression pain is less sensitive to the drugs typically used in the treatment of neuropathic pain (e.g., tricyclic antidepressants, anticonvulsants).

The symptoms of CMN depend on the kind of nerve impinged. Small, superficial, purely sensory nerves will present with burning pain in a discrete area served by this nerve. Mixed nerves may give paresthesias, loss of muscle function, and sometimes, when long lasting, muscle atrophy. Suprascapular nerve entrapment may give atrophy of supra- and infraspinatus muscles without any pain [10].

Providing there is timely recognition, CMN is usually reversible. Patients with a better prognosis may undergo neurosurgical decompression, while patients in poor general condition will need to rely on nerve blocks or pharmacological treatment. The pain is only partially sensitive to opioids, and higher doses of these drugs are usually needed, especially when NSAIDs are contraindicated. Injection of local anaesthetics and methylprednisolone is another option. It is thought that topically injected methylprednisolone acts not only as a local anti-inflammatory agent but also acts through suppression of ectopic discharges [11] (Table 14.1).

Table 14.1 Compression (mono)neuropathies observed in patients with cancer

Compression neuropathy	Clinical picture	Place of entrapment	Treatment
Greater occipital nerve	One sided or two-sided headache	Between the suboccipital muscles (oblique, semispinalis and trapezius)	Injection of first local anaesthetic and later methylprednisolone steroids (40–80 mg)
Supra-scapular nerve	Pain on compression of the supra-scapular area radiating to the tip of the shoulder, shoulder joint immobility, sometimes picture of "frozen shoulder", atrophy of the supra-and infra-spinatus muscles. May be caused by proximal muscle dystrophy due to dexamethazone.	Suprascapular notch, sometimes gleno-hymeral opening	Injection of the vicinity of the suprascapular notch with a mixture of bupivacaine and methylprednisolone 40–80 mg [13–16]. Gentle physiotherapy to mobilise the shoulder i usually indicated. Occupational therapy adjustment of crutches, wheelchairs, household equipment is necessary
Upper lateral cutaneous nerve of the upper arm (from axillary nerve)	This nerve can be compressed by the axillary nodes/tumours. When axillary nerve is compressed, weakness of the deltoid and Teres minor muscles may be apparent. These muscles may be atrophic. Small patch of hyperalgesia may be noticed on the lateral aspect of the skin covering deltoid muscle.	In the axilla	Continuous block has been tried [17]. Radiotherapy to the axillar nodes is indicated and usually effective.
Intercostal nerves	Hyperalgesia in the whole dermatome suggests root compression due to vertebral metastases. Hyperalgesia in only a part of the dermatome may suggest compression of the respective cutaneous branch by spasm of the paraspinal muscles (posterior cutaneous branch) or by nerve damage accompanying rib fracture	Either in the course of vertebral foramen or at the peripheral trajectory of the nerve.	Radiotherapy to vertebral metastases. Five percent lidocaine patch for 12–16 h per day applied directly to the area of hyperalgesia. Intercostal nerve blockade may be highly effective especially when ultrasound is used [18, 19].

(continued)

Table 14.1 (continued)

Compression neuropathy	Clinical picture	Place of entrapment	Treatment
Ramus cutaneous of the XII subcostal nerve.	Pain on movement experienced in the lower part of the chest as well as in the lateral part of the thigh. In these areas there may be a stroke of hyperalgesia. Hyperalgesia may reach as low as the knee. This pain may be apparent when the patient is forced to lie on one side because of lung or liver pathology. Weight loss only, does not explain the mechanism of this EN. Frequently accompanied by the iliohypogastric nerve EN (see below).	The nerve crosses the iliac crest some 8–10 cm posteriorly from the iliac spina. Hence the tender point there.	Injection of bupivacaine and methylprednisolone to the tender point on the iliac crest will differentiate between the higher (paraspinal?) compression or peripheral compression.
Ramus cutaneous of the iliohypoga stric nerve	A stroke of hyperalgesia below this point may be present. Hyperalgesia of the lateral part of public bone suggests involvement of the whole iliohypogastric nerve.	This nerve crosses the iliac crest some 8 cm posteriorly to the tender point of ramus cutaneous of the XII subcostal nerve.	Injection of bupivacaine and methylprednisolone may differentiate the site of compression (see text). Procedure may be difficult in some patients as they not infrequently accumulate quite a lot of fat in this area.
Superior cluneal nerve	This compression can be due to lonlasting supinal positioning when the patient is confined to bed. However, this nerve can get entrapped in the iliolumbar ligament. Hyperalesia of the upper medial area of the buttock may be observed.	7–8 cm from the median line, at the level of L5 processus spinosus.	Injection of bupivacaine and methylprednisolone may be helpful. However, when the points are symmetrical on both sides one should be careful as the pathology of the lumbar vertebrae may result in similar tender points. Relieving of this pain may destabilise the spine and increase the pain.
Lateral cutaneous nerve of the thigh	Syndrome known as meralgia paraesthetica [20–22]. Pain, tingling or burning sensation is observed in the lateral thigh. Hyperalgesia does not extend as far as the knee. May be result of lying flat in bed. May be bilateral.	The nerve is entrapped under the inguinal ligament, usually 2–3 cm medially and below the iliac spina. Tender point is localised there	Injection of bupivacaine and methylprednisolone to the place of tenderness [23–25]. If bilateral, the clinical should think also of the more proximal entrapment in the spine. Five percent lidocaine patch applied to the area of hyperalgesia may be effective.
Obturator nerve	The patient may complain of pain in a small patch at the medial part of the thigh. Hyperalgesia usually may also be found there. Weakness of the adductor muscles usually confirms the diagnosis [26].	Tender point is localised in the upper part of the obturator foramen, below and lateral from the mons pubis.	Injection of bupivacaine and methylprednisolone to the tender point is usually helpful [27, 28]. Accuracy of this block can be increased by ultrasound. The mechanism of this entrapment in patients with cancer is uncertain, so the paravertebral or pelvic nerve compression should be considered [29].
Painful sacrum	This happens in extremely cachexic patients lying whole day in bed. One or more sacral foramina may be extremely painful suggesting extrapment of the cutaneous sacral nerves. Hyperalgesia in the sacral dermatomes may be present.	One or more sacral foramina.	Inject first bupivacaine and 20–30 min later methylprednisolone. Because of lack of space injection of both drugs together may be extremely painful [30].

Adapted from Zylicz [12]

Muscle Wasting and Overuse

There are many reasons why the muscles in cancer patients may became sore and be the origin of pain. First of all, muscles are subject to wasting due to both metabolic changes and atrophy and to specific processes known as cancer cachexia [31, 32]. Weakened, atrophic muscles tend to develop myofascial trigger points (MTPs) [33]. These are painful spots that may pose a considerable problem to the patient. Ischemia and denervation may also contribute to this process. The presence of MTPs has been only rarely reported in cancer patients. In one study [34], myofascial pain was diagnosed in a considerable number of cancer patients. However, the same authors could not confirm this in a subsequent study [35]. In yet another study, myofascial pain with multiple trigger points developed in 45 % of patients with breast cancer 1 year after mastectomy [36].

Another mechanism for muscle ache may be overuse, for example, by patients with wasted muscles who, against all the odds, want to remain ambulant and independent. These pains due to "overuse" can be sensed not only in the muscles but at their insertions to the bones and in the tendons. Cramped, rigid muscles (contractures) may entrap the nerves piercing them, as is the case with the greater occipital nerve which may be the reason for severe occipital headaches [37, 38].

Treatment of this pain is difficult and muscle cramps are notorious for their severity and lack of response to opioids. Instead, local measures aimed at better blood circulation (massage), nourishment, and improvement of muscle length (stretching) are of greater importance.

Skin Pain

Skin is the largest and most richly innervated organ in the human body. When we talk about pain, most of it will be experienced on the skin surface: part of the pain will originate in the deeper structures and organs and will be projected to the skin, but part will originate directly in the skin. Skin wounds, pressure sores, excoriations, inflammatory infiltrations, areas of dysesthesia, edema, and skin stretch may all cause pain. The pain may be localised to a visibly changed area (as in a wound) but may be more generalised and invisible to the naked eye (as in neuropathic pain).

Skin pain can be significant in malnourished patients with atrophic tissues and in patients suffering dehydration. Loss of elasticity of the skin and underlying tissues may be associated with increased skin sensitivity to pain.

Despite the size of a skin and its significance for pain and suffering, there are no comprehensive data on skin pain. All medical knowledge has been divided into thousands of small and local problems and is treated by many different specialists and general practitioners.

Acute skin pain depends on the activation of primary sensory afferent neurons: the C fibres which are sensitive to inflammation. The peripheral administration of drugs as ointments, gels, and creams can potentially increase drug concentrations locally while leading to lower and nontoxic systemic levels of these drugs, which can be translated into fewer adverse systemic effects and fewer drug interactions. Topical drugs may be applied continuously, and there is usually no need for drug titration. Their absorption is usually reduced through normal, non-inflamed skin.

Primary sensory afferent neurons can be activated by a range of inflammatory mediators such as prostaglandins, bradykinin, ATP, histamine, and serotonin. The sensitisation of the peripheral nerve endings can be exacerbated by prostaglandins. Inhibiting specific receptors or synthesis of the inflammatory agents interacting with these receptors is a potential target for the treatment of skin pain. Peripheral nerve endings also express a variety of inhibitory receptors, such as opioid, alpha-adrenergic, cholinergic, adenosine, and cannabinoid receptors. Agonists to these receptors are seen as potential targets for drug development. At present, four groups of drugs are used successively in the treatment of pain in everyday practice: local anaesthetics, nonsteroidal anti-inflammatory drugs (NSAIDs), opioids, and capsaicin. Less well known and less often used are alpha-adrenergic drugs, antidepressants, and glutamate receptor antagonists. Local formulations have been actively researched of adenosine agonists, cannabinoid agonists, cholinergic ligands, cytokine antagonists, bradykinin antagonists, ATP antagonists, biogenic amine antagonists, neuropeptide antagonists, and agents that alter the activity of nerve growth factor. Skin pain is an attractive market for the pharmaceutical industry, and many new drugs with better or worse results in clinical studies are becoming licensed each year. Given that activation of sensory neurons involves multiple mediators, combinations of agents targeting different mechanisms are another, yet untested possibility. Topical analgesics represent a promising area for future drug development.

Capsaicin and Its Analogues

Skin pain originates in C fibre sensory afferent neurons, which contain multiple neuropeptides such as calcitonin gene-related peptide (CGRP) and substance P (SP) and mediate different types of pain, including neurogenic inflammation, chemogenic pain, and thermoregulation. Capsaicin, a constituent of red pepper, activates these fibres, and at higher doses, used for a longer time desensitises these neurons, making them physically unavailable for excitation. Capsaicin interacts with vanilloid receptors in the skin. This can be used therapeutically in some types of skin pain and itch [39], especially where other therapies have been ineffective. Capsaicin is not pleasant in its use as the first and nearly obligatory adverse effect is burning skin pain. Capsaicin analogues resiniferatoxin and phorbol-related diterpene are promising new drugs with different qualities from the parent drug [40]. Resiniferatoxin is similar in potency for the induction of pain to the parent drug but is much more effective for desensitisation [41]. The optimisation of ligands for the individual vanilloid receptor subclasses should revolutionise this therapeutic area (see Chap. 5).

Local Anaesthetics

One of the groups of drugs most often used for pain control is that of local anaesthetics. These inactivate the sodium channels in the neurons and thus impair pain conductance [40]. They can be used as injections around the painful site (e.g., before surgical procedures) or as ointments and creams (e.g., before the insertion of an IV cannula) [42–44]. Local anaesthetics are less valuable for the treatment of chronic pain as the skin remains numb and there is a considerable problem with skin sensitisation. Unfortunately, local anaesthetics used systemically are quite toxic. A variation on the same subject is the use of 5 % lidocaine-medicated plasters. This therapy is used to treat postherpetic neuralgia [45–47] and diabetic neuropathy [48] and, in palliative care, is frequently used off-license to treat various painful skin conditions. Local anaesthetics do not cause skin numbness as only a minimal amount of the drug is absorbed. The plasters are well tolerated but need to be removed after 12–16 h. In the remaining 8–12 h when they are not wearing the plaster, patients usually remain pain free. Wearing the plaster for the full 24 h leads to rapid skin sensitisation. The systemic toxicity of this type of drug is also very low. Although the plasters are expensive, they appear to be cost-effective, providing they are used for the licensed indications [49, 50]. The plasters have a pleasant cooling effect on the skin, and it is possible that they exercise an intensive placebo effect, which may be especially strong when used for off-label indications.

Topical Nonsteroidal Anti-inflammatory Drugs (NSAIDs)

Another group of drugs used in topical pain control is topical NSAIDs. These drugs, including diclofenac, ibuprofen, and ketoprofen, can be useful when the skin is inflamed and penetration is increased but are quite useless when the skin is intact and impermeable. Topical NSAIDs can be useful in the treatment of painful joints and structures beneath the skin, such as joints, tendons, muscles, and fasciae [51–53]. Another topical NSAID is benzydamine. Its value is usually in the treatment of inflamed mouth mucous membranes [54–57].

Topical Opioids

Topical opioids were thought to be effective in the treatment of painful wounds. Opioid receptors are among others localised at the nerve endings [58, 59], and early reports suggested that very low doses of morphine applied to the skin under occlusion may be helpful in wound pain for as long as 24 h [60, 61]. Normal skin is impermeable to hydrophilic morphine, and thus this treatment is indicated when the skin is broken or inflamed. Topical, in contrast to systemic, opioids do not cause adverse effects, and their tolerance and potency remain the same for months or even years [62], and these made them especially attractive in treatment. However, in a small controlled trial, topical morphine appeared ineffective in the treatment of painful arterial ulcerations [63]. This was probably related to the specific situation where the disease process destroys nerve endings and makes them unavailable for treatment. Also unresolved is the question of whether opioids impair wound healing or not. Studies in ophthalmology have shown that 1 % topical morphine provides effective analgesia and does not interfere with cornea wound healing [64, 65]. It is unclear whether these findings can be extended to the skin. In general, topical opioids play only a minor role in pain control.

Osteoporosis

There are many reasons why patients with cancer and cancer survivors may suffer from osteoporosis-related pain. Firstly, osteoporosis is highly prevalent in cancer [66]. Most commonly, but not exclusively, osteoporosis is found in patients with prostate and breast cancers [67, 68]. Many factors can contribute to osteoporosis. Some of them are hormone deprivation [69, 70], shortage of vitamin D and sunshine [71, 72], and the use of glucocorticoids [73, 74], as well as other drugs such as opioids [75] and heparin [76]. However, no data on low molecular heparins are available yet. Fractionated heparin was not associated with bone loss in pregnancy, and the newer, low molecular fractionated heparins most probably lack this effect [76]. Finally, lack of movement and disuse, so frequent in patients experiencing pain, undoubtedly contribute to the development of osteoporosis and the exacerbation of pain [77].

Osteoporosis may cause pain in many different ways. First, it can make bone unstable and increase tension in the periosteal membrane, but it may also compromise and destroy the nerve fibres innervating bone [78]. Bone destruction and fractures may further exacerbate pain, especially when the fractured bones compress neurological structures such as the spinal cord and nerves. It must be said that many osteoporotic vertebral fractures stabilise within weeks and do not cause pain after a while. When the fractures remain unstable, pain is more likely. A lot of pain after osteoporotic fracture is caused by the cramped muscles that stabilise the fracture. Relieving this muscle spasm (e.g., with gentle physiotherapy, warmth) may in short term relieve pain but may at the same time destabilise the fracture and cause pain explosion.

Pain due to osteoporosis, especially when any fractured bones are unstable, is difficult to treat with opioids. Opioids by themselves are known to promote osteoporosis [75]. Bisphosphonates are the drug of choice in both the prevention and treatment of osteoporotic fractures [79, 80]. However, longitudinal use of these drugs has been associated with an increase in atypical femoral fractures [81]. Intervention by an orthopaedic surgeon may help both to prevent and to treat fractures [82]. One potentially useful technique is vertebroplasty, whereby fractured vertebrae are filled with cement. This sometimes causes spectacular improvements. However, the technology is very expensive and requires an experienced interventional radiologist, as the most feared complication of the therapy is leakage of cement into the spinal canal [83]. Despite recent clinical trials not confirming the benefits of vertebroplasty [84], a systematic review of vertebroplasty in cancer patients has shown that this technology has the potential to cause significant pain intensity reduction (47–87 %), which needs to be weighed against the risk (2 %) of serious complications [85]. However, many patients with advanced disease are simply not fit enough to undergo vertebroplasty or extensive surgery.

Dexamethasone

Corticosteroids are frequently used in palliative care [86] for different indications. They have been found to be effective in pain due to spinal cord compression, anorexia, weakness, headache, and nausea and vomiting, with a reduction in symptom intensity being achieved in less than 3 days. If the effects are not clear after this time, corticosteroids should be discontinued. Corticosteroids are less effective in controlling the drowsiness or confusional states associated with advanced illness because of cerebral involvement. The main indication, however, is in their use in cases of increased intracranial pressure, as appears in many brain diseases [87]. Most often, dexamethasone, a fluorinated derivative of cortisone, is used. Fluorination of the molecules renders dexamethasone 20–30 times more potent than cortisone and 7 times more potent than prednisolone. The drug is devoid of mineralocorticoid effects, which makes it very useful as a mainly anti-inflammatory agent. However, fluorination of the molecule is responsible for exacerbation of osteoporosis and atrophy of the adrenals, skin, muscles, and virtually all other tissues [88, 89].

Atrophied tissues may also be the cause of severe pain from the skin as well as from muscles, bones, joints, and other structures. Additionally, atrophy of the adrenals makes patients' dexamethasone dependent, and the discontinuation of dexamethasone results in adrenal failure and death. In recent years, it appears to have been shown that the extent of muscle atrophy (and possibly other atrophies) depends on some genetic factors [90]. Indeed, some patients develop muscle atrophy within weeks after dexamethasone; others may take steroids for many months or even years without noticing many adverse effects. Testosterone may counteract the atrophic effects of dexamethasone [91–93], but clinical studies on large numbers of patients are not yet published. Keeping the dose of dexamethasone as low as possible and early discontinuation of the drug before adrenal atrophy are apparently the key issues in the care of cancer patients. This simple action may prevent a lot of pain later in the course of disease. Discontinuation of corticosteroids in the late stages of disease is only practised in patients who are actually dying and actually are not able to swallow.

Osteoarthritis

Osteoarthritis is very common in elderly and will also be common in patients with cancer or cancer survivors. A full-blown arthritis with joint effusion is rare, probably because patients are all immunosuppressed. However, osteoarthritis can be the result of the paraneoplastic phenomenon or infection [94, 95] which, in turn, will respond to the treatment of the background disease. If left untreated, or as the result of disuse it can atrophy (see above). In very painful large joints (e.g., knee), injection of long-acting corticosteroids can be helpful.

Conclusion

Nonmalignant causes of pain in patients with cancer may be prevalent in those patients who deteriorate during the course of disease. These pains should not be seen as just another type of "cancer pain" but should be specifically diagnosed and treated. Among these nonmalignant pains, tissue degeneration and the nerve compression resulting from it are the main causes of pain. Steroids, especially dexamethasone, are useful in the treatment of many symptoms, but this drug, when used for a long time, is responsible for many types of pain.

References

1. Quintner JL, Bove GM. From neuralgia to peripheral neuropathic pain: evolution of a concept. Reg Anesth Pain Med. 2001;26:368–72.
2. Koltzenburg M, Wall PD, McMahon SB. Does the right side know what the left is doing? Trends Neurosci. 1999;22:122–7.
3. Maigne JY, Maigne R, Guerin-Surville H. Anatomic study of the lateral cutaneous rami of the subcostal and iliohypogastric nerves. Surg Radiol Anat. 1986;8:251–6.

4. Prasad S, Galetta S. Trigeminal neuralgia: historical notes and current concepts. Neurologist. 2009;15:87–94.
5. Schestatsky P, Llado-Carbo E, Casanova-Molla J, Alvarez-Blanco S, Valls-Sole J. Small fibre function in patients with meralgia paresthetica. Pain. 2008;139:342–8.
6. Daemen MA, Kurvers HA, Kitslaar PJ, Slaaf DW, Bullens PH, Van den Wildenberg FA. Neurogenic inflammation in an animal model of neuropathic pain. Neurol Res. 1998;20:41–5.
7. Mosconi T, Kruger L. Fixed-diameter polyethylene cuffs applied to the rat sciatic nerve induce a painful neuropathy: ultrastructural morphometric analysis of axonal alterations. Pain. 1996;64:37–57.
8. Polomano RC, Mannes AJ, Clark US, Bennett GJ. A painful peripheral neuropathy in the rat produced by the chemotherapeutic drug, paclitaxel. Pain. 2001;94:293–304.
9. Dellemijn P. Are opioids effective in relieving neuropathic pain? Pain. 1999;80:453–62.
10. Vorster W, Lange CP, Briet RJ, et al. The sensory branch distribution of the suprascapular nerve: an anatomic study. J Shoulder Elbow Surg. 2008;17:500–2.
11. Johansson A, Bennett GJ. Effect of local methylprednisolone on pain in a nerve injury model. A pilot study. Reg Anesth. 1997;22:59–65.
12. Zylicz Z. Entrapment neuropathies. Adv Pall Med. 2010;9:103–8.
13. McCully SP, Suprak DN, Kosek P, Karduna AR. Suprascapular nerve block results in a compensatory increase in deltoid muscle activity. J Biomech. 2007;40:1839–46.
14. Feigl GC, Anderhuber F, Dorn C, Pipam W, Rosmarin W, Likar R. Modified lateral block of the suprascapular nerve: a safe approach and how much to inject? A morphological study. Reg Anesth Pain Med. 2007;32:488–94.
15. Penn J, Zylicz Z. Could shoulder pain be suprascapular nerve entrapment? Eur J Pall Care. 2006;13:98–100.
16. Taskaynatan MA, Yilmaz B, Ozgul A, Yazicioglu K, Kalyon TA. Suprascapular nerve block versus steroid injection for non-specific shoulder pain. Tohoku J Exp Med. 2005;205:19–25.
17. Fewtrell MS, Sapsford DJ, Herrick MJ, Noble-Jamieson G, Russell RI. Continuous axillary nerve block for chronic pain. Arch Dis Child. 1994;70:54–5.
18. Shibata Y, Nishiwaki K. Ultrasound-guided intercostal approach to thoracic paravertebral block. Anesth Analg. 2009;109:996–7.
19. Ben-Ari A, Moreno M, Chelly JE, Bigeleisen PE. Ultrasound-guided paravertebral block using an intercostal approach. Anesth Analg. 2009;109:1691–4.
20. Seror P, Seror R. Meralgia paresthetica: clinical and electrophysiological diagnosis in 120 cases. Muscle Nerve. 2006;33:650–4.
21. Haim A, Pritsch T, Ben-Galim P, Dekel S. Meralgia paresthetica: a retrospective analysis of 79 patients evaluated and treated according to a standard algorithm. Acta Orthop. 2006;77:482–6.
22. Grossman MG, Ducey SA, Nadler SS, Levy AS. Meralgia paresthetica: diagnosis and treatment. J Am Acad Orthop Surg. 2001;9:336–44.
23. Tumber PS, Bhatia A, Chan VW. Ultrasound-guided lateral femoral cutaneous nerve block for meralgia paresthetica. Anesth Analg. 2008;106:1021–2.
24. Moucharafieh R, Wehbe J, Maalouf G. Meralgia paresthetica: a result of tight new trendy low cut trousers ('taille basse'). Int J Surg. 2008;6:164–8.
25. Mayne A, Delire V, Collard E, Randour P, Joucken K, Buche M. Possible treatment for meralgia paresthetica after coronary bypass operations. J Thorac Cardiovasc Surg. 1992;104:1489–90.
26. Waldman SD. Obturator neuralgia. In: Atlas of uncommon pain syndromes. Philadelphia: Saunders-Elsevier; 2008.
27. Vasilev SA. Obturator nerve injury: a review of management options. Gynecol Oncol. 1994;53:152–5.
28. Fujiwara Y, Sato Y, Kitayama M, Shibata Y, Komatsu T, Hirota K. Obturator nerve block using ultrasound guidance. Anesth Analg. 2007;105:888–9.
29. Rogers LR, Borkowski GP, Albers JW, Levin KH, Barohn RJ, Mitsumoto H. Obturator mononeuropathy caused by pelvic cancer: six cases. Neurology. 1993;43:1489–92.
30. Lewis M, Hay EM, Paterson SM, Croft P. Local steroid injections for tennis elbow: does the pain get worse before it gets better? Results from a randomized controlled trial. Clin J Pain. 2005;21:330–4.
31. Donohoe CL, Ryan AM, Reynolds JV. Cancer cachexia: mechanisms and clinical implications. Gastroenterol Res Pract. 2011;2011:601434.
32. Fearon K, Strasser F, Anker SD, et al. Definition and classification of cancer cachexia: an international consensus. Lancet Oncol. 2011;12:489–95.
33. Cummings M, Baldry P. Regional myofascial pain: diagnosis and management. Best Pract Res Clin Rheumatol. 2007;21:367–87.
34. Twycross RG, Fairfield S. Pain in far-advanced cancer. Pain. 1982;14:303–10.
35. Twycross R, Harcourt J, Bergl S. A survey of pain in patients with advanced cancer. J Pain Symptom Manage. 1996;12:273–82.
36. Torres Lacomba M, Mayoral del Moral O, Coperias Zazo JL, Gerwin RD, Goni AZ. Incidence of myofascial pain syndrome in breast cancer surgery: a prospective study. Clin J Pain. 2010;26:320–5.
37. Ambrosini A, Vandenheede M, Rossi P, et al. Suboccipital injection with a mixture of rapid- and long-acting steroids in cluster headache: a double-blind placebo-controlled study. Pain. 2005;118:92–6.
38. Afridi SK, Shields KG, Bhola R, Goadsby PJ. Greater occipital nerve injection in primary headache syndromes–prolonged effects from a single injection. Pain. 2006;122:126–9.
39. Mason L, Moore RA, Derry S, Edwards JE, McQuay HJ. Systematic review of topical capsaicin for the treatment of chronic pain. BMJ. 2004;328:991.
40. Sawynok J. Topical and peripherally acting analgesics. Pharmacol Rev. 2003;55:1–20.
41. Iadarola MJ, Mannes AJ. The vanilloid agonist resiniferatoxin for interventional-based pain control. Curr Top Med Chem. 2011;11:2171–9.

42. Vanscheidt W, Sadjadi Z, Lillieborg S. EMLA anaesthetic cream for sharp leg ulcer debridement: a review of the clinical evidence for analgesic efficacy and tolerability. Eur J Dermatol. 2001;11:90–6.

43. Weise KL, Nahata MC. EMLA for painful procedures in infants. J Pediatr Health Care. 2005;19:42–7; quiz 8–9.

44. Lander JA, Weltman BJ, So SS. EMLA and amethocaine for reduction of children's pain associated with needle insertion. Cochrane Database Syst Rev. 2006; (3):CD004236.

45. Wolff RF, Bala MM, Westwood M, Kessels AG, Kleijnen J. 5 % lidocaine-medicated plaster vs other relevant interventions and placebo for post-herpetic neuralgia (PHN): a systematic review. Acta Neurol Scand. 2011;123:295–309.

46. Rehm S, Binder A, Baron R. Post-herpetic neuralgia: 5 % lidocaine medicated plaster, pregabalin, or a combination of both? A randomized, open, clinical effectiveness study. Curr Med Res Opin. 2010;26:1607–19.

47. Garnock-Jones KP, Keating GM. Lidocaine 5 % medicated plaster: a review of its use in postherpetic neuralgia. Drugs. 2009;69:2149–65.

48. Wolff RF, Bala MM, Westwood M, Kessels AG, Kleijnen J. 5 % Lidocaine medicated plaster in painful diabetic peripheral neuropathy (DPN): a systematic review. Swiss Med Wkly. 2010;140:297–306.

49. Liedgens H, Hertel N, Gabriel A, et al. Cost-effectiveness analysis of a lidocaine 5 % medicated plaster compared with gabapentin and pregabalin for treating postherpetic neuralgia: a German perspective. Clin Drug Investig. 2008;28:583–601.

50. Dakin H, Nuijten M, Liedgens H, Nautrup BP. Cost-effectiveness of a lidocaine 5 % medicated plaster relative to gabapentin for postherpetic neuralgia in the United Kingdom. Clin Ther. 2007;29:1491–507.

51. Rovensky J, Micekova D, Gubzova Z, et al. Treatment of knee osteoarthritis with a topical non-steroidal antiinflammatory drug. Results of a randomized, double-blind, placebo-controlled study on the efficacy and safety of a 5 % ibuprofen cream. Drugs Exp Clin Res. 2001;27:209–21.

52. Moore RA. Topical nonsteroidal antiinflammatory drugs are effective in osteoarthritis of the knee. J Rheumatol. 2004;31:1893–5.

53. Biswal S, Medhi B, Pandhi P. Longterm efficacy of topical nonsteroidal antiinflammatory drugs in knee osteoarthritis: metaanalysis of randomized placebo controlled clinical trials. J Rheumatol. 2006;33:1841–4.

54. Kose-Ozkan C, Savaser A, Tas C, Ozkan Y. The development and in vitro evaluation of sustained release tablet formulations of benzydamine hydrochloride and its determination. Comb Chem High Throughput Screen. 2010;13:683–9.

55. Cingi C, Songu M, Ural A, Yildirim M, Erdogmus N, Bal C. Effects of chlorhexidine/benzydamine mouth spray on pain and quality of life in acute viral pharyngitis: a prospective, randomized, double-blind, placebo-controlled, multicenter study. Ear Nose Throat J. 2010;89:546–9.

56. Carlucci G, Iuliani P, Di Federico L. Simultaneous determination of benzydamine hydrochloride and five impurities in an oral collutory as a pharmaceutical formulation by high-performance liquid chromatography. J Chromatogr Sci. 2010;48:854–9.

57. Karavana Hizarcioglu SY, Sezer B, Guneri P, et al. Efficacy of topical benzydamine hydrochloride gel on oral mucosal ulcers: an in vivo animal study. Int J Oral Maxillofac Surg. 2011;40:973–8.

58. Stein C, Schafer M, Machelska H. Attacking pain at its source: new perspectives on opioids. Nat Med. 2003;9:1003–8.

59. Stein C. The control of pain in peripheral tissue by opioids. N Engl J Med. 1995;332:1685–90.

60. Krajnik M, Zylicz Z. Topical morphine for cutaneous cancer pain. Palliat Med. 1997;11:325.

61. Krajnik M, Zylicz Z, Finlay I, Luczak J, van Sorge AA. Potential uses of topical opioids in palliative care–report of 6 cases. Pain. 1999;80:121–5.

62. Stein C, Pfluger M, Yassouridis A, et al. No tolerance to peripheral morphine analgesia in presence of opioid expression in inflamed synovia. J Clin Invest. 1996;98:793–9.

63. Jansen MPM, van der Horst JC, van der Valk PGM, Zylicz Z, van Sorge AA. Lack of analgesic effect from topical morphine in painful arterial leg ulcers. IASP Congress of Pain, Sydney; 2005; 1789:292.

64. Peyman GA, Rahimy MH, Fernandes ML. Effects of morphine on corneal sensitivity and epithelial wound healing: implications for topical ophthalmic analgesia. Br J Ophthalmol. 1994;78:138–41.

65. Stiles J, Honda CN, Krohne SG, Kazacos EA. Effect of topical administration of 1 % morphine sulfate solution on signs of pain and corneal wound healing in dogs. Am J Vet Res. 2003;64:813–8.

66. Reuss-Borst M, Hartmann U, Scheede C, Weiss J. Prevalence of osteoporosis among cancer patients in Germany: prospective data from an oncological rehabilitation clinic. Osteoporos Int. 2011;23:1437–44.

67. Sullivan S, Wagner J, Resnick NM, Nelson J, Perera SK, Greenspan SL. Vertebral fractures and the misclassification of osteoporosis in Men with prostate cancer. J Clin Densitom. 2011;14:348–53.

68. Kalder M, Jager C, Seker-Pektas B, Dinas K, Kyvernitakis I, Hadji P. Breast cancer and bone mineral density: the Marburg breast cancer and osteoporosis trial (MABOT II). Climacteric. 2011;14:352–61.

69. VanderWalde A, Hurria A. Aging and osteoporosis in breast and prostate cancer. CA Cancer J Clin. 2011;61:139–56.

70. Kilbreath S, Refshauge KM, Beith J, et al. Prevention of osteoporosis as a consequence of aromatase inhibitor therapy in postmenopausal women with early breast cancer: rationale and design of a randomized controlled trial. Contemp Clin Trials. 2011;32:704–9.

71. The sunshine D-lemma. Sunlight causes skin cancer, but it also produces vitamin D, a substance that seems to prevent some types of cancer and possibly other diseases. Harvard health letter/from Harvard Medical School. 2008;33:6–7.

72. Kampman E, Slattery ML, Caan B, Potter JD. Calcium, vitamin D, sunshine exposure, dairy products and colon cancer risk (United States). Cancer Causes Control. 2000;11:459–66.

73. Weinstein RS. Clinical practice. Glucocorticoid-induced bone disease. N Engl J Med. 2011;365:62–70.

74. Rackoff PJ, Rosen CJ. Pathogenesis and treatment of glucocorticoid-induced osteoporosis. Drugs Aging. 1998;12:477–84.

75. Daniell HW. Opioid osteoporosis. Arch Intern Med. 2004;164:338; author reply.

76. Lefkou E, Khamashta M, Hampson G, Hunt BJ. Review: Low-molecular-weight heparin-induced osteoporosis and osteoporotic fractures: a myth or an existing entity? Lupus. 2010;19:3–12.

77. Alexandre C, Vico L. Pathophysiology of bone loss in disuse osteoporosis. Joint Bone Spine. 2011;78:572–6.

78. Sevcik MA, Luger NM, Mach DB, et al. Bone cancer pain: the effects of the bisphosphonate Alendronate on pain, skeletal remodeling, tumor growth and tumor necrosis. Pain. 2004;111:169–80.

79. Brown SA, Guise TA. Cancer treatment-related bone disease. Crit Rev Eukaryot Gene Expr. 2009;19:47–60.

80. Lussier D, Huskey AG, Portenoy RK. Adjuvant analgesics in cancer pain management. Oncologist. 2004;9:571–91.

81. Yli-Kyyny T. Bisphosphonates and atypical fractures of femur. J Osteoporos. 2011;2011:754972.

82. Westesson PL. Vertebroplasty–breakthrough in treatment of back pain. Cranio. 2001;19:225.

83. Al-Nakshabandi NA. Percutaneous vertebroplasty complications. Ann Saudi Med. 2011;31:294–7.

84. Buchbinder R, Osborne RH, Ebeling PR, et al. A randomized trial of vertebroplasty for painful osteoporotic vertebral fractures. N Engl J Med. 2009;361:557–68.

85. Chew C, Craig L, Edwards R, Moss J, O'Dwyer PJ. Safety and efficacy of percutaneous vertebroplasty in malignancy: a systematic review. Clin Radiol. 2011;66:63–72.

86. Mercadante S, Fulfaro F, Casuccio A. The use of corticosteroids in home palliative care. Support Care Cancer. 2001;9:386–9.

87. Twycross R. The risks and benefits of corticosteroids in advanced cancer. Drug Saf. 1994;11:163–78.

88. Lesniewska B, Nowak KW, Malendowicz LK. Dexamethasone-induced adrenal cortex atrophy and recovery of the gland from partial, steroid-induced atrophy. Exp Clin Endocrinol. 1992;100:133–9.

89. Malendowicz LK, Nussdorfer GG, Markowska A, Nowak KW. Analysis of the preventive action of ACTH on dexamethasone-induced adrenocortical atrophy in the rat. Cytobios. 1992;71:191–9.

90. Gonnella P, Alamdari N, Tizio S, Aversa Z, Petkova V, Hasselgren PO. C/EBPbeta regulates dexamethasone-induced muscle cell atrophy and expression of atrogin-1 and MuRF1. J Cell Biochem. 2011;112: 1737–48.

91. Qin W, Pan J, Wu Y, Bauman WA, Cardozo C. Protection against dexamethasone-induced muscle atrophy is related to modulation by testosterone of FOXO1 and PGC-1alpha. Biochem Biophys Res Commun. 2010;403:473–8.

92. Jones A, Hwang DJ, Narayanan R, Miller DD, Dalton JT. Effects of a novel selective androgen receptor modulator on dexamethasone-induced and hypogonadism-induced muscle atrophy. Endocrinology. 2010;151:3706–19.

93. Zhao W, Pan J, Zhao Z, Wu Y, Bauman WA, Cardozo CP. Testosterone protects against dexamethasone-induced muscle atrophy, protein degradation and MAFbx upregulation. J Steroid Biochem Mol Biol. 2008;110:125–9.

94. Hueber AJ, Rech J, Kallert S, et al. Paraneoplastic syndrome, infection or arthritis: difficulties in diagnosis. Int J Clin Pract. 2006;60:1310–2.

95. Morel J, Deschamps V, Toussirot E, et al. Characteristics and survival of 26 patients with paraneoplastic arthritis. Ann Rheum Dis. 2008;67:244–7.

Rehabilitation of Cancer Patients, a Forgotten Need?

15

Roberto Casale and Danilo Miotti

Abstract

Disability due to pain in cancer patients may be physical, cognitive, sensory, emotional, developmental, or a combination of these. Pain-related disability in cancer patients is a multifactorial problem that deserves a multifaceted rehabilitation approach. Disability is an umbrella term, covering impairments, activity limitations, and participation restrictions. Therefore, rehabilitation encompasses a series of treatments with the aim of helping people to reenter society with the best possible skills, to live through their lifespan appropriately, to survive in the face of a disabling pathology, and to overcome its handicaps sufficiently to go home and lead as normal a life as possible for as long as possible. The rehabilitation of a cancer patient can be distinguished into at least three broad components: (i) therapies centred on the recovery/improvement of motor system failure or weakness, (ii) physical therapies mostly addressed at the non-pharmacological control of pain, and (iii) occupational therapies used to promote the patient's empowerment and, possibly, to facilitate the patient's return home and to work. Maintenance of motricity and physical therapies to control pain in the last phase of life and during palliation is to be considered more centred on psychophysical aspects rather than on achieving a real improvement in mobility and pain control.

Keywords

Pain • Disability • Rehabilitation • Cancer • Remission phases

R. Casale, MD, PhD (✉)
Department of Clinical Neurophysiology and Pain
Rehabilitation Unit, Foundation Salvatore Maugeri,
Research and Care Institute,
Rehabilitation Institute of Montescano,
Via per Montescano N°31, Montescano 27040, Italy
e-mail: roberto.casale@fsm.it

D. Miotti, MD
Palliative Care and Pain Therapy Unit,
Department of Palliative Care and Pain Medicine ,
Fondazione Salvatore Maugeri – IRCCS,
Via Boezio 28, Pavia 27100, Italy
e-mail: danilo.miotti@fsm.it

M. Hanna, Z. Zylicz (eds.), *Cancer Pain*,
DOI 10.1007/978-0-85729-230-8_15, © Springer-Verlag London 2013

Introduction

About 650 million people live with disabilities of various types, and the number is rising because of the increase in chronic diseases and other causes such as the ageing population, the increased number of cancer survivors, and their longer life expectancy. Rehabilitation has a key role to play in these cases.

Rehabilitation, in a broad sense, encompasses a series of treatments with the aim of helping people to reenter society with the best possible skills, to live through their lifespan appropriately, to survive in the face of a disabling pathology, and to overcome its handicaps sufficiently to go home and lead as normal a life as possible for as long as possible.

Although this is something fully accepted when dealing with disorders such as disabling neurological pathologies or chronic progressive degenerative diseases, the same concept has not yet been fully accepted and consequently not adequately tackled in the setting of cancer-related disability. Indeed, only in 2004 did the rehabilitation of cancer pain gain recognition as an essential part of patients' care (NICE 2004) [1]. Despite this strong position, rehabilitation services are quite often excluded from the management of cancer patients. Indeed, even in the Sheffield model, rehabilitation is considered only as supportive care not reflecting the fact that disability is the major problem in cancer survivors [2].

Pain-Related Disability in Cancer Patients

Disability in cancer patients may be physical, cognitive, sensory, emotional, developmental, or a combination of these. Therefore, disability in cancer patients is a multifactorial problem that deserves a multifaceted approach. Moreover, disability is an umbrella term, covering impairments, activity limitations, and participation restrictions. Impairment in cancer patients is mainly due to the cancer itself and is a problem of body function or structure, while activity limitation and difficulties encountered by an

individual in executing a task or action can have a more complex origin depending not only on the disease itself but also on environmental and external factors; participation restriction is a problem experienced by an individual involved in life situations. Thus, disability is a complex phenomenon, reflecting an interaction between features of a person's body and features of the society in which he or she lives [3]. The rehabilitation of cancer patients must take all these aspects into account.

Disability derives not only from cancer itself but also from its treatments and, more frequently, from the presence of pain-related syndromes. The neurophysiology of cancer pain is a striking example of the complexity of pain as it involves chemotherapy-induced neuropathic pain; iatrogenic radionecrosis and postoperative pain; inflammatory, ischemic, and compressive phenomena; and direct tumour invasion of tissues including nerves and plexuses with a neuropathic component [4, 5]. All this makes the treatment of cancer pain a complex and sometimes unsuccessful challenge.

In the advanced stages of disease, 40–50 % of patients have moderate to severe pain, whereas 25–30 % have very severe or excruciating pain [6]. Indeed, it is pain more than the cancer itself that profoundly affects quality of life and functional autonomy. Poor pain control is a factor determining the quality of life of cancer patients [7]. Indeed, Turk and coworkers demonstrated that the pain in cancer as well as noncancer patients is associated with a high level of perceived disability and a low level of activity [8].

As far as we know, there are no data in literature on the effect of rehabilitation on the underlying disease. One question that must be asked in order to eliminate confusion and define the true role of rehabilitation in cancer patients is whether rehabilitation is a form of palliation or whether it can have a pivotal role in the "medical" management of such patients. In other words, should maintaining maximal physical efficiency, a good level of participation, a satisfactory quality of life, and non-pharmacological, noninvasive control of pain be considered a curative treatment, or, we repeat, should it be termed palliation?

Rehabilitation and occupational therapy have a key role in the holistic management of a patient in any stage of his or her disease [9]. Possibly, this is the most important point in the management of cancer pain, as rehabilitation should be seen as a series of strategies that can be applied differently to the same patient depending on the natural history of the disease: from treatments to improve or maintain motility and reduce pain by means of physical therapies to a more complex form of rehabilitation within the frame of palliative care management.

The rehabilitation of a cancer patient can be distinguished into at least three broad components: (i) therapies centred on the recovery/improvement of motor system failure or weakness, (ii) physical therapies mostly addressed at the non-pharmacological control of pain, and (iii) occupational therapies used to promote the patient's empowerment and, possibly, to facilitate the patient's return home and to work. Maintenance of motricity and physical therapies to control pain in the last phase of life and during palliation is to be considered more centred on psychophysical aspects rather than on achieving a real improvement in motility and pain control (Table 15.1).

The rehabilitation of cancer patients should be tailored to the individual patient as closely as possible because cancer can affect mobility more than pain and vice versa in a very broad variety of combinations. In other words, rehabilitation should be seen as one of the essential components of an integrated management including etiological treatments, palliative treatments, and specific pain treatments [10] (Fig. 15.1).

Rehabilitation in the Early Stages of Cancer

In the early stage of the disease, impairments, activity limitations, and participation restrictions are almost always related to the perception that being "ill with cancer" necessarily implies that normal daily living activities should be reduced and that pain, an indicator of the hypothetical progression of the cancer, can increase with physical activity. This triggers a cascade of events

Table 15.1 Structure, processes, and rehabilitation outcomes

Structure

The operative characteristics of a rehabilitation service consists of a multidisciplinary team who:

    Work together towards shared goals for each patient

    Involve and educate the patient and his/her family

    Have considerable knowledge and skill

    Are able to tackle most of the problems commonly experienced by patients

Working process

Rehabilitation is a reiterative, active, educational, problem-solving process focused on the behaviour (disability) of the patients and has the following components:

    Evaluation – identification of the nature and extent of the patient's problems and what is needed to resolve them

    Establishment of the objectives

    Interventions consisting of treatments aimed at modifying the state of disability or at maintaining the quality of life of the patient

    Reevaluation – with the aim of monitoring the efficacy of the interventions

Outcome

The aims of the rehabilitation processes are:

    To reduce the disability

    Promote functional recovery

    Facilitate the participation of the patient in social and family life

    Reduce the patient's pain and distress

    Reduce the distress of relatives and caregivers

leading to progressive motor deconditioning and the onset of muscle, bone, and joint pains secondary to this deconditioning. No harmful effects on patients with cancer have been reported from moderate exercise. On the contrary, it has been demonstrated that those who exercised regularly had 40–50 % less fatigue, the primary complaint during treatment [11]. This should be clearly explained to the patient. In this initial phase in which patients often undergo surgery and variably invasive treatments, rehabilitation must not be limited only to counteracting the onset of problems related to limited mobility but must also be used as a preparation for the surgical intervention and applied as early as possible in the postoperative phase. Regular rehabilitation with exercise increases muscle strength, joint

Fig. 15.1 Pain rehabilitation of cancer patients: a puzzle that has to be composed by the clinician

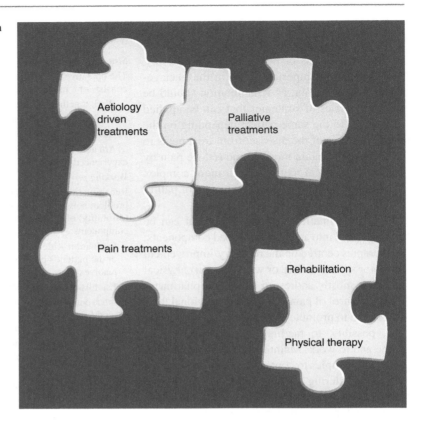

flexibility, and general conditioning, all of which may be impaired by surgery and some therapies. Exercising can help to improve mood, also helping to reduce drug intake against depression that may accompany a cancer diagnosis [12]. One excellent example of this is rehabilitation of the upper limb after radical mastectomy. It is very useful to enter the rehabilitation process early with the aim of preventing a clinical picture of recent onset from becoming chronic through behaviours that cause pain and, therefore, promote lack of activity and inability. In these early phases, physical therapies can be successfully applied not only to maintain physical fitness but also to help control pain alone or in combination with drugs to reduce or postpone the use of morphine or invasive treatments. Under the supervision of a physiotherapist, an effective exercise program can be tailored according to age, sex, and basal physical conditions of the patient and mainly based on an aerobic workout. Examples include walking (outdoors or on a treadmill), soft

jogging, swimming, or bicycling. Yoga and tai chi, though not aerobic, can be recommended as they improve movement and wellness.

However, sometimes the patient does not have enough energy to exercise especially during aggressive chemotherapy or radiating therapy (see "Rehabilitation During Relapses"). In these cases, a moderate daily activity such as gardening or a simple outdoor walking can also provide useful physical workouts.

Finally, exercise helps control weight, as studies have shown that gaining weight during and after treatment raises the risk of a cancer recurrence, particularly breast, colon, and prostate cancers [13].

Rehabilitation During Remission Phases

Remission is the phase in which rehabilitation may be most incisive since it is able to influence any motor impairments, activity limitations, and participation restrictions. In this phase, when

Table 15.2 Physical modalities

Bed, bath, and walking supports
Position instruction
Physical therapy
Energy conservation
Pacing of activities
Massage
Heat and/or ice
Transcutaneous electrical nerve stimulation (TENS)
Acupuncture or acupressure
Ultrasonic stimulation

surgical or chemical treatments have arrested the progress of the disease, the impairment is mainly due to the cancer itself and to the sequelae of the various treatments applied and is a specific problem of body function or structure, while activity limitation and difficulties encountered by an individual in executing a task or action are mainly due to the reduced motor activity and/or bed rest. Fatigue is often a major problem limiting the patient's activity and thereby restricting the patient's participation and involvement in activities of daily life. Rehabilitation interventions include the use of techniques both to control and relieve pain and to improve function. Physiotherapy and occupational therapy are very important in the management of pain in the cancer patient in remission [14]. The rehabilitation program must be tailored to the individual patient and involve the family and other caregivers in order to guarantee a coordinated approach to the objective of empowerment. As for rehabilitation treatment of pain in general, in the context of cancer, the collaboration of the patient is also fundamental. In remission phases, it is essential to consider integrated programs of physiotherapy and cognitive-behavioural therapies in the management of pain and disability [15].

In this phase, all the rehabilitation strategies shown in Table 15.2 can be used.

Rehabilitation During Relapses

In these stages, rehabilitation must be even more carefully "tailored" to the actual conditions of the patient, with ever greater integration of the rehabilitation and cognitive-behavioural techniques and more involvement of the family and caregivers. Relapses are usually characterised by pain and confinement to bed. The rehabilitation must, therefore, be moved to the "bedside" to enable the patient to preserve the greatest motor capacity possible in relation to the clinical state.

Relapses are often associated with pain and fatigue. In this case, the rehabilitation must provide the instrumental analgesic therapy best suited to the type, intensity, and site of the pain.

Rehabilitation during relapses, as well as in the palliative care setting, should be focused on function rather than on the treatment of single physical impairments. Occupational therapy is also useful to identify and tackle all those tasks that the patient considers fundamental to their own daily activities of living and that they are no longer able to carry out: the aim is to avoid pain-aggravating factors and establish vicarious motor strategies. This aspect is relevant, although of less importance, in the terminal phase of the illness.

Cancer treatments including chemotherapy, radiation energy, as well as drugs can induce anaemia and its subsequent fatigue. The symptom often lessens or disappears when treatment ends, but it sometimes lingers. Indeed, along with pain, the sensation of fatigue is by far the most common – and for many, the most distressing symptom and described as draining, unrelenting exhausted sensation that impedes the ability to enjoy life and carry out daily activities.

Depression and anxiety, inactivity, sleep problems, and nutritional deficiencies can also affect the development of fatigue. In this context, rehabilitation should take into account all of these problems.

Rehabilitation in Long-Term Survivors

Rehabilitation in long-term survivors is essentially based on the concept of empowerment in terms of the ability to make decisions about personal circumstances and positive thinking about the possibility of making changes in their physical and emotional status related to their condition of cancer survivors, increasing their positive self-image and overcoming stigma produced by cancer and associated by surgical procedures.

The patient's engagement in meaningful activities is fundamental and must be tailored to improve his or her self-conception and to gain maximum independency. Graded activity should be focused on increasing tolerance of effort, autonomy, and social integration.

Many patients with cancer lose weight and are unable to eat normally due to long treatment-related effects such as persistent nausea and anorexia. In this context, rehabilitation can be also useful to asses eventual problems in deglutition and in the ergonomic approach to possible physical limitation in carrying the food to the mouth or to chew the food.

In long-term survivors as well as in all other phases of the disease, it is important to balance activity and rest as it is important to conserve energy and undertake only the most important activities at the time when their physical energy is enough to complete the task well before exhaustion [16].

Rehabilitation in the Palliative Care Unit

The rehabilitation of patients in palliative care becomes essentially a "maintenance" with both active and passive rehabilitation in bed and, when possible, in the ward. Rehabilitation in this phase can only rarely be conducted, even temporarily, outside the ward. However, an early referral to the rehabilitation unit can lead to a greater possibility of helping the patients to return to their home or to their preferred place of care. Empowerment of the patient is pivotal in obtaining the best possible strategy. Learning ergonomic strategies, support, and operative instructions for the family and caregivers is essential. Physical analgesic therapies do not usually have a concrete application in this phase. In this and in all the preceding stages, rehabilitation techniques and instrumental therapies can be administered in different combinations.

In these patients, physiotherapy has the purpose to maintain joint excursion, muscle tone, and to control and to correct bed posture. Massages and any kind of soft tissue manipulation

can induce a sensation of well-being in these patients. Heat, more than cold, therapies are most frequently applicable in this phase. The most widely used are presented in the table reporting the NCCN Guidelines for Adult Cancer Pain.

A particular mention should be made of rehabilitation in cancer patients who undergo destructive surgery either to remove the cancer itself or to control pain. In these cases, the surgical procedures can be integrated with physically induced, therapeutic nerve lesions produced by chemical agents (alcohol, phenol) or physical ones (radio frequency, cryoablation, thermocoagulation). Preoperative counselling and management of the psychosocial component should be provided in addition to rehabilitation of the motor disability. Almost all of the interventions described can generally be used independently of the stages of the disease. In these cases, the rehabilitation must be differentiated and very carefully tailored to the individual.

Finally, it should be remembered that sometimes so-called complementary or alternative techniques are added to the set of physical and rehabilitation treatments. Of all the complementary techniques used, only acupuncture, herbal medicines (which in any case contain active ingredients), and hypnosis have received some form of validation. Relaxation techniques, use of music, nonmedical massage, and aromatherapy, although not having any scientific basis, are often enjoyed by the patient and can, therefore, be used in a pragmatic manner in the context of rehabilitation to enhance a sensation of well-being without, however, expecting any objectively demonstrable therapeutic effect. Other strategies suggested to be therapeutic, such as homeopathy, not only do not enter within the sphere of rehabilitation but have never been shown to have therapeutic validity in general and in cancer pain in particular [17].

References

1. National Institute for Clinical Excellence. Guidance on cancer services improving supportive and palliative care for adults with cancer. 2004. http://guidance. nice.org.uk/CSGSP/Guidance.
2. Ahmedzai SH, Walsh TD. Palliative medicine and modern cancer care. Semin Oncol. 2001;27:1–6.

3. WHO. International Classification of Functioning, Disability and Health. Geneva: World Health Organization, 2001. http://www.who.int/topics/disabilities/en/

4. Schmidt BL, Hamamoto DT, Simone DA, Wilcox GL. Mechanism of cancer pain. Mol Interv. 2010;10(3): 164–78.

5. Raphael J, Ahmedzai S, Hester J, Urch C, Barrie J, Williams J, et al. Cancer pain: part 1: pathophysiology; oncological, pharmacological, and psychological treatments: a perspective from the British pain society endorsed by the UK association of palliative medicine and the royal college of general practitioners. Pain Med. 2010;11(5):742–64.

6. Van den Beuken-van Everdingen MH, De Rijke JM, Kessels AG, et al. Prevalence of pain in patients with cancer: a systematic review of the past 40 years. Ann Oncol. 2007;18:1437–49.

7. Cheville AL. Pain management in cancer rehabilitation. Arch Phys Med Rehab. 2001;82:S84–7.

8. Turk DC, Sist TC, Okifuji A, Miner MF, Florio G, Harrison P, et al. Adaptation to metastatic cancer pain, regional/local cancer pain and non-cancer pain: role of psychological and behavioral factors. Pain. 1998; 74(2–3):247–56.

9. Tookman AJ, Hopkins K, Sharpen-von-Heussen K. Rehabilitation in palliative medicine. In: Doyle D, Hanks G, Cherny NI, Calman K, editors. Oxford textbook of Palliative Care. 3rd edition, Oxford, UK: Oxford University Press; vol 14. 2004. pp. 1021–32.

10. Payne R. Chronic pain: challenges in the assessment and management of cancer pain. J Pain Symptom Manag. 2000;19:S12–5.

11. Black B, Herr K, Fine P, Sanders S, Tang X, Bergen-Jackson K, et al. The relationships among pain, non-pain symptoms, and quality of life measures in older adults with cancer receiving hospice care. Pain Med. 2011;12(6):880–9.

12. Craft LL, Vaniterson EH, Helenowski IB, Rademaker AW, Courneya KS. Exercise effects on depressive symptoms in cancer survivors: a systematic review and meta-analysis. Cancer Epidemiol Biomarkers Prev. 2012;21(1):3–19.

13. Davies NJ, Batehup L, Thomas R. The role of diet and physical activity in breast, colorectal, and prostate cancer survivorship: a review of the literature. Br J Cancer. 2011;105 Suppl 1:S52–73.

14. The British Pain Society's. Cancer pain management. 2010. www.britishpainsociety.org/book_cancer_pain. pdf.

15. Swarm R, Abernethy AP, Anghelescu DL, Benedetti C, Blinderman CD, Boston B, et al. NCCN Adult Cancer Pain. J Natl Compr Canc Netw. 2010;8(9):1046–86. http://www.nccn.org/professionals/physician_gls/ pdf/pain.pdf

16. Levy MH, Adolph MD, Back A, Block S, Codada SN, Dalal S, et al. Palliative care. NCCN (National Comprehensive Cancer Network). J Natl Compr Canc Netw. 2012;10(10):1284–309. http://www.nccn.org/professionals/physician_gls/pdf/fatigue.pdf

17. Milazzo S, Ernst E. Newspaper coverage of complementary and alternative therapies for cancer–UK 2002–2004. Support Care Cancer. 2006;14(9): 885–9.

Psychosocial Aspects of Cancer Pain

16

Marijana Braš and Veljko Đorđević

Abstract

Pain is one of the most common and distressing symptoms in cancer patients. Although medications and other methods for cancer pain treatment are available, a significant number of patients suffer from intolerable pain.

Current conceptualisations of cancer pain adopt a biopsychosocial perspective. The patient's emotional experiences, beliefs, and expectations may determine the outcome of treatment and are fully emphasised in the focus of treatment interventions. Complex and disabling pain conditions often require comprehensive pain treatment programs, involving interdisciplinary and multimodal treatment approaches. Psychological/psychiatric aspects have an important place in all phases of treatment, with an important role in research and education. There are many roles that the psychiatrist can perform in the assessment and treatment of patients with cancer pain, and psychological treatment can and should be individually tailored to meet the specific needs of the patient.

Rational polypharmacy is also highly important in the treatment of cancer pain, with antidepressants and anticonvulsants being the most important adjuvant analgesic agents.

Quality of interactions between health professionals and patients, education of professionals about biopsychosocial approaches, communication skills, psychological interventions, and continuing care should all be present. It is also important to help cancer patients communicate more effectively about pain and become more involved in deciding pain management treatment.

Keywords

Total pain • Psychooncology • Depression • Anxiety • Psychotherapy • Antidepressants • Communication skills • Person-centred approach

M. Braš, MD, PhD (biomedicine) (✉) • V. Đorđević, MD, PhD
Department of Psychological Medicine,
University of Zagreb, School of Medicine,
Centre for Palliative Medicine, Medical Ethics and
Communication Skills, Zagreb 10000, Salata 4
e-mail: marijana.bras@kbc-zagreb.hr;
veljko.djordjevic1@zg.t-com.hr

M. Hanna, Z. Zylicz (eds.), *Cancer Pain*,
DOI 10.1007/978-0-85729-230-8_16, © Springer-Verlag London 2013

Introduction

Pain is one of the most feared and distressing symptoms of cancer [1, 2]. An estimated 90 % of patients with cancer experience at least moderate pain at some point in their illness, and almost half do not achieve adequate pain control [3]. Pain is always a subjective experience that disrupts a cancer patient's life by influencing physical, psychological, social, and spiritual aspects [4]. Uncontrolled pain can also contribute to depression, patient refusal to undertake potentially beneficial therapy, and emotional burdens on caregivers [5–7]. Research has demonstrated that despite the effective analgesic therapy and array of treatment modalities currently available, there has not been a significant reduction in the prevalence of pain in patients with cancer [8, 9]. Pain medications are often underutilised because patients are worried about dependency and side effects [10, 11] and because physicians do not understand the extent of a patient's pain [12].

The changing nature of cancer pain requires constant evaluation and frequently changing therapeutic strategies. The interaction of pain with other symptoms of the disease (fatigue, weakness, nausea, vomiting, constipation, decreased cognitive function) increases the negative effect of the pain and creates a vicious circle that is very difficult to treat successfully. The founder of the modern hospice movement Dame Cicely Saunders coined the term "total pain" to characterise the multidimensional nature of the palliative patient's pain experience to include physical, psychological, social, and spiritual factors. All of these elements are sources of suffering for the patients. This term can also be extrapolated to other chronic pain states [13]. We could translate the term "total pain" into the modern concept of "quality of life"; the improvement of which is the ultimate goal of pain management [14]. Physical pain is a major component of total pain. A few patients may suffer pain that is so intense that no communication is possible. Once pain has been relieved with appropriate analgesics, the patient can gradually find communication with family and caregivers possible. Anxiety about the future, body image alteration, and concerns about dependency on others are very important components of the psychological suffering in patients with cancer pain. Unfortunately, a progressive depression can invade the patient, but the depressive state is largely underestimated by caregivers. Social pain is also often present. Family members do not know how to react, what to say, and are fearful of addressing the patient's real worries. An exclusion from professional and social life often also occurs.

The spiritual dimension of the pain is another important component of suffering. The patient fears death, not so much "the end" but the circumstances around the dying process. Religious certainties need to be reconsidered and newly assimilated by the person, and many difficult questions are brought forward, such as "Why is this happening to me?" "What did I do to displease God?". It is clear that such massive, total suffering cannot be endured by one single person, and therefore, patients need to be supported by a multidisciplinary team.

Studies of the brain in cancer pain play an important role in the rapid development of "personalised medicine" in cancer pain patients because the information on the structure and function of the brain in patients with pain disorders could help in predicting response to specific therapeutic interventions (both pharmacological and psychotherapeutic).

Common Psychological Problems in Patients with Cancer Pain

Psychological aspects and psychosocial interventions in cancer pain treatment are important aspects of psychooncology, a discipline covering the continuum of care from prevention through treatment to survivorship or death and bereavement. In the everyday clinical practice of cancer pain management, it is important to recognise individual strength and coping skills in the patient and their family, the personality structure of the patient and his/her level of distress. Therefore, it is necessary to identify vulnerable individuals through various psychological and social factors and use these factors as predictors of adequate or inadequate adjustment towards the disease and pain.

Psychological consequences of the diagnosis of cancer and various treatment modalities can be significant and debilitating. There are several common psychiatric disorders accompanying and complicating the experience of cancer pain that can be the focus of psychiatric treatment. These include depression, anxiety, adjustment disorders, sleep disorders, somatoform disorders, substance-related disorders, delirium, and dementia. Psychiatrists must also deal with various issues ranging from suicidal ideations, lack of social support, personality disorders, grief, bereavement, spiritual issues, etc. We must note that these disorders may arise in family members too.

Depression and Cancer Pain

A significant number of patients with cancer suffer from depressive disorder. Major depressive disorder is estimated to occur in 10–25 % of patients with cancer. Depressive symptoms range from 7 to 21 % in one systematic review [15] to as high as 58 % in another [16]. During the past two decades, a small body of research has accumulated that suggests a relationship between pain and mood disturbance in patients with cancer. Depressive symptoms and perceived emotional distress are significantly more frequent in pain patients than in patients without pain [17, 18]. Gerbershagen et al. studied health-related quality of life in patients with prostate cancer both with and without pain. They found that depressive symptoms are significantly more frequent in pain patients than in patients without pain [19]. Another study compared patients with and without pain who were matched by site and progression of disease [20]. Patients with pain scored higher on measures of depression as well as anxiety, hostility, and somatisation. For patients with progressive life-threatening diseases, pain can add greatly to the debilitating effects of the disease and foster hopelessness and fear [21].

The negative impact of cancer pain is not culture specific. The presence of depression worsens other medical illnesses, interferes with therapy, and has a causal link to higher pain intensity, longer duration of pain, reduced life control, use of passive coping strategies, and intensive behavioural changes. Depression impairs the ability to communicate, find meaning, and have a functioning family life and drastically impairs a patient's quality of life. It is associated with the aggravation of cancer pain and other symptoms. It is important to note that the highest risk factor of depression in the context of oncologic patients is suicidal behaviour and ideations. It is crucial to understand that depression must not be regarded as a normal reaction and needs to be treated thoroughly.

Anxiety Disorders

There is a high prevalence of treatable anxiety disorders among patients with cancer. Anxiety syndromes, defined by instruments like the Hospital Anxiety and Depression Scales (HADS), are found in 15–28 % [22]. When measured with a semi-structured interview, anxiety syndromes range as follows: generalised anxiety disorder, 1.7–2.3 %; adjustment disorder with anxious mood, 3.9–4.2 %; phobic disorder, 6.9 %; and panic disorder, 1.3 % [23]. Anxiety and pain can be understood within a multidimensional framework that accounts for somatic, emotional, cognitive, and behavioural aspects of these conditions. As two bodily alarms, pain and anxiety are strongly linked, so activities that reduce anxiety can significantly reduce the pain, and analgesic treatment might reduce the anxiety that is intensified by the pain [24]. In patients with cancer pain, the entire spectrum of anxiety disorders is present, including generalised anxiety disorder, adjustment disorder with anxiety symptoms, obsessive-compulsive disorder, phobic disorders, panic disorder, and PTSD. Patients who have cancer or treatment-related pain are more likely to be anxious than cancer patients without pain.

Patients with cancer pain and anxiety cause difficult diagnostic dilemmas because some degree of anxiety is a normal response to having a severe medical illness. Furthermore, the somatic symptoms of anxiety often overlap with symptoms related to underlying disease processes or treatment effects. Fear caused by intolerable pain, resulting in invalidity and low functional capacity, is more present than fear caused by the threat of death. The degree of disruption in a patient's life is often the critical factor in distinguishing normal from maladaptive anxiety. Anxiety strongly influences pain behaviour. Making an accurate diagnosis will help guide anxiety treatment, and screening instruments can facilitate the recognition of those patients in need of further assessment. There are a variety of psychopharmacologic, psychotherapeutic, and complementary/alternative treatments available. A comprehensive approach to care includes these approaches in an individualised way.

Among the chronic emotional reactions, the most common are suffering and demoralisation. Suffering is often used as a synonym of pain, although these terms are quite distinct. Deeper understanding of suffering lies in the paradigm that a human being is a person with integrity and identity. Suffering is not a universal reaction; it is deeply personal and cannot be predicted. Furthermore, suffering as a reaction does not imply an underlying psychiatric disorder.

If suffering is the outward symptom of disintegration of the component parts that make up a "self," we must try to reintegrate the person by using open questions techniques, active listening in order to obtain the patients' life story which may be helpful in reintegration.

Demoralisation is manifested as individual and specific reactions among heavily ill patients, characterised by anxiety and inability to perceive any positive outcome in the future. In the demoralised state there is an inability to plan and cope with the future, while the depressive patient is characterised by both anhedonia and lack of motivation. Skills appropriate for alleviating demoralisation include empathy, open questions methods, the giving of information and encouragement, and adapting appropriate coping mechanisms. Treatment of demoralisation includes the active symptom management of pain and related physical symptoms, examination of role, preservation of dignity and self-worth, acceptance of change, and the restoration of meaning. Interpersonal psychotherapy, dignity-conserving therapy, and meaning-centred psychotherapies are useful applied techniques to restore morale in the seriously ill [25–27].

The Role of a Liaison Psychiatrist in Patients with Chronic Pain

The psychiatrist is an important member of the multidisciplinary team for the management of cancer pain. The liaison psychiatrist has to help other members of the team understand the psychological dimensions of pain in each patient and to educate other health professionals about specific therapeutic interventions that they may implement later on their own. In the assessment of patients, it is extremely important to conduct good psychiatric interviews during one or more meetings. Pain diaries, different scales of pain, other psychological instruments, the evaluation of the experience of the disease, and behaviours associated with pain are all important elements in the process of assessment of pain. It is also important to analyse the response to disease and cancer pain by others and the impact of cancer pain on work, family, and the social functioning of patients [28]. A relationship between patient and therapist that is based on partnership, trust, and empathy is extremely important in ensuring safe and effective treatment. Comorbid psychiatric disorders should be treated by the integrative way, i.e., by the combination of pharmacological agents, and psychotherapeutic and sociotherapeutic interventions.

Psychosocial Interventions

Pain therapy that addresses only one component of the pain experience might be destined to fail. Interventions that address the multidimensional aspect of pain by relieving the patient's physical burden, psychological disturbance, and emotional distress are more likely to lead to long-term benefits. In the last few years, psychological interventions have also emerged as a useful adjunct to pharmacological approaches to cancer pain management. They can enhance patients' sense of self-efficacy in their own abilities to control pain. Increased self-efficacy for pain control has been linked to lower psychological distress, less interference of pain with daily activities, and improved quality of life. Psychological interventions teach patients skills that can be applied to many of the day-to-day challenges of living with persistent pain, such as coping with pain flares, managing emotional reactions to pain (e.g., anxiety, fear, depression), and maintaining an active and rewarding life despite having pain. Psychological interventions and pain medications may have synergistic effects for cancer patients and produce multiple benefits that may not be achieved by pain medication alone. Psychological interventions may offer a viable pain management option for patients who respond poorly or have difficulty tolerating pain medications. In the process of planning the individually tailored psychosocial interventions, it is important to define the patient's personality structure; current issues (the reason for intervention); the patient's situation, i.e., life story; the patient's perception of the cancer and any specific meaning they give it (e.g., if they view it as a punishment or similar); life events or situations associated with the current event; coping mechanisms with distress caused by the disease and pain; modalities of treatment; and finally past behavioural patterns. These elements should all be used as possible predictors for the current issue.

Psychotherapeutic Intervention

A psychotherapeutic intervention includes a further spectrum of strategies that have the shared goal of understanding a patient and raising unspoken problems. These are psychoeducative sessions with the patients, individual and group psychotherapy, consultation with other members of the team, family therapy, and more. Their aim in the treatment process is to alleviate and resolve problems and reach psychological balance. In patients with cancer pain, it is necessary to have both a careful evaluation of indications and a wide choice of tools for psychotherapeutic intervention.

The Psychodynamic Approach

A psychodynamic approach to patients with cancer pain emphasises the importance of individual differences in patients on the basis of their development, intrapsychological conflicts, interpersonal differences, and their level of ability to adapt to a chronic illness. Psychodynamic psychotherapy emphasises the need to search for unconscious conflict that contributes to and supports the development of psychological disorders in therapeutic alliance with the therapist.

Cognitive Behavioural Therapy (CBT)

Cognitive behavioural therapy or supportive counselling involves using therapeutic techniques to help the patient obtain a sense of motivation, better acceptance, and improved self-esteem. The initial task is to assess maladaptive conditions and consequent behavioural patterns. Cognitive behavioural models of chronic pain emphasise the importance of pain-related cognitions and patient-held beliefs affecting pain adjustment [29]. The therapist's role is one of support, acceptance, and facilitation of interaction – this interaction should be directive without being coercive. Pain is rooted in our sociocultural context and belief system [30], and beliefs about cause, control, duration, outcome, and blame are especially important. Although certain cognitions and beliefs may be adaptive and help patients to cope with the experience of pain, others may actually contribute to increased pain and affective distress. Identification of adaptive and maladaptive pain-related beliefs and cognitions might improve our understanding of individual responses to chronic pain and contribute to more effective treatment interventions [31]. The belief that pain is understandable has been associated with better treatment compliance and use of adaptive coping strategies, while the belief that pain is mysterious has been associated with greater use of catastrophising [32]. Several studies have demonstrated the impact of pain cognition on patients' pain experience, disability, distress, nonadherence, and outcome of treatment [33].

Biofeedback, Relaxation Techniques, and Medical Hypnosis

Biofeedback, relaxation techniques, and medical hypnosis are very common components in the treatment of patients with chronic pain; they all share common features and are often combined. All these techniques emphasise the active involvement of patients in treatment and their personal responsibility in this process. Biofeedback can be used to train the patient to relax specific tense muscles, to lessen autonomic arousal, and to promote general relaxation by providing biological information (such as skin temperature) by means of a monitoring device. These devices are used in conjunction with other techniques such as relaxation exercises to achieve the desired effect. The role of biofeedback is limited in pain control, but it can be an adjunct to conventional pain therapy, contributing to helping the patient gain some control over the pain. Another intervention that has been found useful in the treatment of cancer pain is hypnosis. Hypnosis as an adjuvant to other cancer pain treatment is helpful in a significant number of patients. It is a skill that should be taught by a qualified therapist.

Relaxation exercises can be useful in assisting the patient to promote muscle relaxation, improve blood flow to a painful part, as well as to reduce anxiety. Several techniques may be employed including progressive muscle relaxation, rhythmic breathing, and guided imagery. These can be used individually or in combination and should be individually tailored to the patient's needs and preferences. Any of these techniques can be enhanced through the use of music or recorded tapes that take the patient through the process step by step. It is important to choose music or other recordings that the patient finds appealing for them to be successful.

Psychoeducation is an extremely important part of treating patients with cancer pain, being particularly suitable because it can be implemented at all levels (individual, group/through a multimedia presentation) and by all health professionals. During psychoeducation the patient can gradually take control of the situation and learns skills to maintain that control.

The "Family Disease"

A family member's disease affects other members and translates into the "family disease."

After the diagnosis, it is crucial to involve the family as primary caregivers in order to surpass several obstacles such as diet, compliance, and resolving issues concerning possible death or invalidity.

The family has a difficult time with the suffering of one of its members. This is a basis for interventions aiming to reestablish functional relationship patterns in family dynamics.

Palliative Care Units

A recent and welcome development in the care of cancer pain patients is the palliative care unit. It has been observed that when patients enter a palliative care unit (hospice), the control of pain improves significantly. One probable contributing factor is the high priority hospices give to psychosocial and spiritual issues. A palliative care unit is able to provide multidimensional care that requires a multidisciplinary team approach.

The establishment of palliative care units should be encouraged in all communities, and there is a growing emphasis on palliative care as a supportive approach involving pain and symptom management throughout the course of the patient's experience with cancer, not just when the end of life is near and all tumour treatment options have been exhausted.

Psychopharmacotherapy

In patients with cancer pain, the liaison psychiatrist will prescribe psychopharmacological treatment either as adjuvant (additional) analgesic therapy or as a specific therapy for the treatment of psychiatric comorbidity. Compliance to drug therapy (compliance) is an important issue for a large number of patients with cancer pain, particularly the problem of properly taking opioid medications. Medications may have a number of meanings to the patient, and some psychoeducational interventions can contribute to better patient compliance.

The treatment of psychiatric comorbidity disorders includes drugs indicated for those disorders, but one must be very careful of their safety and tolerability. This is especially due to the fact that patients with cancer pain are already suffering from a serious somatic illness and often take a number other drugs with possible adverse interactions [34].

The term "adjuvant analgesics" describes those psychotropic drugs whose primary indication is not pain. However, they act as analgesics in certain conditions, in addition to treatment of psychiatric comorbidity. Psychotropic drugs as adjuvant therapy are becoming an increasingly important group of drugs, useful because they might cause the possible reduction in dose of opioids and other analgesics but also because of their proven efficacy in treating certain painful entities, particularly neuropathic pain and fibromyalgia. Despite the high prevalence of psychiatric disorders among patients with cancer, only a few studies have explored the use of psychopharmacologic agents in treatment. Clinical practice shows the effectiveness of antidepressants for anxiety, adjustment and depression disorders, psychiatric disorders due to a specific drug or general medical condition, as well as for pain management in patients with cancer. Antidepressants reduce potential side effects of (neo) adjuvant therapy such as insomnia and anorexia. While prescribing antidepressants, we must be aware of possible pharmacokinetic interactions and follow the rules of rational polypharmacy. Due to a highly specific response to antidepressants, several lines of therapy must be undertaken to reach a therapeutic response. Generally, these drugs have a good profile of tolerability, and various authors recommend the early use of antidepressants in depressive states. Some antidepressants and mood stabilisers have been proven as analgesics, especially for the neuropathic component of cancer pain, and there is a need for deep knowledge regarding their optimal prescribing where possible unpleasant interactions can be expected, particularly in combination with analgesics. In addition to effects on the pain pathways, comorbid psychiatric disorders may worsen the perception of pain, interfere with ways of coping, and cause additional morbidity. This is why antidepressants reduce pain when it is a symptom of PTSD or depression, as well as reduce depression if it is caused by pain. Antidepressants reduce other symptoms associated with chronic pain (appetite, sleep, etc.) which significantly contribute to overall distress, psychological morbidity, and physical disability [35]. Tricyclic antidepressants (TCA) are often used for neuropathic pain but have many side effects such as sedation, constipation, dry mouth, urinary retention, postural hypotension, tachycardia, and cardiovascular side effects. Selective serotonin reuptake inhibitors (SSRIs) are generally better tolerated and safer than TCAs, but they are not as effective in eliminating chronic pain as TCAs, and their use makes sense only if the pain is a symptom of the psychiatric disorder. Chronic pain syndromes accompanied by depression are much more effectively cured with antidepressants with a dual effect on noradrenergic and serotonergic receptors (venlafaxine, duloxetine, mirtazapine). This has an explanation in the pathophysiology of pain, as these transmitters are important both in the pathogenesis of depression and in the pain perception, due to the descending control of pain. Bupropion (dopamine reuptake inhibitor and NA) has a good analgesic potential of a unique profile of possible side effects and has been proven to be effective in reducing fatigue in cancer patients. Serotonin modulators (trazodone, nefazodone) are useful in treating insomnia with a pronounced analgesic effect [36]. Some anticonvulsants also have analgesic effects for certain categories of neuropathic pain and are useful in treating some psychiatric disorders.

Today, in the treatment of chronic pain, the focus is on the so-called rational polypharmacy.

Communication Skills

One of the key elements to improve cancer pain treatment is the inclusion of the patient in decision-making through communication with health care professionals. Pain management in cancer care could be improved through better physician-patient communication, particularly with respect to encouraging and facilitating patient involvement in discussing their pain experiences, options for pain relief, and concerns about medication. If patients talk more openly about these issues, physicians might gain a better understanding of how to provide more personalised care focused on the patient's unique pain control needs. Through adequate communication we can educate the patient and reinforce his or her active role in treatment. Generally speaking, communication skills have been associated with positive treatment outcomes, including the patients' satisfaction, better compliance, and fewer complaints. Communication is a fundamental part of the physician-patient-family triad, and it is a key for the success of the medical team. Research across other clinical contexts has shown that clinicians give more information, achieve a better understanding of the patient's perspective, are more supportive, and are more accommodating when patients ask questions, express concerns, state their preferences, and make requests [37–39].

Clinician-patient communication skills training promotes person-centred care by all the members of the oncology treatment team. For patients, improved decision-making, adherence to treatments, and overall psychosocial adjustment result from such skill development [40].

Past decades have shown significant efforts to refocus medicine on the person of the patient, the clinician, and the members of the community at large, with a relational emphasis [41–43]. Structural features of the treatment of the person include the coverage of both ill and positive aspects of health, the person's experience and values, and both risk and protective factors. This is achieved through the use of descriptive categories, dimensions, and narratives and the cultivation of patient-family-clinician partnerships. This achieves shared diagnostic understanding and shared commitment to care. What is crucial is a renewed commitment to the clinician-patient relationship, optimising clinical communication and building an effective dialogue among clinicians, patients, and families, while respecting the diversity of their perspectives. Person-centred medicine is to a large extent relationship-centred medicine [44, 45].

Conclusion

Cancer pain is a complex phenomenon which is always personal and associated with the social, cultural, biological, and spiritual legacy of the patient. Although medications and other methods used in cancer pain treatment are available, a significant number of patients suffer from intolerable pain. When evaluating the pain, one must be aware that intensive fear, depression, and fatigue often result in overwhelming pain. Furthermore, the pain itself translates into the family, impairing the caregivers. In patients suffering from comorbid psychiatric disorder, there is higher intensity and prevalence of cancer pain. Optimal pain relief is not possible if all dimensions of "total pain" are not addressed. The concept of "total pain" should be the driving force leading to the standardisation of pain definition, intervention, and evaluation for cancer patients. There are a number of multidisciplinary programs and protocols for treating patients with cancer pain today, in which the liaison psychiatrist has an important place. The primary goal of the multidisciplinary treatment is to improve the patient's level of functioning, while reducing the frequency and intensity of pain, and increase quality of life. The role of the health care professional is based on the ability to help the patient to overcome all these components of total pain, by using empathy, medical knowledge in pain management, and communications skills. Adequate communication skills are prerequisite to overcoming the barriers in cancer pain treatment.

References

1. Bruera E, Kim HN. Cancer pain. JAMA. 2003; 290:2476–9.
2. Foley KM. Advances in cancer pain. Arch Neurol. 1999;56:413–6.
3. Patrick DL, Ferketich SL, Frame PS, et al. National Institutes of Health State-of-the-Science conference statement: symptom management in cancer: pain, depression, and fatigue, July 15–17, 2002. J Natl Cancer Inst. 2003;95:1110–7.
4. Foley KM. Pain assessment and cancer pain syndromes. In: Doyle D, Hanks G, MacDonald N, editors. Textbook of palliative medicine. 2nd ed. Oxford: Oxford University Press; 1998. p. 310–31.
5. Ferrell BR, Grant M, Chan J, Ahn C, Ferrell BA. The impact of cancer pain education on family caregivers of elderly patients. Oncol Nurs Forum. 1995;22:1211–8.
6. Grov EK, Fossa SD, Sorebo O, Dahl AA. Primary caregivers of cancer patients in the palliative phase: a path analysis of variables influencing their burden. Soc Sci Med. 2006;63:2429–39.
7. Higginson IJ, Gao W. Caregiver assessment of patients with advanced cancer: concordance with patients, effect of burden and positivity. Health Qual Life Outcomes. 2008;6:42.
8. Vainio A, Aveinen A. Prevalence of symptoms among patients with advanced cancer: an international collaborative study. J Pain Symptom Manage. 1996;12:3–10.

9. Ahmedzai S. Recent clinical trials of pain control: impact on quality of life. Eur J Cancer. 1995; 31:S2–7.

10. Potter VT, Wiseman CE, Dunn SM, Boyle FM. Patient barriers to optimal cancer pain control. Psychooncology. 2003;12:153–60.

11. Ward SE, Goldberg N, Miller-McCauley V, et al. Patient-related barriers to management of cancer pain. Pain. 1993;52:319–24.

12. Cleeland CS. Barriers to the management of cancer pain. Oncology (Williston Park). 1987;1:19–26.

13. Saunders CM. The management of terminal disease. London: Arnold; 1978.

14. Felce D, Perry J. Quality of life: its definition and measurement. Res Dev Disabil. 1995;16:51–74.

15. Pirl WF. Evidence report on the occurrence, assessment, and treatment of depression in cancer patients. J Natl Cancer Inst Monogr. 2004; (32):32–9.

16. Massie MJ. Prevalence of depression in patients with cancer. J Natl Cancer Inst Monogr. 2004; (32):57–71.

17. Chapman CR, Gavrin J. Suffering: the contributions of persistent pain. Lancet. 1999;353:2233–7.

18. Georgesen J, Dungan JM. Managing spiritual distress in patients with advanced cancer pain. Cancer Nurs. 1996;19:376–83.

19. Gerbershagen HJ, Ozgur E, Straub K, et al. Prevalence, severity, and chronicity of pain and general health-related quality of life in patients with localized prostate cancer. Eur J Pain. 2008;12:339–50.

20. Ahles TA, Blanchard EB, Ruckdeschel JC. Multidimensional nature of cancer pain. Pain. 1983; 17:277–88.

21. Glover J, Dibble SL, Dodd MJ. Mood states of oncology outpatients: does pain make a difference? J Pain Symptom Manage. 1995;10:120–8.

22. Kerrihard T, Breitbart W, Dent R, Strout D. Anxiety in patients with cancer and human immunodeficiency virus. Semin Clin Neuropsychiatry. 1999;4: 114–32.

23. Stark DP, House A. Anxiety in cancer patients. Br J Cancer. 2000;83:1261–7.

24. Symreng I, Fishman SM. Anxiety and pain. In: Pain clinical updates. Settle: International Association for the Study of Pain; 2004. p. 1–6.

25. Breitbart W. Reframing hope: meaning-centered care for patients near the end of life. Interview by Karen S. Heller. J Palliat Med. 2003;6:979–88.

26. Chochinov HM. Dignity-conserving care-a new model for palliative care: helping the patient feel valued. JAMA. 2002;287:2253–60.

27. Donnelly JM, Kornblith AB, Fleishman S, et al. A pilot study of interpersonal psychotherapy by telephone with cancer patients and their partners. Psychooncology. 2000;9:44–56.

28. Braš M, Fingler M, Filaković P. Chronic pain. In: Gregurek R et al., editors. Liaison psychiatry. Psychiatric and psychological problems in somatic medicine (in Croatian). Zagreb: Školska knjiga; 2006. p. 101–12.

29. Meagher RB. Cognitive-behavioral therapy in health psychology. In: Millon T, Green C, Meagher R,

editors. Handbook of clinical health psychology. New York: Plenum Press; 1982.

30. Boothby JL, Thorn BE, Stroud MW, Jensen MP. Coping with pain. In: Gatchel RJ, Turk DC, editors. Psychosocial factors in pain: clinical perspective. New York: Guilford Press; 1999.

31. Lame IE, Peters ML, Vlaeyen JWS, Kleef M, Patijn J. Quality of life in chronic pain is more associated with beliefs about pain, than with pain intensity. Eur J Pain. 2005;9:15–24.

32. Jensen MP, Turner JA, Romano JM, Lawler BK. Relationship of pain specific beliefs to chronic pain adjustment. Pain. 1994;57:361–9.

33. Stroud MW, Thorn BE, Jensen MP, Boothby JL. The relation between pain beliefs, negative thoughts, and psychosocial functioning in chronic pain patients. Pain. 2000;84:347–52.

34. Braš M. Antidepressants in the treatment of chronic pain, in psychooncology and palliative medicine. In: Mihaljević-Peleš A, Šagud M, editors. Antidepressants in clinical practice (in Croatian). Zagreb: Medicinska naklada; 2009. p. 41–54.

35. Leo RJ, Barkin RL. Antidepressant use in chronic pain management: is there evidence of a role for duloxetine? Prim Care Companion J Clin Psychiatry. 2003;5:118–23.

36. Leo RJ. Clinical manual of pain management in psychiatry. Arlington: American Psychiatric Publishing Inc.; 2007.

37. Hines SC, Moss AH, McKenzie JM. Prolong life and prolonging death: communication's role in difficulty dialysis decisions. Health Commun. 1997;9(4): 369–87.

38. Kravitz RL, Epstein RM, Feldman MD, et al. Influence of patients' requests for direct-to-consumer advertised antidepressants: a randomized controlled trial. JAMA. 2005;293:1995–2002.

39. Street Jr RL, Richardson MN, Cox V, Suarez-Almazor ME. (Mis)understanding in patient-health care provider communication about total knee replacement. Arthritis Rheum. 2009;61:100–7.

40. DiMatteo MR, Giordani PJ, Lepper HS, Croghan TW. Patient adherence and medical treatment outcomes: a meta-analysis. Med Care. 2002;40:794–811.

41. Miles A, Loughlin M, Polychronis A. Evidence-based healthcare, clinical knowledge and the rise of personalised medicine. J Eval Clin Pract. 2008;14: 621–49.

42. Miles A. On a medicine for the whole person: away from scientist reductionism and towards the embrace of complex clinical practice. J Eval Clin Pract. 2009;15:941–9.

43. Tasman A. Presidential address: the doctor-patient relationship. Am J Psychiatry. 2000;157:1763–8.

44. Mezzich JE, Snaedal J, Van Weel C, Heath I. Person-centered medicine: a conceptual exploration. Int J Integr Care. 2010;10(Suppl):e002.

45. Mezzich JE, Snaedal J, van Weel C, Botbol M, Salloum IM. Introduction to person-centered medicine: from concepts to practice. J Eval Clin Pract. 2010;17(2):330–2.

Spiritual Care and Pain in Cancer

17

Carlo Leget

Abstract

Cancer pain is a multidimensional phenomenon in which meaning is a central element. Therefore, pain treatment should focus on the whole person, and be given by caregivers who are aware of the healing impact of their role. Spiritual care focuses on the aspect of meaning, purpose, and connectedness in cancer pain. Spiritual care may be religious of nature, but not necessarily so. In the normal development of the spiritual process of cancer patients, six phases can be distinguished: sense of finiteness and mortality, loss of grip, loss of meaning, grief, experience of new meaning, and integration of old and new meaningfulness.

According to a consensus-based guideline on spiritual care published in 2010 in the Netherlands, three levels of spiritual care are distinguished. Spiritual care starts with attention, openness, and attentiveness. Although this is the basis of good care in general, it can become spiritual care if there is trust and willingness to engage with one another on an existential level. Attention may develop into accompaniment which may take different forms, depending on one's personality, background, and profession. Sometimes patients can have a spiritual crisis. Then, referral and intervention by a chaplain of trained psychosocial caregiver is needed.

Keywords

Spiritual • Existential • Religious • Care • Pain • Suffering • Cancer

C. Leget, PhD
Ethics of Care,
University of Humanistic Studies,
Kromme Nieuwegracht 29,
Utrecht 3512 HD,
The Netherlands
e-mail: c.leget@uvh.nl

Introduction

Globally speaking, there are two ways of approaching the relationship between spiritual care and pain caused by cancer. The first takes its starting point at medical care and tries to incorporate the

M. Hanna, Z. Zylicz (eds.), *Cancer Pain*,
DOI 10.1007/978-0-85729-230-8_17, © Springer-Verlag London 2013

spiritual. In the medical world, this is the most common way of working. Cancer is considered to be primarily a physical disease, which requires physical treatment. Of course human beings are more than physical beings, so good care requires good communication and psychosocial support. Sometimes this does involve attention to the spiritual dimension of the process. But the primary focus is on the medical dimension of the process: curative treatment and pain reduction.

The second way of approaching the relationship between spiritual care and cancer pain starts from the opposite direction. According to this approach, having cancer is seen as a life event, an existential issue that affects human beings as meaning-giving subjects. Cancer affects the whole person, with all the dimensions that belong to human life. It confronts one with the universal vulnerability and mortality of human beings. This approach takes its starting point in the spiritual dimension and tries to incorporate the physical story of malignant disease into this bigger picture.

In Tibetan Buddhism, for instance, one's own suffering is interpreted as an opportunity for spiritual development and growth towards becoming a more compassionate and loving human being [1]. In Roman Catholicism, one's pain and suffering are interpreted as opportunities to follow the example of Christ and grow in love towards God and one's neighbours [2]. A patient once told me that she refused to undergo chemotherapy for her breast cancer because she "wanted to understand the story that her body was trying to tell her by confronting her with this disease, instead of suppressing the voice of her body." In each of these three approaches, pain and suffering are interpreted within a larger framework surpassing both the limits of medical science and even life on earth.

Speaking in global schemes may help to remind us that the world can be described and interpreted in different ways, just like the patients we meet have different ways of making sense of what is happening to them. In the medical world, the regular way of interpreting a disease like cancer and all the pain that is involved leads to an instrumental view of spiritual care; spiritual care is seen as positive so long as it is helpful in reducing pain, or making it more bearable, just as psychosocial help is employed to relieve suffering and promote comfort. This instrumental approach, however, is unsatisfying when viewed from within a spiritual framework. From a spiritual perspective, spirituality is seen not as adjuvant to traditional medical care, but as something meaningful in and of itself, and in fact provides an overarching view of the world and the disease.

These two ways of approaching pain in cancer lead us directly to a fundamental feature of spiritual care: Both what counts as "spiritual" and what counts as "good care" depend on the time and culture in which one lives. This also goes for the third subject of this chapter, the concept of pain. Therefore, in this contribution, we will constantly be aware of the importance to clarify keywords like spirituality, pain, and care and develop our insights from there.

Spirituality

Defining spirituality is far from easy. One for the most widespread misconceptions concerning the concept "spiritual" is that it is more or less the same as "religious." The cause of this misunderstanding is clear: In the Western world, institutionalised religion has been the place where spiritual issues have been dealt with for ages – and is still so for many patients. But the world changes, and at present many people in the developed world no longer consider themselves to have any religious affiliations. Many of them, however, do consider themselves to be spiritual beings. Others consider themselves to be religious but dislike the term spiritual. A third group avoids both terms, religion and spirituality, but are struggling with the very same questions that the first group calls spiritual.

Consulting dictionaries, experts, or scientific papers does not seem of much help here. Definitions vary considerably. Some definitions are so elaborate and wide that they seem to cover our entire life [3]. Others are so technical and formal that they raise many questions [4]. Is spirituality then "a sort of giant conceptual sponge, absorbing a lavish and apparently inexhaustible range of items," as one eloquent critic put it [5]? Or is it an essential feature of spirituality to be transcendent and escape from what we can pin down, define, or frame?

In any case, achieving a solid understanding of the subject can be a great challenge for people who are trained in scientific methods that focus on understanding the material dimension of reality by means of reduction and research. Nowhere is the gulf between scientists and scholars, medicine, and the humanities, wider than with regard to the subject of spirituality. What we share with our patients is that the way we approach spirituality depends on the way we interpret the world and live our life. Our concept of spirituality and the words we choose to express it are closely related to our life history. Even experts on the subject cannot escape from this, as discussions about spiritual care show [6].

If we take a pragmatic approach – and this route can also be defended if we take the cultural relativity of our subject seriously – we may take a look at the definition of spiritual care proposed at the Consensus Conference in the United Sates in 2009 [7] or the European working definition that was proposed in 2010 [8]. According to the European working definition, spirituality can be defined as:

> the dynamic dimension of human life that relates to the way persons (individual and community) experience, express and/or seek meaning, purpose and transcendence, and the way they connect to the moment, to self, to others, to nature, to the significant and/or the sacred. (p. 88)

In order to help understand what this formal definition means, a comment is added:
The spiritual field is multidimensional:
Existential challenges (e.g. questions concerning identity, meaning, suffering and death, guilt and shame, reconciliation and forgiveness, freedom and responsibility, hope and despair, love and joy).
Value based considerations and attitudes (what is most important for each person, such as relations to oneself, family, friends, work, things nature, art and culture, ethics and morals, and life itself).

Religious considerations and foundations (faith, beliefs and practices, the relationship with God or the ultimate).

If we try to find the essence of all this, we might say that spirituality is about establishing connections, connections between words and thoughts (meanings), actions (purpose), and connection with that which surpasses our grip (what is "transcendent"). Perhaps Dan Sulmasy is right when he concludes, "One's spirituality may be defined simply as the characteristics and qualities of one's relationship with the transcendent (p.14)" [9].

Consequently, it is easy to see that spiritual issues come to the fore when the normal course of life is suddenly disrupted by a life-threatening disease like cancer. Many connections (future, purpose in life, confidence in one's body, attachment to loved ones) are challenged, and this challenge has destabilising effects. The question is, however, how these spiritual issues are related to pain caused by the malignant disease.

Pain

Is there something like spiritual pain that can be addressed specifically? Is there a spiritual approach to pain next to a physical and psychosocial one? Or should we rather consider pain a multidimensional phenomenon, which always comprises meaning, and thus a spiritual dimension? The answer to these questions is far reaching. It is decisive in knowing whether it is good to split the care for cancer patients and allocate different parts to different professionals.

Any answer to questions like these, however, depends on one's conception of pain. Two important thinkers in the medical world that have had a significant impact on the way many caregivers think about pain and suffering are Dame Cicely Saunders and Eric Cassell. Despite the many differences between the two, a common idea they propose is seeing pain as something that regards the entire person.

The British nurse, social worker, and physician Cicely Saunders has had great influence on new approaches to pain, by introducing the concept of "total pain" [10]. Saunders considered listening to the patient experiences as crucial in order to understand the multifaceted nature of suffering. Her concept of "total pain" incorporates physical, psychological, social, emotional, and spiritual elements [11].

By focusing on the patient as a unique person with a unique biography, she was able to understand the various layers comprising one's experience of pain (what does it mean, e.g., if one is still awaking from nightmares about a war that has been over for more than decennia?). In doing this, she developed a key to unlocking the complexity of the phenomenon. As a result, it became clear that pain should often be addressed using multiple interventions and by more than one discipline.

The New York-based physician Eric Cassell arrives at a similar point of view, with a slightly different terminology, but with a same patient-centred approach [12]. In Cassell's view, physicians are still too focused on pain relief and too little on suffering. Suffering is more than an affliction of the body. It is an affliction of the person. By focusing on the person, physicians can contribute to the relief of suffering – in its entirety – significantly.

Cassell's approach can be summarised in three points. Firstly, the historical dualism of mind and body should be rejected, because it considers suffering as either subjective and thus not truly "real," i.e., not within the domain of medicine, and not identified with bodily pain.

Because of this, the total suffering of an individual (including spiritual pain) is not addressed, and as a consequence, total suffering increases. Instead of the anachronistic dualism between mind and body, Cassell proposes to focus on the person as the subject that one has to deal in order to address pain, rather than specific treatment of a localised disease.

Secondly, suffering can be defined as "the state of severe distress associated with events that threaten the intactness of the person." As with all serious diseases, cancer does threaten the intactness of the person, and as this person is uniquely composed of various elements, the ways in which people suffer are almost infinite.

Cassell lists a number of factors that for each patient co create a unique way of suffering: one's past, life experiences, family, cultural background, roles, relationship with self, political orientation, activities, regular behaviours, relation with one's body, secret life, perceived future and a transcendent dimension. All these aspects of personhood are susceptible to damage and loss, and the way people perceive this is mediated by meaning. There may be, however, contradictions in the different levels of meaning. As Cassell puts it:

> For example, in a patient who was receiving chemotherapy, the word "chemotherapy" could be shown to elicit simultaneously a cognitive meaning that included his beliefs about the cellular mechanism of drug action, the emotion of fear, the body sensation of nausea, and the transcendent feeling that God would protect him. (p. 36)

Cassell's reflections on pain and suffering – originating from his clinical experience, scientific research, and philosophical reflection – are essentially based on taking seriously the complex and unique way people, as meaning-giving creatures, undergo pain.

This leads to the third point he makes: There is only one way of taking good care of the patient and that is by opening up to the patient personally. Cassell puts it very strongly: The physician *is* the treatment. What he means is not that physicians are gurus or more important than nurses, social workers, or chaplains – any health-care professional may stand in this role – but that the active presence of the physician (opening up, listening, looking, touching, being interested, etc.) is a part of the treatment itself.

Care

If the ideas of physicians like Saunders and Cassell are taken seriously, care for patients with cancer becomes more than an effort to fix or repair what has been broken. Care is essentially a relationship between two people, and much of what care is able to achieve – in terms of well-being, comfort, and healing – is dependent on the quality of this relationship [13].

In fact, we now have two reasons why spiritual care for cancer patients should be integrated and embedded into the larger picture of a caring relationship. Firstly, spirituality is a dimension of human life that is related to the way people make sense of what happens to them, which in turn is related to everything they are and do. Secondly, when caregivers focus on their patients as whole persons, they cannot isolate the spiritual dimension from the rest of what constitutes a human person. But what then is the role of the healthcare professional? And what does spiritual care look like?

In 2010, a national consensus-based guideline on spiritual care for patients suffering from cancer was published in the Netherlands, as a common point of reference for caregivers [14]. In this guideline, three levels of spiritual care are distinguished. We will use this guideline as a framework for reflecting on spiritual care.

First Level: Attention

The first, most general, and basic level of spiritual care is attention. Attention is a crucial aspect of care, as we have seen in the previous paragraph. Being attentive enables one to be open to noticing what is important to the patient. The kind of attention that is meant here, however, is more than just being concentrated and focused. Because the spiritual dimension of the process is often beneath the surface of awareness and language, a significant amount of time is required to build the relationship between caregiver and patient. Similarly, this relationship must be based on trust and confidence, in order to allow the patient to feel secure enough to disclose what maybe – at the base level – is concerning them. What is framed as attention in the guideline is closely related to the concept of "presence" – as it is referred to in other writings. Being present is defined as "a shared encounter or encounters marked by intentionality or the deliberate ideation and purposeful action of care that went beyond medical treatment, giving attention to emotional, social, and spiritual needs" [15].

With this, we touch upon an important question: Is it enough to limit spiritual care to cancer patients to what they themselves explicitly formulate as "spiritual pain" or do we have to take it more broadly? In the first case, one could proceed by a tick box, questionnaire approach; in the second case, one would need other strategies. An example from clinical practice, reported by a chaplain in an academic hospital, may help to understand what is at stake here [16]:

> I was asked to visit a woman who had heard the day before that there was no longer any treatment available for her and that she should reckon with the fact that she might die in a couple of months. She said: "I don't know why I asked you to come I don't have any questions." And so we were sitting there. In silence. After a while she thanked me and asked if I could return the next day. During that second encounter she told me that in the silence that we had shared the day before, for the first time she had been given the space to reflect on her coming death and the loneliness that had followed upon the bad news. Physicians, nurses and also relatives, she told me, were mostly busy with practical affairs; because there was a lot to be managed before she could go home to die there....

This example shows that spiritual care can never be reduced to making an inventory of spiritual needs, firstly, because there is a big difference between needs that are felt and needs that are expressed [17] – good care focuses on the whole person including the nonrational and nonverbal parts – and, secondly, because sometimes patients need some additional time, time shared by a sensitive caregiver, to become aware of what is going on in their inner space. That suggests that the quality of the relationship between the patient and the caregiver is a crucial factor for the quality of the spiritual support that can be given. Good patient care is care with patience.

Nevertheless, a number of – sometimes quick – instruments have been developed to focus the attention of caregivers on the spiritual issues of a patient with a life-threatening disease [18]. Some of these instruments explicitly deal with the assessment of spiritual issues [19]. Three of the most widely used instruments for spiritual history taking are known by their acronyms: HOPE [20], FICA [21], and SPIRIT [22], of which the FICA tool is the only one that is validated [23].

These instruments are very short lists of questions that focus on the belief of the patient (personal, institutional, communal, practical) and its impact on care. They are designed to be used by non-chaplains and are not time intensive.

Instruments like these are just that: instruments. It depends on the person and skill of the user as to whether they are meaningful, helpful, or harmful. Taking a spiritual history requires more than simply ticking boxes. It is the opening up of a conversational space that gives patients a confidential and attentive place to tell their story and share their existential concerns. For this reason, some people prefer a simple tool like the one launched by the Mount Vernon Cancer Network in 2007. This is limited to three open questions [24]:

How do you make sense of what is happening to you?

What sources of strength do you look to when life is difficult?

Would you find it helpful to talk to someone who could help you explore the issues of spirituality/faith?

Second Level: Accompaniment

The second level of spiritual care is accompaniment. Of course, the second level presupposes the first. Spiritual care can only be realised upon the basis of a relationship in which people feel comfortable enough to share their inner and intimate thoughts and feelings. But accompaniment requires more than just being present and listening. The spiritual dimension of pain is always part of a process and can only be interpreted correctly within that process. One of the frightening aspects of having cancer can be that one's framework of interpreting the world is not helpful anymore. There can be a huge experience of loss, which is in a way a process of grief. This experience is frightening because it is disorienting. It is important to know that this process of disorientation – when it occurs, because not all patients are familiar with it – is a normal process. There is nothing pathological about it, and it should not be confused with a clinical depression. Nor should

caregivers hasten to solve of fix it. Normally within a certain period (days to weeks to months, depending on the person), new elements of sense and meaning appear, and one gradually discovers new possibilities of living with one's disease.

In the Dutch guideline for spiritual care, six phases are distinguished in the normal development of the spiritual process of cancer patients:

Sense of finiteness and mortality: Patients diagnosed with cancer face an existential threat. Some panic immediately. Others experience an intense feeling of loneliness. And sometimes, this existential fear gradually increases when the disease and treatment have more and more impact on the patient's life and context.

Loss of grip: The sense of finiteness may lead to the experience that all grip is lost. The system of meaning that had been functioning so far, and which reckoned with living a long life is no longer effective. Patients struggle with negative emotions like fear, panic, and depressive moods. Because the patient feels isolated, relatives often feel unable to support them.

Loss of meaning: The loss of a future is often experienced as unreasonable and unjust. Making plans seems senseless and realising plans seems no longer possible. Normally after a few days, the emotional impact of the shock gradually decreases. The patient experiences that death is not imminent.

Grief: When the shock decreases one becomes more and more aware of what one will have to let go of eventually. One starts grieving about having to say goodbye to loved ones, plans, and life in general.

Experience of meaning: After awhile most patients experience sudden and unexpected moments of meaningfulness. These moments are often characterised by a sense of being part of something greater. Experiences like this cannot be produced or made on purpose. They suddenly appear, often after a period of time in which the patient has become more familiar with the thought that life is finite. Often patients do not know how to speak about these new experiences of meaningfulness. The words are lacking or they feel embarrassed about it.

Integration of old and new meaningfulness: Whenever patients learn to live with their new situation and new experiences of meaningfulness, often a shift takes place. Patients feel more embedded in a bigger whole and become more open to accept the finiteness of life. They are more focused on living in the moment. Priorities shift and people worry less about what the outside world thinks of them and become more focused on what is really important to them in life. This may result in feelings of more confidence and hope, although still fear and resistance may play a large role.

The six phases of a spiritual process as sketched above do not apply to each and every patient. There are big differences among patients, ranging from people with a preexisting (spiritual) lifestyle that is close to the sixth phase to people who skip phases, fall back, or remain stuck in places that cause great pain and suffering. Of course, differences in age, character, and social and cultural context also play an important role. The benefit of this outline of the spiritual process is that it provides us with an overall framework that helps interpret the process of individual patients.

This second level of care for spiritual aspects of pain is not reserved for chaplains or spiritual caregivers. Every professional or voluntary caregiver can contribute to giving spiritual care and accompaniment. Often the patient chooses whom to share their intimate thoughts with, just like in ordinary life.

Accompaniment may take different forms according to the profession one has and the kind of relationship one has with the patient. Different patients have different sources of inspiration and meaning. Some patients have a style of spirituality that is emotional, and they find comfort in enjoying nature, music, literature, arts, or expressing themselves in creative ways. Others find sources of inspiration in contemplation and study. A third group is more practically oriented and finds inspiration in meditation, rituals, and doing good things for other people. These same three orientations can be found among people who have an explicitly religious ("vertical") spirituality in which the relationship with a higher being is central, to people who have a more secular less explicitly religious spirituality. Whatever the form in which spirituality is experienced, it is always about being related and connected in such a way that the pain and suffering is framed in a meaningful context.

Accompaniment may be done in various ways. Apart from general rules such as respecting the patient (being nonjudgemental) and respecting the limits of one's professional and private self, there are a few basic rules:

A certain familiarity with one's own spirituality

An attitude of authenticity (being yourself) and sympathy

Open questions and a real interest in what it means for the patients

A noninterventionist mode of working: patience, attunement, following, availability, and no proselytising [25]

Apart from a conversation with open questions, accompaniment can be done with the help of various interpretative frameworks in which different dimensions of spirituality are distinguished. Examples of these are the 7×7 model developed by George Fitchett which has been proven to be a useful tool for chaplains [26] and the *ars moriendi* tool – based on the medieval tradition, and not limited to palliative care – in which five domains are distinguished, which is used by nurses, physicians, and chaplains [27].

Third Level: Crisis Intervention

Not all patients ask for accompaniment. Usually, the normal development of the spiritual process of cancer patients develops without serious problems. But sometimes, things go wrong. Patients can be suddenly stuck in the middle of a horrible black period that is close to clinical depression. Sometimes they are so scared that special help is needed. This is where the guidelines suggest a third level: one of crisis intervention.

Signals of an existential or spiritual crisis can be given off by both patients themselves and the people around them. Signals include certain expressions of patients ("what is it all good for?"), changes in normal behaviour (sudden depressive moods, a lack of planning for the future, anger), somatising (more often by men than by women), isolation, and a desperate longing to die. Of course, signals are not evidence, and only by exploring these possible indications can a decision be made that these symptoms amount to a crisis.

There are two types of factors that have been identified as leading to spiritual crises. The first type is patient-related factors, such as a history with one of more periods of clinical depression, a history with one or more psychic traumas that have been treated insufficiently, suicide attempts, strong fear of being punished in a next life, a high level of striving for perfection in combination with the feeling that achievement in life has been realised, refusal to allow oneself to emotionally react to one's situation, and a great tension between one's ideas about reality and one's actual situation.

The second type of factors is related to the environment of the patient. These are directly related to the way care is provided:

Patients are confronted with their situation against their will, because others think it is better for them. Although often springing from good intentions ("It is better when patients do not deny their situation"), these confrontations are counterproductive, violent and are often not motivated by knowledge of the spiritual process as sketched above.

Patients are not given the opportunity to really deal with their struggles. This can be induced by many factors: The disease proceeds too fast, there are too many visitors, the family or caregivers are afraid of the emotional side of the process, or the spiritual dimension is silenced out of a misguided attempt to protect the patient.

The patient considers the way he is treated or cared for as disrespectful of his autonomy, independence, or dignity.

The patient has insufficient social support.

There is a serious illness of the patient's child or partner which gives the patient the feeling that he cannot complete his task in life.

In contrast to accompaniment, the actual crisis intervention itself is the domain of trained chaplains, spiritual caregivers, or professionals trained in the psychosocial dimension of care. All other caregivers and volunteers, however, play a very important role in observing and reporting when a spiritual crisis is at stake.

Conclusion and Ethical Consideration

Spiritual care is an important element of good care for cancer patients. What it looks like and how intense it is differ in each and every patient. The reason for this is not only that the patient differs, but the quality of the process also depends on the relationship between the caregiver and the patient. A more fundamental reason is that we live in a multicultural society in which we no longer share a common spiritual background or framework. That means that we constantly have to find out in what language and in what way we can address the spiritual needs of patients. This state of affairs may induce the temptation to try to get a grip on the spiritual part of cancer care in terms of transparency and control. I want to conclude this contribution with an ethical consideration which focuses on this temptation.

When spiritual care is integrated in a multidisciplinary approach, the question arises as to what extent information about the spirituality of the patient should be reported and exchanged in a way that is similar to information on other subjects. A golden rule of course is that patients themselves are the first to decide what information about their intimate concerns may be shared with others. In general, and when patients are not able to decide for themselves, the rule mandates that only that information is shared that is necessary for taking good care of the patient. Of course, general rules do not solve all ethical problems that may arise. But they can help us sail between the Scylla of a scrupulous respect for privacy that leads to patient isolation and the Charybdis of a total "Big Brother" transparency. Care for the spiritual dimension of cancer pain and suffering is also care for a respectful and humanising space in the health-care system.

Summary

Spiritual care is more than religious care: It is about meaning, purpose, and connectedness of patients who are in a vulnerable and uncertain position.

Pain is a multidimensional phenomenon in which meaning is a central element. Pain treatment should be focused by caregivers on the whole person, by caregivers who are aware of the healing impact of their role.

In the normal development of the spiritual process of cancer patients, six phases can be distinguished: sense of finiteness and mortality, loss of grip, loss of meaning, grief, experience of new meaning, and integration of old and new meaningfulness.

Spiritual care starts with attention, openness, and attentiveness. This is the basis of good care in general, but it can become spiritual care if there is trust and willingness to engage with one another.

Attention may develop into accompaniment which may take different forms, depending on one's personality, background, and profession.

Sometimes patients can have a spiritual crisis. Then, referral and intervention by a chaplain of trained psychosocial caregiver is needed.

References

1. Rinpoche S. The Tibetan book of living and dying: revised and updated. San Francisco: Harper Collins Publishers; 2002.
2. Pope John Paul II. Salvifici Doloris. Apostolic Letter on the Christian Meaning of Human Suffering. Boston MA: St Paul Editions; 1984.
3. Tanyi AR. Towards clarification of the meaning of spirituality. J Adv Nurs. 2002;39:500–9.
4. Waaijman K. Spirituality: forms, foundations, methods. Leuven: Peeters; 2002.
5. Paley J. Spirituality and nursing: a reductionist approach. Nurs Philos. 2008;9:2–18.
6. Nolan S. In defence of the indefensible: an alternative to John Paley's reductionist, atheistic, psychological alternative to spirituality. Nurs Philos. 2009;10:203–13.
7. Puchalski CM, Ferrell B, Virani R, et al. Improving the quality of spiritual care as a dimension of palliative care: the report of the Consensus Conference. J Palliat Med. 2009;12:885–904.
8. Nolan S, Saltmarsh P, Leget C. Spiritual care in palliative care: working towards an EAPC Task Force. Eur J Pall Care. 2011;18:86–9.
9. Sulmasy D. The rebirth of the clinic. An introduction to spirituality in health care. Washington, D.C.: Georgetown University Press; 2006.
10. Clark D. "Total pain", disciplinary power and the body in the work of Cicely Saunders, 1958–1967. Soc Sci Med. 1999;49:727–36.
11. Saunders C. Care of patients suffering from terminal illness at St. Joseph's Hospice, Hackney, London. Nurs Mirror. 1964;14:vii–x.
12. Cassell E. The nature of suffering and the goals of medicine. 2nd ed. Oxford: University Press; 2004.
13. Van Heijst A. Professional loving care. Leuven: Peeters; 2011.
14. Leget C, et al. Richtlijn Spirituele zorg. In: Palliatieve Zorg: Richtlijnen voor de Praktijk. Utrecht: VIKC; 2010. p. 637–62.
15. Daaleman TP et al. An exploratory study of spiritual care at the end of life. Ann Fam Med. 2008;6:406–11.
16. Van Meurs J. Geestelijke Begeleiding in het Algemeen Ziekenhuis. MA thesis. Radboud University Nijmegen, 2011. p. 54–5.
17. Narayanasamy A. Recognising spiritual needs. In: McSherry W, Ross L, editors. Spiritual assessment in healthcare practice. Penrith: M&K Publishing; 2010. p. 37–55.
18. Holloway M, et al. Spiritual care at the end of life: a systematic review of the literature. 2011. http://www.dh.gov.uk/publications. Accessed 8 Mar 2011.
19. McSherry W. Spiritual assessment: definition, categorisation and features. In: McSherry W, Ross L, editors. Spiritual assessment in healthcare practice. Penrith: M&K Publishing; 2010. p. 57–78.
20. Anandarajah G, Hight E. Spirituality and medical practice: using the HOPE questions as a practical tool for spiritual assessment. Am Fam Physician. 2001;63:81–8.
21. Puchalski CM. Spirituality and end-of-life care: a time for listening and caring. J Palliat Med. 2002;5:289–94.
22. Maugans TA. The SPIRITual history. Arch Fam Med. 1996;5:11–6.
23. Puchalski CM. The spiritual history: an essential element of patient-centered care. In: McSherry W, Ross L, editors. Spiritual assessment in healthcare practice. Penrith: M&K Publishing; 2010. p. 93–7.
24. Holloway M et al. Spiritual Care at the End of Life, Department of Health United Kingdom, Published to DH website, in electronic PDF format only. http://www.dh.gov.uk/publications, 2011. p. 92.
25. Baart A, Vosman F. Relationship based care and recognition. Part one: sketching good care from the theory of presence and five entries. In: Leget C, Gastmans C, Verkerk M, editors. Compassion and recognition: an ethical discussion. Leuven: Peeters; 2011.
26. Fitchett G, Handzo G. Spiritual assessment, screening and intervention. In: Holland J, editor. Psycho-oncology. New York: Oxford University Press; 1998. p. 790–808.
27. Leget C. Retrieving the Ars moriendi tradition. Med Health Care Philos. 2007;10:313–9.

Interventional Techniques in Cancer Pain: Critical Appraisal

18

Vittorio Schweiger, Enrico Polati, Antonella Paladini, and Giustino Varrassi

Abstract

Modern understanding of the pathophysiology of pain associated with cancer, accompanied with the improved survival rate of cancer patients, should lead to a new a critical appraisal of the role of interventional techniques used to emolliate cancer pain. A critical appraisal with evidence-based analysis will confirm that some techniques can have a better outcome than just pharmacological therapy.

Celiac plexus blocks, neuraxial infusions, and vertebroplasty have been used with good analgesic efficacy as well as good overall improved outcomes for cancer pain patients. Interventional therapy should be planned as part of a comprehensive multimodal approach in cancer pain management that encompasses pharmacological, psychological, and behavioral therapy in equal measures and not as either or modality or, even worse, when all other treatment has failed.

Keywords

Interventional therapy • Celiac plexus • Percutaneous cordotomy • Vertebroplasty • Cancer pain

V. Schweiger, PhD • E. Polati, DR
Department of Anaesthesia and Intensive Care,
Pain Therapy Centre,
Policlinico G.B. Rossi,
Piazzale Scuro 10, Verona 37126, Italy
e-mail: vittorio.schweiger@ospedaleuniverona.it;
enrico.polati@ospedaleuniverona.it

A. Paladini, DR
Department of Anaesthesiology,
Intensive Care and Pain Medicine,
Ospedale San Savatore,
University of L'Aquila – Italy,
Via Vetoio, 1 – Coppito,
L'Aquila, Abruzzo 67010, Italy
e-mail: antopaladini@gmail.com

G. Varrassi, DR, PhD, FIPP (✉)
Asl Teramo – National Health Care Service,
Circ. Ragusa, 1, Teramo, Abruzzo 64100, Italy
e-mail: giuvarr@gmail.com

M. Hanna, Z. Zylicz (eds.), *Cancer Pain*,
DOI 10.1007/978-0-85729-230-8_18, © Springer-Verlag London 2013

Introduction

Cancer pain management continues to be a significant global problem despite increased awareness, improved knowledge, understanding of pain pathophysiology, and standardised treatment guidelines of this distressing and debilitating symptom [1]. The complexed mechanisms (look at Chap. 5) that play a role in initiating and sustaining pain in cancer, combined with the dynamic nature of this disease, adds to the challenges that physicians, who encounter pain syndromes associated with cancer, face. The utilisation of "interventional therapies for pain associated with cancer" has fluctuated significantly over the last few decades. The rate of their use also varies from one cancer centre, where their use is considered and occasionally used, to other centres where they are never considered and never used. Invariably interventional, whether anaesthetics or surgical, modalities have been considered only when comprehensive medical pharmacological therapy titrated to maximum doses fails to provide an appropriate level of analgesia, or side effects associated with these therapies impair the ability to increase the doses to obtain appropriate therapeutic effects in patients [2]. However, since the aims of cancer pain therapy are to optimise pain control, minimise side effects, equally is to enhance functional abilities, physical as well as psychological well-being and improve quality of life. Considering all the above, a new and radical appraisal for the role and timing of those interventional therapies should take place. The vast improvement in survival rate from cancer should encourage a new critical appraisal of the role of interventional therapy (look at Chap. 3), since paradoxically this has been accompanied by the actual increase in the prevalence of pain secondary to cancer therapy and the apparent increase in opioid adverse effects (look at Chap. 10). Interventional therapy should be planned as part of a comprehensive multimodal approach in cancer pain management that encompasses pharmacological, psychological, and behavioral therapy in equal measures and not as either or modality or, even worse, when all failed treatment. Neuroablative techniques act at different levels by interrupting the transmission of painful stimuli irreversibly, employing chemical, mechanical, and thermal means. The main neuroablative techniques used in refractory cancer pain are percutaneous cervical cordotomy and celiac and hypogastric neurolytic plexus blocks.

Neurolytic Celiac Plexus Block (NCPB)

Pancreatic carcinoma is one of the most significant causes of cancer death, because of its rates of incidence and poor prognosis. Unfortunately, at diagnosis, only 7.5 % of patients present with a lesion without local infiltration or distant metastases. Of these patients, there is a 15.2 % survival rate after 5 years. The presence at diagnosis of local lesions or distant metastases dramatically reduces this survival percentage to 6.3 and 1.6 %, respectively [3]. Pancreatic cancer pain occurs in 72 % of patients affected by head lesions, while it occurs in 87 % of patients with body-tail cancer [4]. Pain is present in 30 % of patients with confined cancer, in 60 % of those with locally spread cancer, and in 80 % of those with advanced-stage disease [5]. The pain is configured, especially in the early stages, with the typical pattern of visceral celiac pain, located in the epigastric and/or hypochondriacal region, sometimes radiating bilaterally to the back. It is accentuated by the supine and chaired by the squatting position, intermittent and/or continuous type, described as oppressive, constricting, throbbing, or stabbing. In advanced stages, visceral-somatic pain may appear, which can be explained by widespread invasion of the retroperitoneum. Pain can also occur by compression or infiltration of the lower intercostal nerves, in this case defined as visceral-neurogenic. A referred-type pain may arise in the shoulder by infiltration of the central wall of the diaphragm innervated from the phrenic nerve [6]. The neurolysis of the high abdomen pain pathways is a valuable treatment for this distressing pain syndrome. The first splanchnic nerve neurolysis was introduced by the German surgeon Max Kappis in 1914. Since then, many techniques have been proposed in order to perform selective block of splanchnic nerves or of the celiac plexus. Among these, we must remember the Moore's posterior retrocrural splanchnicectomy, performed at the level of the vertebral body of L1; the Boas splanchnicectomy, performed at the level of the vertebral body of T12; the transcrural CT-guided technique, introduced by Singler in 1982; and the transaortic celiac plexus block, introduced by Ischia in 1983. The anterior approach to the celiac plexus, experienced by Wendling in 1918, was improved by Montero-Matamala in 1988 by employing CT and sonography. Recent proposals of alternative techniques to destroy splanchnic pain afferents should be mentioned, in particular the thoracoscopic or laparoscopic splanchnicectomy and the endoscopic-ultrasonographic celiac plexus neurolysis performed by trans-gastric approach (EUS-NCPB).

Anatomical Recalls

The pain afferents from high abdominal viscera (pancreas, liver, gallbladder, adrenal, kidney, and gastrointestinal tract from the gastroesophageal junction to the colic splenic flexure) are carried by nerve fibres that enter the context of the celiac plexus and splanchnic nerves. Celiac plexus consists of nerve fibres and a variable number of ganglia that constitute a dense nerve network embracing the anterior wall of the abdominal aorta in the precrural compartment, which is always located closed to celiac arterial trunk. This vessel has a variable position with respect to the bony landmarks of the spine, ranging from the vertebral body of T12 to vertebral body of L2 [7]. In particular, the relationship assessment with the bony landmarks showed that in 27 % of cases the celiac trunk prolongs the lower portion of the vertebral body of T12, in 18 % of cases is located between T12 and L1, in 23 % lies in the upper portion of L1, and in 21 % in the middle portion of L1. However, extreme locations like the middle portion of T12 (6 %) and the top of L2 (2 %) are possible. The splanchnic nerves, greater (GSN) and lesser (LSN), originate from the thoracic sympathetic chain. From the

retrocrural space, they pass, along the anterolateral portion of the vertebral bodies, into the abdominal cavity to make contact with the celiac plexus. The greater splanchnic nerve originates from the union of four to five roots which radiate from the 6th, 7th, 8th, and 9th thoracic ganglia of the sympathetic trunk. Sometimes, it can even get a root from the 4th to 5th ganglia and more rarely by the 10th. In some cases, the number of roots can be reduced by one or two. In the latter case, recent anatomical studies revealed that the superior root arises from the thoracic segments at the level of T6 (21 %), T5 (18 %), or T4 (16 %), while the lower root originates mainly from T9 (34 %) or T10 (26 %) [8]. The highest root, which usually shows more consistency, descends obliquely and a little forward, laterally of the vertebral bodies. Successive roots usually reach the upper portion of T11, where the nerve is completely formed. By crossing the diaphragm, in the section between the medial and intermediate pillars, the abdominal cavity is reached. The lesser splanchnic nerve consists of small branches emerging from the 10th, 11th, and 12th thoracic ganglion and passes through the diaphragm between the medial and intermediate column to join the celiac plexus. In some cases, the lesser splanchnic can merge with the greater. Root filaments from 11th and 12th ganglion may form a third splanchnic nerve (least splanchnic nerve) which sends its fibres mainly in the renal plexus [7].

Effects of Neurolytic Solutions on the Nervous Structures

The administration of absolute alcohol in contact with the nerve structures can produce extensive tissue damage. The substance causes the extraction of cholesterol, phospholipids, and cerebrosides and precipitation of lipo- and mucoproteins. The application of alcohol on peripheral nerve fibres triggers the Wallerian degeneration, characterised by axonal disruption, retraction, and hydrolysis of the myelin sheath [9]. Although ethanol has been widely used in neurolytic procedures for pain relief, the exact concentration required to produce sufficient lesion has never been clearly determined. Gaston Labat used alcohol with a 33.3 % concentration for neurolysis reporting satisfactory results, but not all the observations published later reported as favourable impressions. The concentration commonly used in pain therapy and available on the market is 95 %. However, the high concentration can cause significant pain and a burning sensation at the time of injection. For this reason, the administration is usually preceded by the injection of local anaesthetic.

Instruments

The most percutaneous techniques can be performed with a small instrument that consists of an image intensifier, a radiolucent operating table, long needles with stylet, local anaesthetic, and neurolytic solution. Special techniques require the use of CT or ultrasound to determine the route and avoid needle puncture of intraabdominal organs. On the broader debate on which kind of radiological guidance is recommended in this context is discussed below. The needles generally used are 18 G and 15 cm of length. Thinner needles are used in other approaches, such as in the anterior procedure. For the posterior approach, robust needles are necessary, because the operator should drive the needle exactly to the target structure, and not be driven by the flexible needle somewhere else. The techniques are usually performed in the awake patient with possible mild sedation/anxiolysis.

Percutaneous Techniques

The target areas for celiac axis destruction are the splanchnic nerves and/or the celiac ganglia. The splanchnic nerves may be reached percutaneously via a posterior route with two needles according to the classic retrocrural technique [10] or at a more cephalad level, as described by Boas [11]. The celiac ganglia may be reached by different techniques, with one needle via the anterior route [12, 13], with two needles [14], or one needle [15] via the posterior root.

Posterior Percutaneous Splanchnicectomy

The splanchnic nerves can be reached percutaneously only with a posterior approach. The retrocrural approaches to the splanchnic nerves are the classic ones described by Bridenbaugh and Moore in 1964 [16] and the bilateral chemical splanchnicectomy described by Boas in 1978 [11]. The classic retrocrural approach according to Moore's technique requires placing the needles, with skin entry point at 5–7 cm from the midline just below the edge of the 12th rib and the injection of the neurolytic solution in the retrocrural space at the anterolateral portion of the L1 vertebral body. The target is reached by crawling against the bone, with the right needle positioned more deeply than the left by about 1.5–2 cm. Once the needles are properly positioned (after the administration of contrast dye, a "butterfly" image from an anteroposterior and "wedge" image from a lateral view are obtained under fluoroscopy), 15–20 ml of absolute alcohol with 4–5 ml of local anaesthetic for each needle is injected (Fig. 18.1a, b). The local anaesthetic injection has the dual purpose of minimising the pain of neurolysis and of highlighting any incorrect needle position. The bilateral chemical splanchnicectomy described by Boas differs from the classic retrocrural technique for the more cephalad position of the needle, between the middle third and upper third of the vertebral body of T12. The needles, inserted to make contact with the vertebral body, are then pushed by the loss of resistance technique in the anterolateral compartment of the vertebral body, laterally to the parietal pleura, inferiorly to diaphragmatic crura insertion. After obtaining the latero-lateral fluoroscopic image of contrast dye that covers the anterolateral compartment of the vertebral body and anteroposterior with two fusiform spaced lines (Fig. 18.2a, b), neurolytic solution is injected with a smaller volume, consisting of approximately 8–10 ml of absolute alcohol per wire.

Celiac Plexus Block

The destruction of the celiac plexus requires the injection of the neurolytic solution in the precrural compartment behind the celiac arterial trunk

Fig. 18.1 (**a**) Moore's technique: "butterfly" image from an anteroposterior view. (**b**) Moore's technique: "wedge" image from a lateral view

Fig. 18.2 (**a**) Boas's technique: latero-lateral view of contrast dye that covers the anterolateral compartment of the vertebral body. (**b**) Boas's technique: anteroposterior view with two fusiform spaced lines

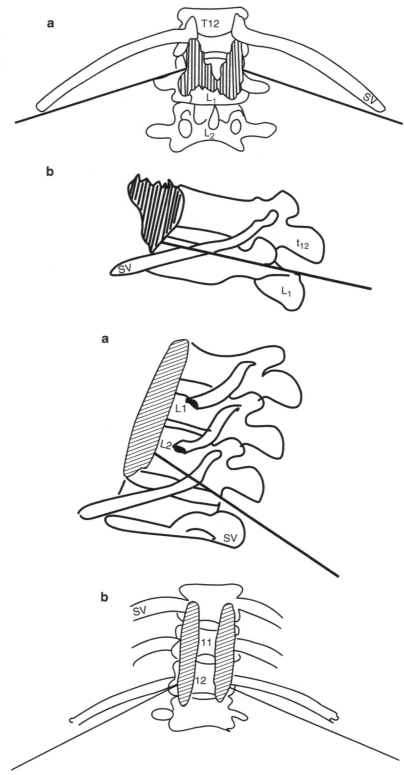

and the anterior wall of the aorta. The plexus can be achieved either percutaneously by a posterior approach with one or two needles or with a single needle by an anterior approach. The transcrural CT-guided posterior technique, proposed by Singler in 1982, involves placing the needles in the proximity of the celiac ganglia, anterolaterally to the aorta, caudally to the diaphragm, which is deliberately crossed to reach the target. CT guide is essential to place the needles at the origin of the celiac artery and to prevent accidental punctures of vascular structures or renal injuries. The volume of neurolytic solution is usually of 25 ml for each needle [14]. The use of a single needle has been postulated in the modified Singler's technique, where the entry point is 4–6 cm to the left of the midline, in the lower portion of the vertebral body of L1 with a final position in the anterolateral portion of the aorta, in a preaortic compartment. The block is performed with the patient in lateral position [17]. The posterior approach can also be achieved by the transaortic technique described by Ischia in 1983. The approach uses a single needle introduced about 6 cm to the left of the midline which is advanced crawling the lateral face of the vertebral body corresponding to the position which is projected the celiac trunk. The needle is then advanced trough the vessel from side to side, to reach the target area in front of the aorta. After verifying the correct position of the tip of the needle by injection of contrast dye (Fig. 18.3a, b), 20 ml of neurolytic solution is injected [15]. The posterior trans-discal approach involves the insertion of two needles through the intervertebral disc under fluoroscopic or CT guidance and their positioning in the anterolateral or lateral segment of the aorta to prevent intra-abdominal organ injuries [18]. The celiac plexus destruction by the anterior approach with single needle under ultrasound or CT guidance requires the passage of a thin needle through the abdominal viscera. The target area is located between the celiac artery and the emergence of the superior mesenteric artery. The block is performed with the patient in the supine position, because it is better tolerated by patients with severe abdominal pain [12, 13].

Other Techniques

Splanchnic nerves and celiac plexus can also be destroyed adopting other techniques. The chemical splanchnicectomy has long been used to complement the surgical treatment of unresectable pancreatic cancer. The technique involves instillation by the surgeon of 20 ml (50 % alcohol) on each side of the abdominal aorta at the level of celiac axis using 20 or 22 G spinal needle [19]. The video-assisted thoracoscopic splanchnicectomy consists in surgical ligation with clips of one or both splanchnic nerves. The procedure is performed under general anaesthesia with selective bronchial intubation and unilateral pulmonary exclusion. The use of thoracic drainage in the postoperative period is not considered essential by the authors [20]. The celiac plexus block can be performed even by laparoscopy. The procedure requires general anaesthesia and induction of a pneumoperitoneum. It consists in surgical exposition of the plexus and the injection of 20 ml of 50 % alcohol in the periaortic adipose tissue bilaterally using a 23 gauge needle under direct vision [21]. The celiac plexus can also be reached endoscopically using a transgastric ultrasound probe equipped with a thin needle. The ultrasound view of the plexus and adjacent vessels (with the use of colour Doppler) would identify the nerve structures and reach celiac ganglia via transgastric puncture [22]. This technique has been popular in the last 10 years, but its results and its future developments are still under evaluation [23].

Side Effects and Complications

Side effects are common to all techniques, due to sympathetic denervation. The most notable side effects are transient postural hypotension (60–90 %) and hyperperistalsis bowel with diarrhoea (40 %). Generally, these effects, which are a sign of block success, are transient and disappear within a few days (1–4 days). Sometimes the diarrhoea can last longer and become a source

Fig. 18.3 (**a**) Ischia's technique: anteroposterior view with correct placement of contrast dye. (**b**) Ischia's technique: latero-lateral view with correct placement of contrast dye

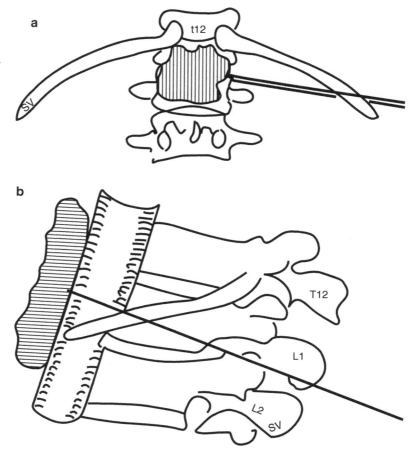

of discomfort for the patient. The percutaneous techniques have a few complications in common. The only frequent complication is transient pain in site of injection (90 %). Infrequent complications are shoulder pain, numbness, difficult ejaculation, diaphragmatic paralysis, and pneumothorax. The most important but extremely rare neurological complication is paraplegia. It has been reported with both classic retrocrural and transaortic techniques and we know of only 11 confirmed cases. The complication may be caused to the damage of the artery of Adamkiewicz (vasospasm by neurolytic solution, intramural injection, extramural compression of the substance injected into the retrocrural space, thrombosis, spasm). It was also assumed the direct inadvertent injection of neurolytic substance in subarachnoid compartment [24].

Outcomes

On the effectiveness of NCPB in treating pancreatic cancer pain, the debate was lively and contrasted from the earliest years. The first articles are dated in the mid-1960s, when Bridenbaugh, Moore, and Campbell firstly published on percutaneous posterior splanchnicectomy. The largest series published until the early 1990s showed that NCPB had a very high effectiveness in providing long-lasting pain relief [24]. Nevertheless, the real efficacy of this technique was heavily doubted. In 1990, the lack of data from controlled trials made Sharfman and Walsh suggest that the published series on NCPB does not prove the effectiveness of the procedure in regards to providing acute or long-term analgesia. They also questioned the indications for its use, suggesting there are investigations required into its long-term morbidity and to clarify that it is more efficacious than other methods of treating pancreatic cancer pain [25]. This observation has stimulated all subsequent experiences. A first prospective study, conducted using the three posterior percutaneous techniques, did not show significantly different results in a pain relief. However, it was first established as the blockades were able to abolish completely, until death, the pain from pancreatic cancer in 10–24 % of patients when used alone and in 80–90 % if associated with other treatments [26]. In addition, it was clearly highlighted that an early performance of the block resulted more effective than a later one, as stated, even recently, by other authors [27]. Finally, it was emphasised that the complications of the intervention were in most cases negligible and transient.

Other important contributions come from three key studies. Mercadante and coworkers demonstrated that opioids were effective for treating patients with pancreatic cancer pain, although the neurolytic block can reduce drug consumption and, ultimately, the side effects, including constipation [28]. Lillemoe and coworkers demonstrated that splanchnicectomy performed early in the course of surgery was effective in pain treatment and even improve survival of patients [19]. Kawamata and coworkers, finally, pointed out that the block execution is able to prevent the deterioration of the patient quality of life with regard to lower incidence of drug-related adverse effects. However, all the data were derived from a small sample of patients and are not statistically significant [29]. These findings encouraged further clinical trials. A prospective study compared the anaesthetic with the neurolytic block using the Boas's technique and showed how neurolysis is able to abolish the visceral component of pain from pancreatic cancer. It also seemed to guarantee a complete pain relief in 15 % of treated patients. In other patients, it reduced significantly the consumption of analgesic drugs up to death. The reduction in drug consumption was accompanied by a statistically significant reduction of adverse effects related to drug therapy. The study also confirmed negligible

and transient complications related to the methodology [30]. Some questions, however, remained unanswered. In particular, it was not yet clear whether some radiological parameters can indicate if the celiac axis had been completely destroyed (a prerequisite for obtaining complete pain relief) and whether these parameters could be detected with a simple radiological device, such as fluoroscopy, or require more complex and expensive instruments. Correlating X-ray images obtained with fluoroscopy and CT results for pain relief, we could detect that for bilateral Boas splanchnicectomy and transaortic neurolysis, CT images showed a close correlation with the abolition of celiac pain. It also demonstrated how CT guidance was not necessary for bilateral splanchnicectomy (where we noted a good correlation between fluoroscopic and CT images). In the transaortic block, the fluoroscopic guidance could be considered sufficient to evaluate the block success if the anatomical location of the target (which has variability, as mentioned above) is performed prior block execution using the diagnostic CT scan with contrast dye, performed in all patients during their diagnostic workup [31].

The conclusions reached by Kawamata were not shared by others. In particular, critics questioned the possibility of routine employment of CT guide as a tool to prevent the most feared complication, although rare, which is paraplegia [32]. In fact, the damage induced to anterior spinal artery (which is believed to be one of the most relevant mechanisms of spinal cord ischemia) would not be preventable with either TAC or with fluoroscopy, as the Adamkiewicz artery is not detectable by none of these radiological investigations during block execution [33]. The question is, however, still debated. A balance on clinical efficacy of NCPB, in the light of the available literature in the late 1990s, has allowed us to draw some important conclusions. The block ensures pain relief in 10–24 % of patients alone and 80–90 % if associated with other treatments. Complications related to the different techniques are rare and transient. The procedure ensures a reduction in the consumption of drugs, does not necessarily require expensive radiological procedures, and is more effective if performed early, when celiac pain occurs, and before the onset of extraceliacal somatic pain, which is not abolished by neurolysis of visceral afferents [34].

In considering the various posterior percutaneous techniques, focus is needed on the classic retrocrural technique introduced by Moore. It also requires a very high amount of neurolytic (50 ml total) and has completely unpredictable distribution that does not allow to assess the total destruction of the celiac axis. The transaortic technique may be exposed to incomplete destruction of the celiac plexus for the different positions they take on the aorta and the celiac trunk respect to bony landmarks. If these abnormalities were also analysed and identified a priori, the distortion of the preaortic area induced by the tumour may account for the anomalous distribution of neurolytic solution and lack of satisfactory pain relief. When the preaortic compartment is infiltrated by cancer, the chances of getting a correct picture of the spread of radiological contrast by fluoroscopy and by CT are also very reduced. Moreover, an appropriate spread of the neurolytic with the achievement of all the preaortic ganglia is seriously hampered. It is likely that the same factor represents a limit by performing a neurolytic celiac plexus block using the anterior echo or CT-guided technique [35].

Finally, to return to the Boas's technique, it is reasonable to conclude that the incomplete destruction of splanchnic nerves may be due to difficulties in correct placement of needles, impaired spread of the neurolytic solution, or presence of anatomic variables in the composition of splanchnic nerves themselves. These observations are the main reasons for the doubts of some operators on the effectiveness of the different percutaneous techniques, especially when compared to other methods of treatment of celiac pain such as intraoperative surgical, thoracoscopic splanchnicectomy or conventional drug therapy. Some authors have judged the results unsatisfactory and in any case lower than those reported in the literature with respect to the open splanchnicectomy [36]. Others have shown that it is not possible to define the impact of NCPB on the quality of life, especially in relation to other therapeutic options [37, 38]. Other authors, finally, while attributing

significant results to neurolytic procedures in terms of pain relief, reduction of analgesic drugs consumption, and related constipation, still consider these techniques only additional therapeutic modalities to be used in selected patients [39–41].

So, what are the prospects for an improvement in pain relief following splanchnic and celiac denervation? Some news may come from the evaluation of technical changes based on new acquisitions. In this context, the anatomical observations on the origin of the greater splanchnic nerve at the level of T6 or even T4 dermatomal level that is normally not reached by the posterior percutaneous neurolytic techniques could provide a convincing explanation for the failure to obtain adequate analgesia that occurs in some cases. To do this, a change to classical Boas's posterior bilateral splanchnicectomy has been considered, to running a higher level approach (T11–T10), in order to allow neurolytic spread of up to vertebral bodies of T5–T6 (Fig. 18.4a–c). Preliminary data on 75 of the 191 treated patients were encouraging and have demonstrated pain relief until death in 68 % of cases. Of these patients, 35.3 % had not complained of any pain until death, while 64.7 % complained of pain of different types (somatic, neurogenic) in the period between the block execution and death. The mortality of the procedure was none. Complications were injection site pain (60 % of patients), transient hypotension (90 % of patients), and pneumothorax (10 % of patients). This latter event did not require placement of a drainage given the small size and predominantly anterior positioning of the collection [42]. Finally, new studies are needed to clarify the impact of the NCPB on patients' quality of life. In a prospective randomised study on 100 patients affected with irresectable pancreatic cancer and referred to our pain relief centre for pancreatic cancer pain, we performed neurolytic and anaesthetic bilateral splanchnic block. The study showed that the consumption of analgesic drugs has been lower in the group treated with neurolytic block. Likewise, this group showed the best scores for the quality of life of patients compared with the anaesthetic control group [24].

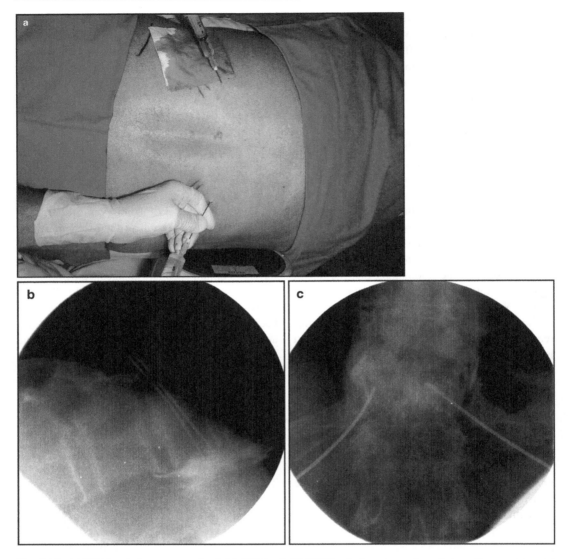

Fig. 18.4 (**a**) PPBS technique: approach at T11–T10 level. (**b**) PPBS technique: latero-lateral view of contrast dye. (**c**) PPBS technique: anteroposterior view of contrast dye

Conclusions

Neurolytic celiac plexus block (NCPB) includes different techniques. With respect to new approaches, such as celiac plexus block performed using ultrasound-guided endoscopy, judgment is suspended for the small numbers of published series. The percutaneous techniques were introduced a long time ago, and their effectiveness and safety in the treatment of pain from pancreatic cancer have been extensively delin-eated, although complete pain relief without additional treatments is obtained until death only in a minority of patients. However, the benefits found are the reduction of general analgesic consumption, which has a positive impact on quality of life. At present, none of the available techniques are able to achieve the total destruction of the splanchnic-celiac axis, which is a key point for obtaining complete relief of visceral pain. A more rostral approach to the splanchnic nerves at a level of T11–T10 obtained with the bilateral posterior percutaneous splanchnicectomy (PPBS) has been shown to produce, if properly executed, the complete destruction of the splanchnic axis in a higher percentage of patients. This preliminary data needs to be confirmed by further observations. Finally, the different procedures always require a thorough knowledge of regional anatomy and ability to correctly interpret radiological images. Current acquirements do not allow us to establish with certainty what is the best radiological guidance to perform posterior percutaneous blocks or if more expensive devices like CT scan are necessary to avoid major complications related to technique. Recent randomised studies and a Cochrane Database Systematic Review have confirmed the effectiveness of celiac plexus blockade in various cancer pain syndromes regardless of the techniques used. When compared with optimum medication, those studies supported the clinical impression of reduced side effects from medications and a better outcome overall [37, 43, 44].

Hypogastric Superior Plexus Block

Hypogastric plexus is located in the retroperitoneal space under the aortic bifurcation, corresponding to the space between the L4 and L5 lumbar and the first sacral vertebral bodies on the median line (sacral promontory). This plexus results from the union of the aortic plexus with 3rd and 4th lumbar splanchnic nerves, and it prolongs downwards with the inferior hypogastric plexus. It receives ramifications from the near orthosympathetic chain. The plexus receives afferent nerve fibres exclusively from the pelvic viscera. The neurolytic block is performed with the patient in the prone position, under fluoroscopic guidance. The insertion points of the two 18 G needles are located approximately 5–7 cm from the midline, bilaterally at the L4–L5 intervertebral space. From the point of insertion, the needles are directed towards the midline and downwards. After having made contact with the vertebral body, the needle is slightly advanced to reach the correct position in the anterolateral

portion of the intervertebral space between L5 and S1. After the injection of the dye, it is important to verify its correct spread and to inject a local anaesthetic solution (10 ml through each needle). Then, if no neurological deficit occurs, the neurolytic solution (8–15 ml of alcohol or phenol for each needle) is injected. This block is performed to treat visceral cancer pain originated from pelvic organs in a far advanced stage of the disease. The studies published to date have shown a reduction in painful symptoms and a reduction of analgesics consumption in treated patients [45–47].

Neuraxial Infusions

The use of the spinal route to administer drugs, particularly opioids, gains considerable popularity in the 1980s following the discovery of opioid receptors in the spinal cord. It was observed in some patients with advanced cancer who could not tolerate systemically administered opioids due to severe side effects responded better to spinally administered opioids with significantly reduced doses [48]. The type of infusions has varied from centre to centre and from simple percutaneous epidural catheter to a full implantable epidural or intrathecal infusion pumps. The fully implanted systems carry less risk of infection and have lower maintenance, but the operation is more prolonged and there are cost implications [49].

Recent randomised controlled trials of spinal infusions have highlighted an overall improvement in pain relief and less drug-related side effects compared with medical therapy for fully implanted systems, particularly in relation to the degree of sedation that was associated with systemic opioids [50–52].

The most commonly used drugs are opioids, in combination with local anaesthetics. Morphine has been the opioid of choice as it is the most used and studied, with Bupivacaine as the local anaesthetic commonly used in this combination, and generally patients who respond to spinal morphine are those who only partially respond to systemic morphine and/or are limited by dose-related side effects. Other compounds have been used spinally with varying degrees of efficacy, alpha-2 agonists (clonidine), and ziconotide [52]. Intraventricular opioids have been used in selective cancer pain patients with good results, though the complexity of this procedure and the rapid development of tolerance would make this route impractical for most cancer patients.

Percutaneous Cervical Cordotomy (PCC)

The idea of working on the anterior lateral quadrant of the spinal cord came to Spiller. He observed a patient with a tuberculoma compressing this part of the spinal cord and noted the onset of analgesia in the contralateral hemisoma. This was the reason he performed an open surgical section of this quadrant in order to relieve pain [53]. In 1963, Mullan et al. [54] developed the first percutaneous technique, using a needle to place a radioactive probe in the anterolateral quadrant of the spinal cord in order to obtain its progressive destruction. Analgesia in the contralateral lower limb was obtained within a week and then in the entire hemisoma. However, if the patient survived for more than 2 months, continuing the effect of the radioactive material on the spinal cord, paresis appeared firstly ipsilateral and then contralateral. Injuries resulting from this procedure were not easily controlled. However, this was the demonstration the anterolateral quadrant of the spinal cord was achievable by a lateral percutaneous approach. A substantial improvement occurred in 1965 when Rosomoff firstly employed radio frequencies that produced the lesion in few seconds after the placement of an electrode in the anterolateral quadrant of the spinal cord [55]. This was the beginning of the modern percutaneous cervical cordotomy. Immediately after, it was improved by Mullan [56] who introduced myelography and neurophysiological stimulations in order to check the correct placement of the electrode. Finally, during the 80s, Ischia extended the procedure to different kinds of oncological pain and further improved the technique, with a more precise myelographic images interpretation, leading to an easier

identification of the spinal target [57–60]. Also a more precise interpretation of the neurological tests and of the parameters to establish a correct execution of cordotomy was achieved [57–60]. The aim of this technique is to destroy the lateral spinothalamic tract, which represents the main ascending nociceptive pathway of the spinal cord. PCC is performed in the laterocervical region between C1 and C2, where the fibres of the lateral spinothalamic tract are closely compacted in the anterolateral quadrant of the spinal cord.

The operation is performed under local anaesthesia in awake and cooperative patients in the supine position. A 18 G needle is introduced immediately below the mastoid process. Skin, soft tissues, and muscular plane are passed through, until the yellow ligament is reached by the needle, in the interlaminar space between C1 and C2. Then, the epidural and the subarachnoidal spaces are reached. The optimal position of the needle is anteriorly to the ipsilateral dentate ligament. At this level, the myelographic images, obtained by injecting 1 ml of a lipophilic dye emulsified with 4 ml of spinal fluid, highlight the landmarks that guide the execution of the cordotomy. The top edge of the spinal cord, the two dentate ligaments, and the dural sac are the areas which gather most of the injected dye (Fig. 18.5). The lateral spinothalamic tract (spinal cord target) is located a few mm anteriorly to the ipsilateral dentate ligament. After having aligned the guide needle with the spinal cord target, a thin electrode needle is inserted (Figs. 18.6 and 18.7). The correct positioning of the needle is then confirmed by motor and sensory electrophysiological stimulations. Motor stimulations (2–5 Hz; 0.5–1 V) confirm the position of the electrode in the anterolateral quadrant of the spinal cord by evoking homolateral trapezium and sternocleidomastoid muscular contractions. Sensory stimulations (75–100 Hz; 0.05–0.1 V) must elicit intense thermal (hot or cold) sensations, on the side affected by pain. The onset of intense muscular contractions in the ipsilateral hemisoma indicates a wrong position of the electrode in the corticospinal tract. After obtaining correct myelographic images and electrophysiological stimulations, an ablation can be performed by delivering electric intensity of 50 μA for a

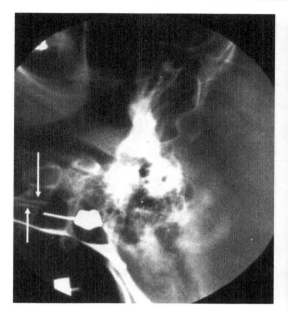

Fig. 18.5 Fluoroscopic image of top edge of the spinal cord (*downward arrow*), dentate ligaments (*upward arrow*), and dural sac after injection of contrast dye

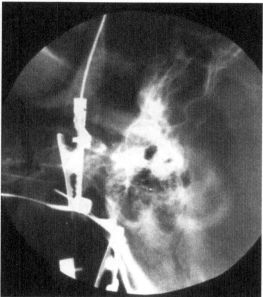

Fig. 18.7 Fluoroscopy performed to confirm correct electrode position

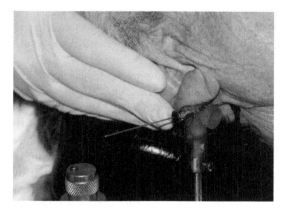

Fig. 18.6 The electrode is introduced into the spinal cord

period ranging from 3 to 10 s (Fig. 18.8). A proper execution of cordotomy must achieve:

- Deep pinch analgesia contralaterally to the lesion (from C3 to S5), with preservation of tactile and proprioceptional sensitivity
- A Claude Bernard-Horner syndrome with an ipsilateral sympathetic block

If these signs are present, the interruption of the nociception contralaterally to the ablation is confirmed, and it usually persists till the death of

the patient [57–60]. In about 80 % of cases, it is accompanied by a complete abolition of pain on the treated side. However, since cordotomy is technically difficult to perform, in order to obtain these rates of success, prolonged training of the operator is absolutely required. In fact, the success rate is directly proportional to the experience and skill of the operator, as well as the incidence of complications is inversely proportional to them (Fig. 18.1).

In some patients, who undergo cordotomy, pain may persist or appear. In this setting, it is important to distinguish the site of the pain:

- *Pain ipsilaterally to cordotomy* (untreated side). When pain is already present bilaterally before cordotomy, it is obvious that on the untreated side (ipsilaterally to cordotomy) pain may still be present; it is also well known that in the course of the disease, pain can often appear ipsilaterally as a consequence of spreading of neoplastic disease. In both cases, pain is easily controlled with drugs, and only in few patients a bilateral cordotomy is required. A bilateral cordotomy may be required in cases of "low," abdominal or pelvic-sacral pain. In some patients, in post-cordotomy, pain may

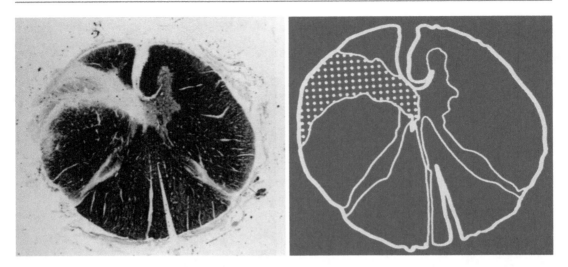

Fig. 18.8 Result of a left cordotomy performed in a patient with unilateral pain from C6 to T8

appear contralaterally to the original site. Such pain, defined as mirror pain, is not completely explained from a physiopathological point of view [61–63]. It occurs in approximately 5 % of treated patients. While in some cases this pain regresses spontaneously after a few days, in others, it is difficult to treat and it requires treatment with centrally acting drugs (opioids, tricyclic antidepressants, anticonvulsants) that interfere with the mechanisms of pain modulation.

• *Pain contralaterally to cordotomy* (treated side). In this situation, it is essential to distinguish if pain is present in a deep analgesia zone or not. In the first case, we are dealing with a non-nociceptive pain, often due to a deafferentation cancer pain, which may persist immediately after cordotomy or appear later in the time course of the disease. The two main predictors of this type of pain are the presence of neurogenic pain before cordotomy and the length of patient survival. The incidence of this type of pain is limited to a minority of patients (about 10–15 %). The treatment consists of the use of centrally acting drugs (opioids, tricyclic antidepressants, anticonvulsants). In some cases, neuroinvasive techniques, that include epidural and subarachnoidal administration of local anaesthetics and other analgesic

drugs, may be useful. The second case results from an incomplete ablation of the lateral spinothalamic tract. The incidence of this depends on the skill of the operator. In our series, the incomplete ablation occurred at a frequency of less than 3 % in 850 performed cordotomies (Fig. 18.9).

In considering complications, it is important to distinguish transient adverse effects and permanent complications. The first consists in fever, headache/neck pain, orthostatic hypotension, urinary retention, and weakness/fatigue. They are quite frequent and regress spontaneously within a few days. The latter are mainly represented by motor dysfunctions (incidence of paralysis between 0 and 15 % in different series), bladder dysfunctions (urinary retention in 2–18 % of cases), and by respiratory disorders. The influence of the procedure on the respiratory function is due to the section of reticular spinal fibres running in the most ventral portion of the anterior lateral quadrant. Cordotomy can cause changes in respiratory function of varying degrees, depending on the extent of injury to the spinal cord. In the case of unilateral cordotomy, these alterations, consisting mainly in small changes in vital capacity, maximum vital capacity and strength of respiratory muscles, are clinically silent and detectable only through functional

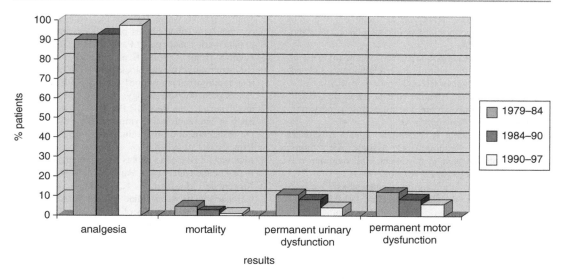

Fig. 18.9 Results and complications of cervical percutaneous cordotomy in our series (1979–1997, 850 patients)

tests. Alterations of the same type but of higher entity appear after bilateral cordotomy, particularly if associated with high levels of analgesia. The bilateral destruction of the reticular spinal fibres, instead, causes the onset of the Ondine's syndrome (sleep apnoea) [59]. Operative mortality ranges between 0 and 5 %. Again, this is dependent on the skill and experience of the operator, which is statistically significantly correlated to the presence of severe respiratory failure ($PaO_2 < 60$ mmHg) and the performance status of the patient. In our series, with careful selection of patients undergoing to this procedure, operative mortality has been reduced to less than 1 %.

Recent assessments of the role of percutaneous cordotomy have highlighted its usefulness in selective cases [64], though it has never been tested in critical study format.

Vertebroplasty

Painful pathological fractures of vertebra that do not respond to the conservative therapies of medications, TENS or steroid epidurals can be considered for fixation by cemented vertebroplasty. Open studies in myeloma and metastatic cancers report pain relief that is often complete in around 80 % of patients [65–67]. Cement leak is the

commonest risk at around 5 %, and complications from this are rare but serious [68].

Other Neurosurgical Procedures

A variety of neurosurgical techniques, including dorsal rhizotomy, pituitary ablation, and cingulotomy, can be used to ablate central and peripheral nociceptive pathways. The use of these destructive techniques has declined primarily because of advances in both pharmacotherapy and nonablative techniques.

References

1. Krakauer EL et al. Opioid inaccessibility and its human consequences: reports from the field. J Pain Palliat Care Pharmacother. 2010;24(3):239–43.
2. Kim PS. Interventional cancer pain therapies. Semin Oncol. 2005;32(2):194–9.
3. Greene FL. Pancreatic cancer staging. In: Greene FL, Page DL, Fleming ID, Fritz A, Balch CM, Haller DG, Morrow M, editors. AJCC cancer staging handbook. 6th ed. New York: Springer; 2002. p. 179–88.
4. Freelove R, Walling AD. Pancreatic cancer. Diagnosis and management. Am Fam Physician. 2006;73: 485–92.
5. Ceyhan GO, Michalski CW, Demir IE, et al. Pancreatic pain. Best Pract Res Clin Gastroenterol. 2008;22: 31–44.

6. Polati E, Finco G, Rigo V, et al. Treatment of pain in advanced-stage intra-abdominal neoplasms. Chir Ital. 1993;45:77–84.

7. Plexuses of the autonomic nervous system. In: Warwick R, Williams PL, editors. Gray's anatomy. 35th ed. Edinburg: Longman Group Ltd; 1973. p. 1077.

8. Naidoo N, Partab P, Pather N, et al. Thoracic splanchnic nerves: implications for splanchnic denervation. J Anat. 2001;199(5):585–90.

9. Subhash J, Gupta R. Neurolytic agents in clinical practice. In: Waldman SD, Winnie AP, editors. Interventional pain management. Philadelphia: W.B Saunders Company; 1996. p. 167–70.

10. Kappis M. Erfahrungen mit localanesthesie bie bauchoperationen. Verh Dtsch Ges Chir. 1914;43:87–9.

11. Boas RA. Sympathetic blocks in clinical practice. Int Anesthesiol Clin. 1978;4:149–82.

12. Montero Matamala A, Vidal Lopez F, Inaraja Martinez L. The percutaneous anterior approach to the celiac plexus using CT guidance. Pain. 1988;34:285–8.

13. Montero Matamala A, Vidal Lopez F, Aguilar Sanchez JL, et al. Percutaneous anterior approach to the celiac plexus using ultrasound. Br J Anaesth. 1989;62: 637–40.

14. Singler RC. An improved technique for alcohol neurolysis of the celiac plexus. Anesthesiology. 1982;56:137–41.

15. Ischia S, Luzzani A, Ischia A, et al. A new approach to the neurolytic celiac plexus block: the transaortic technique. Pain. 1983;16:333–41.

16. Bridenbaugh LD, Moore DC, Campbell DD. Management of upper abdominal cancer pain: treatment with celiac plexus block with alcohol. JAMA. 1964;190:877–80.

17. Hilgier M, Rykowsky JJ. One needle transcrural celiac plexus block. Single shot or continuous technique, or both. Reg Anesth. 1994;4:277.

18. Ina H, Kitoh T, Kobayashi M, et al. New technique for the neurolytic celiac plexus block: the transintervertebral disc approach. Anesthesiology. 1996;85:212–7.

19. Lillemoe KD, Cameron JL, Kaufman HS, et al. Chemical splanchnicectomy in patients with unresectable pancreatic cancer. A prospective randomized trial. Ann Surg. 1993;217:447–57.

20. Melki J, Rivière J, Roullée N, et al. Thoracic splanchnicectomy under video-thoracoscopy. Presse Med. 1993;26:1095–7.

21. Strong VE, Dalal KM, Malhotra VT, et al. Initial report of laparoscopic celiac plexus block for pain relief in patients with unresectable pancreatic cancer. J Am Coll Surg. 2006;203:129–31.

22. Wiersema MJ, Wiersema LM. Endosonography guided celiac plexus neurolysis. Gastrointest Endosc. 1996;44:656–62.

23. Penman ID, Rosch T. EUS 2008 Working Group document: evaluation of EUS-guided celiac plexus neurolysis/block. Gastrointest Endosc. 2009;69:S28–31.

24. Polati E, Luzzani A, Schweiger V, et al. The role of neurolytic celiac plexus block in the treatment of pancreatic cancer pain. Transplant Proc. 2008;40:1200–4.

25. Sharfman WH, Walsh TD. Has the analgesic efficacy of neurolytic celiac plexus block been demonstrated in pancreatic cancer pain? Pain. 1990;41:267–71.

26. Ischia S, Ischia A, Polati E, et al. Three posterior percutaneous celiac plexus block techniques. A prospective, randomized study in 61 patients with pancreatic cancer pain. Anesthesiology. 1992;76:534–40.

27. de Oliveira R, dos Reis MP, Prado WA. The effects of early or late neurolytic sympathetic plexus block on the management of abdominal or pelvic cancer pain. Pain. 2004;110:400–8.

28. Mercadante S. Celiac plexus block versus analgesics in pancreatic cancer pain. Pain. 1993;52:187–92.

29. Kawamata M, Ishitani K, Ishikawa K, et al. Comparison between celiac plexus block and morphine treatment on quality of life in patients with pancreatic cancer pain. Pain. 1996;64:527–602.

30. Polati E, Finco G, Gottin L, et al. Prospective randomized double blind trial of neurolytic coeliac plexus block in patients with pancreatic cancer. Br J Surg. 1998;85:199–201.

31. Ischia S, Polati E, Finco G, et al. 1998 Labat Lecture: the role of neurolytic celiac plexus block in pancreatic cancer pain management: do we have the answers? Reg Anesth Pain Med. 1998;23:611–4.

32. Moore DC. Computed tomography eliminates paraplegia and/or death from neurolytic celiac plexus block. Reg Anesth Pain Med. 1999;24:483–4.

33. Ischia S, Polati E. Reply to Dr. Moore. Reg Anesth Pain Med. 1999;24:484–6.

34. Ischia S, Polati E, Finco G, et al. Celiac block for the treatment of pancreatic pain. Curr Rev Pain. 2000;4(2):127–33.

35. De Cicco M, Matovic M, Bortolussi R, et al. Celiac plexus block: injectate spread and pain relief in patients with regional anatomic distortions. Anesthesiology. 2001;94:561–5.

36. Patrick DL, Ferketich SL, Frame PS, et al. National Institutes of Health State-of-the-Science Conference Statement: Symptom management in cancer: pain, depression, and fatigue, July 15-17, 2002. J Natl Cancer Inst. 2003;95(15):1110–7.

37. Wong GY, Schroeder DR, Carns PE, et al. Effect of neurolytic celiac plexus block on pain relief, quality of life and survival in patients with unresectable pancreatic cancer. A randomized controlled trial. JAMA. 2004;291:1092–9.

38. Staats PS, Hekmat H, Sauter P, et al. The effects of alcohol celiac plexus block, pain and mood on longevity in patients with unresectable pancreatic cancer: a double-blind, randomized, placebo-control study. Pain Med. 2001;2:28–34.

39. Yan BM, Meyers RP. Neurolytic celiac plexus block for pain control in unresectable pancreatic cancer. Am J Gastroenterol. 2007;102:430–8.

40. Noble M, Gress FG. Techniques and results of neurolysis in chronic pancreatitis and pancreatic cancer pain. Curr Gastroenterol Rep. 2006;8:99–103.

41. Carrol I. Celiac plexus block for visceral pain. Curr Pain Headache Rep. 2006;10:20–5.

42. Ischia S, Schweiger V, Ceola M. Splanchnic vs celiac lesion. Sofia: International Forum on Pain Medicine; 2005. p. 83.

43. Arcidiacono PG, Calori G, Carrara S, et al. Celiac plexus block for pancreatic cancer pain in adults. Cochrane Database Syst Rev. 2011;(3):CD007519.

44. Rykowski JJ, Hilgier M. Efficacy of neurolytic celiac plexus block in varying locations of pancreatic cancer. Anesthesiology. 2000;92:347–54.

45. Plancarte R, Amescua C, Patt RB, et al. Superior hypogastric plexus block for pelvic cancer pain. Anesthesiology. 1990;73:326–9.

46. De Leon-Casasola OA, Kent E, Lema MJ. Neurolytic superior hypogastric plexus block for chronic pelvic pain associated with cancer. Pain. 1993;54: 145–51.

47. Plancarte R, de Leon-Casasola OA, El-Helaly M. Neurolytic superior hypogastric plexus block for chronic pain associated with cancer. Reg Anesth Pain Med. 1997;22:562–8.

48. Baker L, Lee M, Regnard C, Crack L, Callin S. Evolving spinal analgesia practice in palliative care. Palliat Med. 2004;18:507–15.

49. Williams JE, Louw G, Towlerton G. Intrathecal pumps for giving opioids in chronic pain: a systematic review. Health Technol Assess. 2000;4(32):iii–iv, 1–65.

50. Smith TJ, Coyne PJ, Staats PS, et al. An implantable drug delivery system (IDSS) for refractory cancer pain provides sustained pain control, less drug related toxicity and possibly better survival compared with comprehensive medical management (CMM). Ann Oncol. 2005;16:825–33.

51. Smith TJ, Staats PS, Deer T, Implantable drug delivery systems study group, et al. Randomised clinical trial of an implantable drug delivery system compared with comprehensive medical management for refractory cancer pain; impact on pain, drug related toxicity and survival. J Clin Oncol. 2002;20:4040–9.

52. Staats P, Yearwood T, Wallace MS, et al. Intrathecal ziconotide in the treatment of refractory pain in patients with cancer or AIDS. JAMA. 2004;291: 63–70.

53. Spiller WG, Martin E. The treatment of persistent pain of organic origin in the lower part of the body by division of the anterolateral column of the spinal cord. JAMA. 1912;58:1489–90.

54. Mullan S, Harper PV, Hekmatpanah J, et al. Percutaneous interruption of spinal-pain tracts by means of a strontium needle. J Neurosurg. 1963;20: 931–9.

55. Rosomoff HL, Carroll F, Brown J, et al. Percutaneous radiofrequency cervical cordotomy: technique. J Neurosurg. 1965;23:639–44.

56. Mullan S. Percutaneous cordotomy. J Neurosurg. 1971;35:360–6.

57. Ischia S, Luzzani A, Ischia A, et al. Role of unilateral percutaneous cervical cordotomy in the treatment of neoplastic vertebral pain. Pain. 1984;19:123–31.

58. Ischia S, Luzzani A, Ischia A, et al. Subarachnoid neurolytic block (L5-S1) and unilateral percutaneous cordotomy in the treatment of pain secondary to pelvic malignant disease. Pain. 1984;20:139–49.

59. Ischia S, Luzzani A, Ischia A, et al. Bilateral percutaneous cervical cordotomy: immediate and long-term results in 36 patients with neoplastic disease. J Neurol Neurosurg Psychiatry. 1984;47:141–7.

60. Ischia S, Ischia A, Luzzani A, et al. Results up to death in the treatment of persistent cervico-thoracic (Pancoast) and thoracic malignant pain by percutaneous cervical cordotomy. Pain. 1985;21:339–55.

61. Bowsher D. Contralateral mirror-image pain following anterolateral cordotomy. Pain. 1988;88:63–5.

62. Nagaro T, Amakawa K, Kimura S, et al. Reference of pain following percutaneous cervical cordotomy. Pain. 1993;53:205–11.

63. Ischia S, Polati E, Finco G, et al. Referred pain in cancer patients: effects of percutaneous cervical cordotomy. In: Vecchiet L, Albe-Fessard D, Lindblom U, Giamberardino MA, editors. New trends in referred pain and hyperalgesia. Amsterdam: Elsevier Science Publisher; 1993. p. 403–8.

64. Crul BJP, Blok LM, Van Egmond J, Van Dongen RTM. The present role of percutaneous cervical cordotomy for the treatment of cancer pain. J Headache Pain. 2005;6(1):24–9.

65. Gangi A, Guth S, Imbert JP, et al. Percutaneous vertebroplasty: indications, technique, and results. Radiographics. 2003;23(2):e10.

66. Dudeney S, Lieberman IH, Reinhardt MK, et al. Kyphoplasty in the treatment of osteolytic vertebral compression fractures as a result of multiple myeloma. J Clin Oncol. 2002;20(9):2382–7.

67. Fourney DR, Schomer DF, Nader R, et al. Percutaneous vertebroplasty and kyphoplasty for painful vertebral body fractures in cancer patients. J Neurosurg. 2003;98(1):21–30.

68. Hentschel SJ, Burton AW, Fourney DR, et al. Percutaneous vertebroplasty and kyphoplasty performed at a cancer center: refuting proposed contraindications. J Neurosurg Spine. 2005;2(4):436–40.

Access to Opioid Analgesics: Essential for Quality Cancer Care

19

Willem Scholten

Abstract

Many cancer patients suffer moderate to severe pain, but owing to a focus on the prevention of abuse of and dependence on drugs, medical access to opioid analgesics has been neglected. Today, opioid analgesics are not readily available for medical use in many parts of the world. The World Health Organization (WHO) estimates that 5.5 billion people (83 % of the world's population) live in countries with low to non-existent access to controlled medicines and have inadequate access to treatment for moderate to severe pain. Although some have been advocating for improved pain management for several decades, only recently has the inadequate access to and availability of opioid analgesics become an internationally recognised problem.

Measuring opioid analgesic consumption is possible using data from the International Narcotics Control Board. This requires aggregation of the various opioid analgesics expressed in "mg morphine equivalents". For determining the level of consumption that will be adequate in a country, its per capita consumption can be compared with the consumption level in most developed countries by calculating the Adequacy of Consumption Measure (ACM). A correction of the need for opioid analgesics depending on the morbidity level in a country is possible by using HIV, cancer, and injuries as a proxy, but this has its limitations owing to the unreliability of health statistics in some countries.

Independent of the method, all methods show that there is a huge disparity between countries: the difference between the countries with the highest and lowest ACM in 2006 was 40,000 folds.

W. Scholten
Consultant – Medicines and Controlled Substances,
Chemin du Lignolet 18A,
1260 Nyon, Switzerland
e-mail: wk.scholten@bluewin.ch

M. Hanna, Z. Zylicz (eds.), *Cancer Pain*,
DOI 10.1007/978-0-85729-230-8_19, © Springer-Verlag London 2013

The World Health Organization defined availability, accessibility, and affordability as the key areas of concern around controlled medicines. These three terms relate to the questions: "Is the medicine present in the pharmacy?", "Is it possible to obtain the medicines from the pharmacy?" and "Has the patient sufficient means to buy it?" If these conditions are not met, the patient's pain will not be managed. A variety of barriers can be at the root of limited availability, accessibility, and affordability. Four categories of barriers can be distinguished: legislative and policy barriers, knowledge barriers, attitudes barriers, and economic barriers.

The World Health Organization established the Access to Controlled Medicines Programme (ACMP), which developed a number of documents to guide policy makers and health-care professionals to improve access to opioid analgesics and other controlled medicines. The ACMP and a number of NGOs also provide support to countries that want to improve access to controlled medicines e.g. by organising workshops and reviewing (draft) legislation. Moreover, international organisations of health-care professionals also called for adequate access to pain medicines and treatment of pain.

In order to ensure that "effective pain control measures will be available universally to all cancer patients in pain" by 2020, we will need to record our progress toward and analyse the barriers to adequate pain management. Access to opioid analgesics is essential for quality cancer care because by treating the pain, we improve the patient's quality of life in one important aspect of his or her disease.

Keywords

Access to medicines • Opioid analgesics • Statistics • Barriers • International

Introduction

Many cancer patients suffer moderate to severe pain. Opium is known for centuries and morphine since 1803, when it was isolated for the first time by Sertürner. Yet, for a long time it has not been recognised in society that access to and availability of opioid analgesics is essential for relieving this pain. Among health-care professionals, a focus on treatment of cancer itself used to be the norm, and as they considered pain often a symptom, the treatment of pain was, and still is, often neglected. During the past half a century, this coincided with emphasis in drug control policies to prevent abuse and diversion of substances that can cause dependence, such as opioid analgesics, rather than to acknowledge that there is also a medical need for these substances. It rendered opioid analgesics less and less readily available for medical treatment. Harsh situations from all over the world, resulting from inadequate pain relief, were described [1].

In 1989, the International Narcotics Control Board (INCB) drew attention to some governments' overreaction to the drug abuse problem when "...the reaction of some legislators and administrators to the fear of drug abuse developing or spreading has led to the enactment of laws and regulations that may, in some cases, unduly impede the availability of opiates" [2]. The Pain and Policy Studies Group at the University of Wisconsin has been a lonely advocate for adequate access to opioid analgesics since the end of the 1980s, but in recent years both international governmental and nongovernmental organisations requested that the situation improve (see section, International Developments Toward Adequate Access for All). Today, with the rising importance of noncommunicable diseases because of ageing populations, the inadequate access and availability of opioid analgesics has become an internationally recognised problem.

Opioid analgesics are not the only medicines that are made from substances that are controlled under the international drug control conventions, and other controlled medicines face similar problems [3]. For the treatment of moderate and severe cancer pain, opioid analgesics are the only effective medicines. This chapter will focus on their availability, accessibility, and, to a lesser extent, the affordability around the world.

Extent of the Non-availability of Opioid Analgesics

In 2009, 94 % of all the morphine used for medical purposes were used by only 27.7 % of the world population [4]. The World Health Organization (WHO) estimates that 5.5 billion people (83 % of the world's population) live in countries with low to nonexistent access to controlled medicines and have inadequate access to treatment for moderate to severe pain. This includes 5.5 million terminal cancer patients annually and furthermore 1 million end-stage HIV/AIDS patients and 0.8 million patients suffering injuries caused by accidents and violence. In addition to this, it includes patients with chronic illnesses, patients recovering from surgery, women in labour (110 million births each year), and paediatric patients. Several of these categories are hard to quantify due to lack of data [5].

The INCB is an international UN body responsible, inter alia, for the collection of statistics of production, imports, exports, and consumption of opioid analgesics. As countries cannot import or export these substances without a license and both the importing and exporting countries need to submit the amounts to the INCB, the international statistics on the consumption of opioids analgesics are relatively reliable. They are published annually and submission of these data to INCB is mandatory for the countries [6, 7].

However, for all other variables that one would need for measuring the adequacy of pain treatment in a direct way by calculating the need of all patients regardless of their disease, global health statistics do not exist. Therefore, if we want to measure the adequacy of opioid consumption around the world, other approaches are needed.

Per Capita Consumption

Opioid analgesic consumption per capita in morphine equivalents is an absolute presentation of the level of use. A presentation on a per capita basis allows the comparison of the consumption levels of countries with different population sizes. For totalising the various opioids in use, their amount used needs to be converted into "morphine equivalents" using ratios according their equipotent weights (e.g., 1 mg of fentanyl being as potent as 100 mg of morphine, 1 mg fentanyl counts for 100 mg morphine equivalents). This can best be standardised by using the Defined Daily Dose (DDD) as established by the World Health Organization [8], which is a universal unit for the quantity of a medicine. It is designed for statistical purposes. By using the DDD, one avoids the problem that various handbooks present different equipotencies. By representing the total use of strong opioid analgesics instead of separate opioids, it is possible to compare countries that use different opioids to treat pain.

The Pain and Policy Studies Group (PPSG) of the Paul Carbone Cancer Center, University of Wisconsin, presents at its website[1] the total and per capita consumption of separate opioids and of the total of opioids for all countries where data are available from the INCB, and they are presented in various ways, including tables, graphs, and motion charts. These data go back as far as to 1980 and are annually updated. PPSG states now at its website that it uses the same conversion method.

The per capita consumption is a neutral presentation of the consumption level. However, it does not give any information if the consumption is sufficient or not to treat all pain adequately, or even if there is overconsumption.

---

[1] http://www.painpolicy.wisc.edu/

Adequate Treatment Level

Theoretically there would be two methods to determine whether the consumption level is adequate: one is to list all the many diseases that come with moderate and severe pain and should be treated with opioids. For each condition, there should be a trial or survey what the average use per patient is or should be in order to let the pain disappear or be bearable. This should be multiplied with the prevalence for each condition, and then all these conditions and diseases need to be totalised for the need for opioids. This calculated total need can then be compared to the actual use for opioids in a country, region, or globally. However, these data hardly exist and it is obvious that collecting them for all these conditions is a hopeless task.

Another method is to hold a survey among patients, asking whether their pain is addressed and if it is well addressed. It was done for the Netherlands through a meta-analysis [9]. However, to compare between many countries, again, it seems to be a hopeless task.

Therefore, a different method was followed by Seya et al. [10]. They developed the Adequacy of Consumption Measure for strong opioids (ACM). This is a morbidity corrected measure related to per capita consumption of strong opioids. As a standard for adequate per capita consumption, they took the opioid consumption of the top 20 countries of the Human Development Index (HDI), whereas this average is set equal to 100 %. An ACM of 100 % and higher is considered to be adequate. Thus, the method assumes that the average consumption level in the most developed countries is about right. In fact the method has several assumptions: One is that the most developed countries are closest to adequate treatment of pain and the second is that this is best represented by taking the top 20; taking the top 10 would put the benchmark very high and taking, e.g., the top 30 (or include even more countries) in the benchmark would bring it very quickly down and would not leave a challenge for countries where treatment is not adequate. In fact, there is some support for the choice of the top 20: the study by Bekkering mentioned above found that 43 % of chronic noncancer pain patients report not to receive pain treatment and that 79 % of patients believe their pain is inadequately treated [9]. This is the same order as the 51 % of adequacy found for the Netherlands by Seya, meaning that the country needs to double its opium consumption for being adequate. Therefore, both studies seem to be congruent and therefore using the top 20 as a benchmark is plausible, although not validated in full.

A third assumption relates to the morbidity correction, which attributes a higher need for opioid analgesics to countries with a higher cancer incidence, a higher HIV prevalence, and/or a higher level of lethal injuries. The prevalence of these three diseases is in fact a proxy for total morbidity, and it acknowledges that countries with a higher morbidity level have a higher need for opioid analgesics.

The HDI is published annually by the United Nations Development Programme (UNDP). It takes into account standard of living, life expectancy, and education [11] and is therefore a broader index than the country income level annually published by the World Bank. Using the top 20 HDI has a consequence that the standard is not fixed, but shifts over time with the dynamics of the development of countries (each year countries drop off from the top 20 and new countries enter) and with changing opinions about the best practice of treatment of pain. The composition of the top 20 changed considerable during the global financial crisis that started in 2008, and per capita opioid consumption in more developed countries is still increasing. Therefore, a country that increased its absolute per capita consumption from 1 year to another may still have decreased its ACM if it did not keep pace with the developments in the most developed countries.

The method developed by Seya et al. is sensitive for the low quality of health statistics around the world. Underreporting of cancer mortality or HIV mortality is a problem in many countries and leads to a too optimistic level of adequacy. A way to circumvent this disadvantage would be to leave out the morbidity correction and to calculate adequacy by expressing a country's per capita consumption and relating this to the per capita consumption of the top 20 HDI.

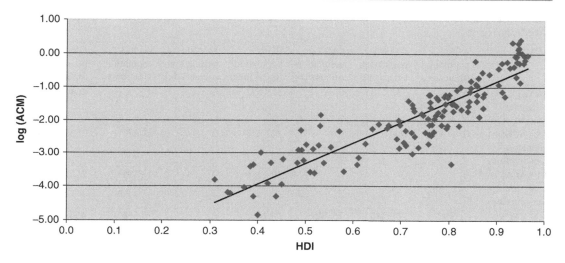

Fig. 19.1 Relation between the log (ACM) and the Human Development Index (HDI) for 139 countries (function formula: log (ACM)=−6.4113+6.200 × HDI; N=139; correlation coefficient: 0.895; p value: <0.0001) (From Seya et al. [9])

Global Situation

Whatever method is used, all methods show that there is a huge disparity between countries. Seya et al. determined the ACM for 145 countries and related it to the Human Development Index (Fig. 19.1).

The difference in ACM 2006 between Canada and Malawi (which were the countries with the highest and lowest ACM in 2006) was 40,000 times. However, as the graph shows, disparity between countries of the same level of development is often also high and also the ACM is relatively low in some highly developed countries.

Seya et al. also calculated how many people live in each WHO region and in the world at various levels of access (Table 19.1). Worldwide 4.7 billion people live in countries with virtually no access to opioid analgesics, while only 464 million live in countries with adequate access.

Availability, Accessibility, and Affordability

For analysing the situation with regard to the use of opioids in a country, the World Health Organization defined availability, accessibility, and affordability of controlled medicines. These three terms are derived from economic and health-economic theory. For controlled medicines, the World Health Organization uses the following definitions [12]:

- *Availability* is the degree to which a medicine is present at distribution points in a defined area for the population living in that area at the moment of need.
- *Accessibility* is the degree to which a medicine is obtainable for those who need it at the moment of need with the least possible regulatory, social, or psychological barriers.
- *Affordability* is the degree to which a medicine is obtainable for those who need it at the moment of need at a cost that does not expose them to the risk of serious negative consequences such as not being able to satisfy other basic human needs.

Or, said in simpler terms: is the medicine present in the pharmacy? Is it possible to obtain the medicines from the pharmacy? And: has the patient sufficient means to buy it? All these three conditions need to be fulfilled in order that the patient is able to benefit the medicines: even if opioids are present in the nearest pharmacy (available), if the doctor is not willing to prescribe or the authorities prevent prescribing

Table 19.1 Number of people (in thousands) living in countries, according to Adequacy of Consumption Measure (ACM) and region

ACM	AFRO population (thousands)	AMRO population (thousands)	EMRO population (thousands)	EURO population (thousands)	SEARO population (thousands)	WPRO population (thousands)	Global population in thousands (%)
ACM≥1 (adequate consumption)	0	335,418	0	128,622	0	0	464,040 (7 %)
0.3≤ACM<1 (moderate consumption)	0	0	0	227,658	0	24,670	252,328 (4 %)
0.1≤ACM <0.3 (low consumption)	0	0	0	127,390	0	127,953	255,343 (4 %)
0.03≤ACM <0.1 (very low consumption)	1,338	206,346	76,506	94,160	0	78,566	456,916 (7 %)
ACM<0.03 (virtually no consumption)	502,501	303,900	399,919	283,081	1,718,985	1,510,365	4,718,751 (72 %)
No data	269,953	49,280	63,858	25,944	2,063	21,810	432,908 (7 %)
Total	773,792	894,944	540,283	886,855	1,721,048	1,763,364	6,580,286 (100 %)

From Seya et al. [9]

(inaccessible), or if the patient does not have the money for it (unaffordable), the pain will not be relieved. It is possible to measure availability, accessibility, and affordability or aspects of these variables separately, although measuring does not always result in a figure, but rather in a list of medicines, a list of restrictions, etc.

Others define five dimensions under the larger concept of access to health-care; availability, accessibility, affordability, adequacy, and acceptability [13] or affordability, availability, accessibility, accommodation, and acceptability [14, 15].

Availability was measured by Cherny et al. in their almost worldwide surveys on barriers for access to opioid analgesics by showing which opioids were admitted to the market by the authorities. The first one relates to the WHO European region (also including the Commonwealth of Independent States) [16]. The second study covers the rest of the world except for Canada and the USA. For India, it analyses all its states separately (publication under preparation). *Accessibility* is also included in the surveys by Cherny et al. mentioned above by exploring which restrictions exist on prescribing and dispensing of opioid analgesics.

The methods used for measuring *affordability* of opioid analgesics are not any different from those for other medicines. However, there are several difficulties in measuring this variable. Just comparing the cost of treatment is not a good indicator, as income levels, exchange rate to one currency taken as a standard and purchasing power vary over time and between countries. It will be clear that the impact of the need for a treatment that costs $ 1 per day is much different for a worker in a high-income country than for workers in low-income countries. Therefore, it is important to adjust for the local income and the price level. The WHO-HAI methodology expresses affordability of a treatment as the number of days' wages of the lowest-paid unskilled government worker required to purchase the treatment [17]. The lowest rank of government worker was taken because it was considered to be a decent wage. However, this is not true for all countries; in some countries wages are that low that the lowest-paid unskilled government worker needs a second job to survive.

Niëns et al. measured affordability of a treatment by the percentage of people that fall into poverty if they pay for that treatment. For this purpose they use the World Bank limits for poverty of US$ 1.25 and US$ 2.00 (purchasing power parity). For example, using the poverty line of US$ 2.00 means that if the daily cost of a (chronic) treatment is y dollars, everybody with a daily wage below US$ (2.00+y) will fall into poverty if he has to pay for that treatment. Thus, the percentage of people falling into poverty can be calculated from the distribution of wage levels by taking the percentage of the population that earns less than US$ (2.00+y) per day [18]. The advantage of this method is that it is freed from a number of arbitrary standards and that the outcomes can be compared over country boundaries.

Barriers

A variety of barriers can be at the root of limited availability, accessibility, and affordability. In practice, in all countries barriers exist that limit access to controlled medicines including to opioid analgesics. In many countries, these barriers are severe enough to prevent for most patients that they will have adequate treatment when in need. Four categories of barriers can be distinguished:
• Legislative and policy barriers
• Knowledge barriers
• Attitude barriers
• Economic barriers

These barriers will be described now and examples will be given. It is important to realise that often many barriers exist simultaneously and that therefore the problem of inadequate treatment can only truly be dissolved if all barriers are removed. However, in many cases, it is not easy to dissolve the barriers as some barriers interact and maintain each other. (An example is described below, under Attitude Barriers.)

Legislative and Policy Barriers

Substances that potentially can be abused are regulated internationally by three international treaties, including the Single Convention on Narcotic Drugs, 1961, as amended by the 1972 Protocol, which is the most relevant treaty for opioid analgesics [6, 19, 20]. This convention is based on the principle that the substances listed in its annexes ("schedules") are prohibited to be possessed, manufactured, and handled in several other ways. Health-care professionals are exempt from (parts of) this prohibition and companies that manufacture or trade these medicines can be licensed. Patients to whom the controlled medicines were prescribed are also allowed to possess the medicines. Countries that signed the convention (almost all countries in the world) obliged themselves to implement it in their national law. The requirements from the conventions are a minimum: the parties to the treaties are allowed to apply stricter rules.

Furthermore, the convention has a complex system to control international trade: countries need to submit estimates to the INCB in advance of the calendar year for the amount of each substance that they expect to import. For the actual transfer from one country to the other, the importing country needs to issue an import license, and one copy of this license needs to be sent to the exporting country, which checks the balance of the estimate for the substance involved; if the balance is positive, it issues an export license. Often countries do not estimate high enough and then run out of stock in the course of the year, but they can submit a supplementary estimate in order to avoid that exports will be blocked.

There are two ways how this international system of drug control often derails. At the international level many countries are not able to apply the estimate system well and cannot or do not import opioids for this reason. In order to guide the countries how to develop the annual estimates, the World Health Organization and the INCB developed the Guide on Estimating Requirements for Substances under International Control [21].

At the national level, the too strict implementation is often the problem. Restrictions that countries add to the obligations from the conventions can be many. Examples are [12]:
• Legal maximum daily dosage (e.g., dosages as low as 75 mg/day).
• Legal limitation of the duration for which opioid analgesics may be prescribed to a very short period (e.g., as short as 1 day).

- Limitation to certain conditions (e.g., prescription is allowed only for terminal cancer patients).
- Limitation to certain medical specialists (e.g., in one country palliative care physicians are not allowed to prescribe opioids and need to refer to general practitioners; in another country only surgeons, oncologists, and gynaecologists were allowed to prescribe opioids until recently).
- Pharmacists and physicians are not allowed to dispense and to deliver if they are not in the possession of an additional license for controlled medicines.
- Opioid analgesics are dispensed by the police at the police station.
- Obligation to use special prescription forms, sometimes in duplicate, triplicate, or quadruplicate and sometimes hard to obtain or to be obtained against a fee.

Administrative barriers are due to these legislative barriers. In some countries, the authorities in charge of drug control are located in ministries such as the Ministry of Justice, and responsible officers are sometimes unaware that the substances they have to regulate are also used as medicines, while the Ministry of Health has little power to influence the situation. In other countries no policies are in place for availability of medicines, cancer control or HIV, and so on, thus affecting the ability to treat patients with these diseases for their pain.

Knowledge Barriers

Knowledge on the use of opioid analgesics is also problematic in some countries, in particular where opioids are not readily available. Furthermore, many schools of medicines and of pharmacy have very limited time included in their curricula for the treatment of pain.

It is in such a situation almost impossible to become an experienced prescriber. Furthermore, many text and handbooks recommend relatively high initial dosages and do not describe how to titrate the dosage to address the pain adequately. In such a situation, physicians when trying out

the use of opioids based on the recommendations in the handbooks may prescribe too high initial dosages or increase it too quickly, with a result that they see their patient intoxicated and they will not easily use opioids again for treating the pain. The new WHO guidelines on persisting pain in children recommend much lower dosages and slow titration [22]. Special attention was given to the lower dosages and a call was made to adapt text- and handbooks [23].

Also, there are false beliefs that pain patients become easily dependent on opioid analgesics. However, not many physicians who prescribe opioids themselves have seen dependence developing from the opioids they initiated. A recent systematic review could not identify convincing evidence for dependence resulting from pain prescriptions and concluded that it is not justified to withhold treatment to patients because of this fear [24].

Attitude Barriers

Attitude barriers are found among health-care workers, patients, and their families, as well as policy makers. They are often related to knowledge barriers. For instance, many doctors have opinions about opioid analgesics without ever prescribing them. Some of them fear for dependence, mix up withdrawal and tolerance with dependence, or fear that their patients will die from opioids. The fact that opioids are not available in many countries makes that these physicians will never be able to experience the actual benefit/risk ratio of opioid analgesia in their patients, and therefore this contributes to the very low demand for opioid analgesics in these countries. But the fact that there is no demand maintains also their unavailability as there is no advantage for manufacturers to try and sell these medicines. In this way, the lack of knowledge and this attitude interact and maintain each other. Other health-care workers tell themselves that neonates do not feel any pain or find it normal that a certain disease or intervention coincides with severe pain.

Similar attitudes that prevent adequate use of opioid analgesics exist among patients and their families; for instance, the myth that one easily becomes dependent or that one will die from the opioids [1]. The fear of becoming dependent exists even in terminal cancer patients. In fact, if prescribed correctly, opioids are safe medicines, but because they are so often only used in end-stage cancer, there is an association between death and morphine use, which is interpreted by many as a causal relationship with morphine as the cause. Although this may be true if the morphine is not dosed correctly, in most cases it is more likely that the disease is the death cause.

Policy makers tend to give priority to the prevention of abuse, dependence, and diversion of opioid medicines. This may easily lead to restriction on the prescription of opioid analgesics, even if there is no proven mechanism that shows a relation between treatment of pain patients and opioid abuse. In the UK the conviction of Harold Shipman, a practitioner who killed over 250 of his patients with injections of diamorphine, leads to the restriction of the validity of a prescription to 30 days, while the amount on a prescription may not exceed 1 month. It is clear that this does not limit physicians' access to opioid medicines, but indeed, every patient needs to consult his practitioner now every month for a new prescription [25]. This is time-consuming, causes frequent absences from work, and in case of patients who are stable on their medication, this may be exaggerated.

In the USA, the national epidemic of overdoses from prescription opioids leads to a campaign in the press and by others to limit patients' access, even though there is evidence that these medicines usually do not originate from patients. While there are insufficient data available to quantify the amounts diverted to nonmedical use from various parts of the drug distribution system, it appears there is significant theft, fraud, and other unlawful conducts [26, 27]. A national population-based survey found that over 70 % of those who have reported using opioids nonmedically admitted that they obtained the drug for free from friends or family members or through theft or purchase [28]. Large quantities of prescription opioids have been sold by illegitimate pain clinics, and overdose has occurred predominantly in persons obtaining opioids from nonmedical

sources [29]. In a study of unintentional overdose fatalities in West Virginia, 63.1 % of the decedents had used pharmaceuticals with no documented prescriptions, and 55.6 % of the decedents were never prescribed opioid analgesics. In addition, 79.3 % of the decedents has used multiple substances, both illicit and prescription drugs ("polydrug use"), which might have contributed to their death, and 21.4 % of the decedents had controlled medicines prescribed by multiple physicians ("doctor shopping") [30]. This study did not determine, however, whether decedents from the latter group were "real" pain patients or people seeking drugs for illicit purposes. Another American study, describing 9,940 cases of overdose deaths, found 51 cases to whom dosages of 100 mg/day or higher of morphine equivalents were prescribed during the first 3 months of a prescription episode, showing an increased risk for this group [31].

Economic Barriers

Economic barriers are not any different for opioid analgesics than for other medicines. High prices and failure to distribute the medicines adequately are common, although morphine is a cheap starting material and can be made available for even USD 0.05 per day per patient. However, some specific additional barriers exist for those medicines which are controlled as drugs. Examples are that low price levels are often related to low markups. If this is the case, pharmacists and distributors often do not want to invest in a legally required wall safe or strongbox. (In some cases, the legal requirements are disproportionate to the amount to be stored.) Also the amount of paperwork can be disproportionate if the amount of medicines is limited, or it can push up the price [1].

Overviews of Barriers

There are various publications that give overviews of the barriers [16, 32] and pricing of opioids [33]. The WHO policy guidelines also provide a checklist to analyse the national situation in a country.

International Developments Toward Adequate Access for All

The World Health Assembly requested from WHO in a resolution to "examine jointly with the International Narcotics Control Board the feasibility of a possible assistance mechanism that would facilitate the adequate treatment of pain using opioid analgesics" [34]. In response, the World Health Organization established the Access to Controlled Medicines Programme (ACMP) [36]. Over the years, the ACMP developed a number of documents to guide policy makers and health-care professionals to improve access to opioid analgesics and other controlled medicines. For example, it planned to develop a series of treatment guidelines on pain, together covering all types of pain, while in the past only cancer pain has been addressed [37, 38]. Currently the evidence-based guidelines on persisting pain in children [22] and a scoping document describing the outlines of similar guidelines for persisting pain in adults have been published [39]. The ACMP also published the WHO policy guidelines Ensuring Balance in National Policies on Controlled Substances, Accessibility and Availability of Controlled Medicines [12]. This document includes a country checklist to identify the specific barriers in specific countries. It is recommended not only for policy makers but also for organisations of health-care workers who want to work on improved access. Jointly with the INCB, the ACMP published their guide on estimating requirements already mentioned above [21]. Although it is intended for use by the competent authorities for the international drug control treaties, it is recommended that other organisations are familiar with this document, in particular in countries where the importations of controlled medicines pose regular problems. In that case the estimate systems may be involved and it happens that health-care professionals guide the authorities how to solve the problem. The ACMP and a number of NGOs provide support to countries that want to improve access to controlled medicines, e.g., by organising workshops and reviewing (draft) legislation.

The INCB continues to advocate for improved access, and in most years its annual report makes recommendations to the countries who are parties to the international drug control treaties. Recently, it published a special report on the availability of internationally controlled medicines [4]. Strange enough, simultaneously the INCB is lobbying since several years among the countries to place ketamine on their national lists of controlled drugs, in this way precipitating a global crisis for anaesthesia similar to the current crisis in analgesia, while WHO assessed that the substance should not be placed under drug control [40–42].

The UN Economic and Social Council [36] and the UN Commission on Narcotic Drugs also called for greater access for patients to these medicines on several occasions [43, 44].

In addition to these diplomatic activities, international organisations of health-care professionals made the call for adequate access to pain medicines and treatment of pain worldwide heard through documents like the Declaration of Montreal, the World Cancer Declaration, the Morphine Manifesto, and the Declaration of Miami [45–48]. Other international projects are the Global Access to Pain Relief Initiative (GAPRI) [49] and the ATOME Project. The latter is a comprehensive EU-funded project ran by ten organisations, including WHO targeting at 12 eastern European countries [50].

Conclusion

"All moderate and severe pain in children should always be addressed. Depending on the situation, the treatment of moderate to severe pain may include non-pharmacological methods, treatment with non-opioid analgesics and with opioid analgesics" is the approach in the new WHO treatment guidelines on persisting pain in children [22]. Although there are no WHO persisting pain guidelines for adults currently, it could be imagined that such a document would not say any different because of the ethical aspect. It should be noticed that the guidelines do not impose to treat with opioids, but it imposes to act. However, in most cases of moderate and severe pain, opioid analgesics are indicated and even inevitable. It is for this reason that access to opioid analgesics is of utmost importance, but in spite of that, it is still a unfulfilled hope for the majority of the world population. Yet, a change has set on by the efforts of international bodies and NGOs. It is likely that many are already working on these issues on the national and local level in many countries. Sooner or later all countries will have to follow when it becomes clear how beneficial and effective pain treatment can be.

In order to ensure that "effective pain control measures will be available universally to all cancer patients in pain" by 2020 (as mentioned in the World Cancer Declaration) [46], we will need to record our progress and analyse the barriers for adequate pain management. Only by doing both, we can work on solutions and ascertain that our efforts are effective. By treating the pain, we accommodate the patient by improving his quality of life on one important aspect of his or her disease, which is the pain, sometimes excruciating. It is for this reason that access to opioid analgesics is essential for quality cancer care. And this is possible.

Key Points

- Access to and availability of opioid analgesics is essential for relieving this pain, yet opioid analgesics are not accessible to 5.5 billion people.
- Each year, 5.5 million terminal cancer patients, 1 million end-stage HIV/AIDS patients, and 0.8 million patients suffering injuries, caused by accidents and violence, are not treated for moderate and severe pain. In addition to this, it includes patients with chronic illnesses, patients recovering from surgery, women in labour (110 million births each year), and paediatric patients.
- Various methods exist to measure the consumption, usually in morphine equivalents. The top 20 countries from the Human Development Index can be used as a benchmark.

- The adequacy of opioid analgesic consumption has a high logarithmic correlation with the Human Development Index (CC=0.895).
- Availability is the degree to which a medicine is present at distribution points in a defined area for the population living in that area at the moment of need.
- Accessibility is the degree to which a medicine is obtainable for those who need it at the moment of need with the least possible regulatory, social, or psychological barriers.
- Affordability is the degree to which a medicine is obtainable for those who need it at the moment of need at a cost that does not expose them to the risk of serious negative consequences such as not being able to satisfy other basic human needs.
- Four categories of barriers can be distinguished: legislative and policy barriers, knowledge barriers, attitudes barriers, and economic barriers.
- In recent years efforts for improvement are undertaken by international bodies (World Health Organization, International Narcotics Control Board, Commission on Narcotic Drugs) and by nongovernmental organisations (International Association for the Study of Pain, Union for International Cancer Control, Pallium India, American Cancer Society). Joint projects as the Global Access to Pain Relief Initiative (GAPRI) and the Access to Opioid Medications in Europe (ATOME) were initiated.

References

1. Krakauer EL, et al. Opioid inaccessibility and its human consequences: reports from the field. J Pain Palliat Care Pharmacother. 2010;24(3):239–43. Accessible at: http://informahealthcare.com/doi/abs/10.3109/153602 88.2010.501852. Accessed 11 Oct 2012.
2. International Narcotics Control Board. Demand for and supply of opiates for medical and scientific needs.

In: Report of the International Narcotics Control Board for 1989. New York: United Nations; 1989.

3. World Health Organization. mhGAP Mental Health Gap Action Programme. Scaling up care for mental, neurological, and substance use disorders. Geneva. 2008. Accessible at: http://whqlibdoc.who.int/publications/2008/9789241596206_eng.pdf. Accessed 12 Oct 2012.

4. International Narcotics Control Board. Report of the International Narcotics Control Board on the availability of internationally controlled drugs: ensuring adequate access for medical and scientific purposes. New York; 2011, E/INCB/2010/1/Supp.1. ISBN 978-92-1-148260-7. Accessible at: http://www.incb.org/documents/Publications/AnnualReports/AR10_Supp_E.pdf. Accessed 11 Oct 2012.

5. World Health Organization. Access to Controlled Medications Programme: improving access to medications under international drug conventions: briefing note. Geneva. 2012. Accessible at: http://www.who.int/entity/medicines/areas/quality_safety/ACMP_BrNote_Genrl_EN_Apr2012.pdf. Accessed 8 June 2013.

6. Single Convention on Narcotic Drugs, 1961, as amended by the Protocol amending the Single Convention on Narcotic Drugs, 1961. In: The International Drug Conventions. United Nations, New York; 2009. ISBN 978 92 1 148248 5. Accessible at: https://www.unodc.org/pdf/convention_1961_en.pdf. Accessed 11 Oct 2012.

7. International Narcotics Control Board. Narcotic drugs: estimated world requirements for 2012 statistics for 2010. New York: United Nations; 2011. E/INCB/2011/2. ISBN 978-92-1-048149-6. http://www.incb.org/documents/Narcotic-Drugs/Technical-Publications/2011/Narcotic_Drugs_Report_2011.pdf. Accessed on 11 Oct 2012.

8. ATC Index with DDDs. WHO Collaborating Centre for Drug Statistics and Methodology. Oslo, 2005.

9. Bekkering GE, et al. Epidemiology of chronic pain and its treatment in the Netherlands. Neth J Med. 2011;69(3):141–52 (Systematic review).

10. Seya MJ, Gelders SFAM, Achara UA, Milani B, Scholten WK. A first comparison between the consumption of and the need for opioid analgesics at country, regional and global level. J Pain Palliat Care Pharmacother. 2011;25:6–18. Accessible at: http://apps.who.int/medicinedocs/documents/s17976en/s17976en.pdf. Accessed 11 Oct 2012.

11. United Nations Development Programme. Human Development Report 2011, Sustainability and equity: a better future for all. New York: United Nations Development Programme; 2011. ISBN 9780230363311. Accessible at: http://www.undp.org/content/dam/undp/library/corporate/HDR/2011%20Global%20HDR/English/HDR_2011_EN_Complete.pdf. Accessed 11 Oct 2012.

12. World Health Organization. Ensuring balance in national policies on controlled substances, guidance for availability and accessibility of controlled medicines. Geneva. 2011. ISBN 978 92 4 156417 5.

Accessible at: http://whqlibdoc.who.int/publications/2011/9789241564175_eng.pdf. Accessed 1 Oct 2012.

13. Obrist B, et al. Access to health care in contexts of livelihood insecurity: a framework for analysis and action. PLoS Med. 2007;4(10):e308. doi:10.1371/journal.pmed.0040308. Available at: http://www.plosmedicine.org/article/info%3Adoi%2F10.1371%2Fjournal.pmed.0040308. Accessed 14 Oct 2012.

14. Penchansky R, Thomas JW. The concept of access: definition and relationship to consumer satisfaction. Med Care. 1981;19(2):127–40. Accessible at: http://www.ncbi.nlm.nih.gov/pubmed/7206846. Accessed 14 Oct 2012.

15. Wyszewianski L. Access to care: remembering old lessons. Health Serv Res. 2002;37(6):1441–3. doi:10.1111/1475-6773.12171. Accessible at: http://www.ncbi.nlm.nih.gov/pmc/articles/PMC1464050/. Accessed 14 Oct 2012.

16. Cherny NI, et al. Formulary availability and regulatory barriers to accessibility of opioids for cancer pain in Europe: a report from the ESMO/EAPC Opioid Policy Initiative. Ann Oncol. 2010;21(3):615–26. Accessible at: http://www.ncbi.nlm.nih.gov/pubmed/20176694. Accessed 14 Oct 2012.

17. Cameron A, et al. Medicines prices, availability and affordability. In: The World Medicines Situation 2011. Geneva: World Health Organization; 2011. Accessible at: http://apps.who.int/medicinedocs/documents/s18065en/s18065en.pdf. Accessed 14 Oct 2012.

18. Niëns LM, et al. Quantifying the impoverishing effects of purchasing medicines: a cross-country comparison of the affordability of medicines in the developing world. PLoS Med. 2010;7(8):e1000333. doi:10.1371/journal.pmed.1000333. Accessible at: http://apps.who.int/medicinedocs/documents/s17402e/s17402e.pdf. Accessed 14 Oct 2012.

19. Convention on Psychotropic Substances, 1971. In: The International Drug Conventions. New York: United Nations; 2009. ISBN 978 92 1 148248 5. Accessible at: https://www.unodc.org/pdf/convention_1971_en.pdf. Accessed 14 Oct 2012.

20. United Nations Convention against Illicit Traffic in Narcotic Drugs and Psychotropic Substances, 1988. In: The International Drug Conventions. New York: United Nations; 2009. ISBN 978 92 1 148248 5. Accessible at: https://www.unodc.org/pdf/convention_1988_en.pdf. Accessed 14 Oct 2012.

21. Guide on estimating requirements for substances under international control, developed by the International Narcotics Control Board and the World Health Organization for use by the Competent National Authorities, International Narcotics Control Board and World Health Organization, Vienna/Geneva. 2012. ISBN 978-92-4-150328-0. Available at: http://whqlibdoc.who.int/publications/2012/9789241503280_eng.pdf. Accessed 14 Oct 2012.

22. World Health Organization. WHO guidelines on the pharmacological treatment of persisting

pain in children with medical illnesses. 2012. Available at: http://whqlibdoc.who.int/publications/2012/9789241548120_Guidelines.pdf. Accessed 14 Oct 2012.

23. Scholten W. Paediatric morphine dosages. WHO Pharmaceuticals Newsletter. 2012;(4):26–28. Accessible at: http://www.who.int/medicines/publications/Newsletter_4_2012.pdf. Accessed 14 Oct 2012.

24. Minozzi S, et al. Systematic review on dependence following treatment with opioid analgesics for pain relief: a systematic review. Addiction. 2013;108(4):688–98. doi:10.1111/j.1360-0443.2012.04005.x.

25. Gallagher CT. New CD regulations will not obstruct "another Shipman" who intends to kill. Pharm J. 2006;277(7407):13–6.

26. Inciardi JA, et al. Mechanisms of prescription drug diversion among drug-involved club and street based populations. Pain Med. 2007;8(2):171–83. doi:10.1111/j.1526-4637.2006.00255.x.

27. Inciardi JA, et al. Diversion of prescription drugs by health workers in Cincinnati Ohio. Subst Use Misuse. 2006;41(2):255–64.

28. Substance Abuse and Mental Health Services Administration, Results from the 2010 National Survey on Drug Use and Health: Summary of National Findings, NSDUH Series H-41, HHS Publication No. (SMA) 11–4658. Rockville: Substance Abuse and Mental Health Services Administration; 2011. Accessible at: http://oas.samhsa.gov/NSDUH/2k10NSDUH/2k10Results.pdf. Accessed 15 Oct 2012.

29. CDC. Vital signs: overdoses of prescription opioid pain relievers – United States, 1999–2008. Morb Mortal Wkly. 2011;60(43):1487–92. Available at: http://www.cdc.gov/mmwr/preview/mmwrhtml/mm6043a4.htm?s_cid=mm6043a4_w. Accessed 2 July 2012.

30. Hall AJ, Logan JE, Toblin RL, et al. Patterns of abuse among unintentional pharmaceutical overdose fatalities. JAMA. 2008;300:2613–20.

31. Dunn KM, et al. Opioid prescriptions for chronic pain and overdose a cohort study. Ann Intern Med. 2010;152:85–92.

32. Milani B, Scholten W. Access to controlled medicines. In: The world medicines situation 2011. 3rd edn. Geneva: World Health Organization; 2011 (Chapter released April 2011). Accessible at: http://www.who.int/entity/medicines/areas/policy/world_medicines_situation/WMS_ch19_wAccess.pdf. Accessed 15 Oct 2012.

33. International Association for Hospice and Palliative Cate, The Opioid Price Watch Project. Accessible at: http://hospicecare.com/resources/opioid-price-watch/. Accessed 8 June 2013.

34. Resolution WHA58.22. Cancer prevention and control. In: Fifty-eighth World Health Assembly, Geneva, 25 May 2005. A copy of the resolution can be found in: http://www.who.int/entity/medicines/areas/quality_safety/Framework_ACMP_withcover.pdf. Accessed 15 Oct 2012.

35. Resolution ECOSOC 2005/25. On treatment of pain using opioid analgesics. New York. 2005. A copy of the resolution can be found in: http://www.who.int/entity/medicines/areas/quality_safety/Framework_ACMP_withcover.pdf. Accessed 15 Oct 2012.

36. Access to Controlled Medications Programme, Framework. Geneva: World Health Organization; 2007. WHO/PSM/QSM/2007.2. Accessible at: http://www.who.int/entity/medicines/areas/quality_safety/Framework_ACMP_withcover.pdf. Accessed 15 Oct 2012.

37. Cancer pain relief with a guide to opioid availability. 2nd edn. Geneva: World Health Organization; 1996. ISBN 9789241544825. Accessible at: http://apps.who.int/iris/bitstream/10665/37896/1/9241544821.pdf. Accessed 15 Oct 2012.

38. Cancer pain relief and palliative care in children. Geneva: World Health Organization; 1998. ISBN 9789241545129. Accessible at: http://apps.who.int/iris/bitstream/10665/42001/1/9241545127.pdf. Accessed 15 Oct 2012.

39. Scoping document for WHO Guidelines for the pharmacological treatment of persisting pain in adults with medical illnesses. Geneva: World Health Organization, Expert Committee on Drug Dependence, 35th Report. Technical Report Series 973, Geneva 2012. ISBN 978-92-4-120973-1. Accessible at: http://www.who.int/entity/medicines/areas/quality_safety/Final_35th_ECDD.pdf. Accessed 15 Oct 2012.

40. International Narcotics Control Board. Report of the International Narcotics Control Board for 2007. New York. 2008. E/INCB/2007/1. ISBN 978-92-1-148224-9. Accessible at: http://www.incb.org/documents/Publications/AnnualReports/AR_07_English.pdf. Accessed 16 Oct 2012.

41. International Narcotics Control Board. Report of the International Narcotics Control Board for 2008. New York. 2009. E/INCB/2008/1. ISBN 978-92-1-148232-4. Accessible at: http://www.incb.org/documents/Publications/AnnualReports/AR_08_English.pdf. Accessed 16 Oct 2012.

42. WHO Expert Committee on Drug Dependence, Thirty-fifth report. WHO Technical Report Series 973. Geneva: World Health Organization; 2012. ISBN 978 92 4 120973 1, ISSN 0250–8737. Accessible at: http://apps.who.int/iris/bitstream/10665/77747/1/WHO_trs_973_eng.pdf. Accessed 8 June 2013.

43. Commission on Narcotic Drugs. Resolution 53/4 Promoting adequate availability of internationally controlled licit drugs for medical and scientific purposes while preventing their diversion and abuse. Report on the fifty-third session (2 December 2009 and 8–12 March 2010). Economic and Social Council, Official Records, 2010, Supplement No. 8. E/CN.7/2010/18. Accessible at: https://www.unodc.org/unodc/en/commissions/CND/session/cnd-documents-index.html. Accessed 16 Oct 2012.

44. Commission on Narcotic Drugs. Resolution 54/6 Promoting adequate availability of internationally controlled narcotic drugs and psychotropic substances

for medical and scientific purposes while preventing their diversion and abuse. In: Report on the fifty-fourth session (2 December 2010 and 21–25 March 2011) Economic and Social Council, Official Records, 2011, Supplement No. 8. United Nations, New York, 2011. E/CN.7/2011/15. Accessible at: https://www.unodc.org/unodc/en/commissions/CND/session/cnd-documents-index.html. Accessed 16 Oct 2012.

45. Declaration of Montréal, declaration that access to pain management is a fundamental human right, Montreal. 2011. Accessible at: http://www.iasp-pain.org/Content/NavigationMenu/Advocacy/DeclarationofMontr233al/default.htm. Accessed 13 Sept 2012.

46. International Union against Cancer. World Cancer Declaration. Clin J Oncol Nurs. 2006;10(6):721–2. Accessible at: http://www.uicc.org/sites/default/files/private/eWCDEC_2.pdf. Accessed 16 Oct 2012.

47. Pallium India, International Association for Hospice and Palliative Care, and the Pain & Policy Studies Group. A morphine manifesto. J Pain Palliat Care Pharmacother. 2012;26(2):144–5. doi:10.3109/15360288.2012.678475. Accessible at: http://informahealthcare.com/doi/abs/10.3109/15360288.2012.678475. Accessed 16 Oct 2012.

48. Declaration of Miami, Joining forces for better pain treatment and promoting pain medicine all over the world. World Institute of Pain, Miami. 2012. Accessible at: http://www.wipfoundation.org/wp-content/uploads/2012/04/electronic-version-declaration-of-miami1.png. Accessed 19 Oct 2012.

49. GAPRI: Global Access To Pain Relief Initiative, Union for International Cancer Control, s.l.a. Accessible at: http://www.uicc.org/sites/default/files/private/120806_eGAPRI_OnePager_Final.pdf. Accessed 17 Oct 2012.

50. Radbruch L, et al. Access to opioid medication in Europe (Letter to the Editor). J Pain Palliat Care Pharmacother. 2012;26:200–1. Accessible at: http://informahealthcare.com/doi/abs/10.3109/15360288.2012.676614. Accessed 17 Oct 2012.

Challenges for Pain Management in the Twenty-First Century

20

Mellar P. Davis

Abstract

Pain occurs in 20 % of the population, 50 % of patients who present with cancer have pain and 70 % of patients with advanced cancer will have acute and chronic pain. Opioids are the standard treatment of choice, but half of patients experience side effects which can reduce quality of life. Chronic pain is the result of central neuroplasticity and hypersensitivity. Within disease entities, there are different pain phenotypes which are generated by distinct mechanisms, and each phenotype in turn has different responses to analgesics. Analgesics such as opioids selectively bias signalling from mu, kappa, and delta receptors. Receptor responses are modulated by homotropic and heterotropic tolerance mechanisms. Combinations of opioids may modulate responses through single receptors or dimers and reestablish nociception in animal models. This is particularly seen with methadone and morphine. Bivalent opioids are reported to reduce psychologic dependence (as measured by reduced conditioned place preference in animal models), improve analgesia, and reduce side effects presumably through interactions on opioid dimers. Multivalent opioid/non-opioid receptor drugs and opioid-monoamine transporter inhibitor bivalent analgesics are available and have advantages compared to opioid monomers, as demonstrated in certain animal models and clinical situations. The key to analgesic development is to target pain phenotypes with selective analgesics initially in animal models then validate results through enrichment designed trials.

Keywords

Analgesics • Pain • Opioids • Phenotype • Dimers

M.P. Davis, MD, FCCP, FAAHPM
Department of Solid Tumor,
Taussig Cancer Institute,
Cleveland Clinic Lerner School of Medicine,
Cleveland Clinic,
9500 Euclid Ave,
Cleveland, OH 44195, USA
e-mail: davism6@ccf.org

Introduction

Pain is a major health problem which substantially reduces quality of life. It has a major impact on economic health-related costs and imparts a significant financial loss to society in terms of absenteeism,

M. Hanna, Z. Zylicz (eds.), *Cancer Pain*,
DOI 10.1007/978-0-85729-230-8_20, © Springer-Verlag London 2013

production loss, and insurance costs. Management with standard analgesics such as opioids and NSAIDs is less than optimal. Opioids are associated with multiple side effects including nausea, vomiting, and psychotomimetic reactions. In a subset of patients, analgesic tolerance and physical tolerance occur, and, in an unfortunate minority, psychologic dependence can develop. NSAIDs have been associated with renal and liver failure, gastrointestinal bleeding, cardiovascular complications, worsened heart failure, and, in a few, confusion [1].

Most analgesic benefits are determined in randomised trials by the differences in the mean pain intensity between groups or the proportion of responders. Meaningful responses are defined as a 30–50 % reduction in pain severity. Most analgesics have a number needed to treat (NNT) of 3–5, which means one out of three individuals at best will have some meaningful reduction in pain [1].

Most newly released opioids, unfortunately, are reformulations of older potent mu agonists as sustained-release, transdermal, intranasal, or buccal opioids, which continue to have the same problems. Other reformulations are attempts to produce abuse deterrent products, as deaths from commercially available opioids are on the rise.

Physicians are woefully ignorant about the pharmacology of opioids and the neurobiology of pain. Most U.S. states do not require continued education in analgesics. Prescribing is usually empiric, rote, and not clinically attuned to the patient's situation, clinical context, or pain mechanism [1].

On the positive side, there is an improved understanding of pain mechanisms and the molecular and anatomical structure of pain pathways. Pain imaging is now possible. The molecular structure of the opioid receptor and signal transduction that result from conformational changes in opioid receptors are now well described. The recent discovery of opioid dimers has stimulated the development of unique multivalent analgesics. This improved understanding in opioid pharmacology will provide avenues to analgesic development in the twenty-first century.

Pain Mechanisms

For many individuals with chronic maladaptive pain, the trigger or initiator of pain is gone, and the present state is the result of neuroplasticity and central amplification of pain [2–4]. Amplification of sensory signals occurs with maladaptive pain due to loss of inhibition, synaptogenesis, increased synaptic efficiency, altered receptor expression, and enhanced excitatory neurotransmitter production. Pain can be spontaneous, generated at CNS sites upstream from the original injury. What was originally nonpainful becomes painful to light touch [5]. The risk of developing maladaptive pain is known to have a significant genetic component [6–8]. Common pain-processing disorders such as migraines, fibromyalgia, irritable bowel syndrome, interstitial cystitis, and temporomandibular joint disease run in families [1].

Nociceptive input triggers a prolonged but reversible increase in neuronal excitability and synaptic efficacy, which is called central sensitisation. Clinically, central sensitisation may cause dynamic tactile allodynia or secondary punctate hyperalgesia in the area around the site of injury. After sensations and enhanced temporal summation (windup), are also manifestations of central sensitisation which can be imaged by functional MRI (fMRI). Important persistent pain-processing disorders are osteoarthritis, musculoskeletal disorders, neuropathic pain, and persistent postoperative pain (postmastectomy or post-thoracotomy pain syndromes). These syndromes respond to central analgesics. Diabetes is associated with persistent neuropathic pain in a subset and in others associated with the loss of sensation. A subset of patients with shingles develop persistent pain, while others experience persistent numbness. Diabetic neuropathy and postherpetic neuropathy have different pain phenotypes within each disease category. And within disease entity, there are different pain phenotypes [1].

Pain assessment is one way to begin to phenotype pain. As an example, five screening questionnaires have been developed for neuropathic pain [9]. These questionnaires have verbal descriptors for pain qualities and abnormal sensations such as paresthesias and dysesthesias. The questionnaires have discriminate properties and are simple and easy to use. Compared to clinical judgment, these questionnaires are very good to excellent measures of neuropathic pain. Two questionnaires, the Neuropathic Pain Syndrome

Inventory and the Neuropathic Pain Scale are able to measure separate dimensions of neuropathic pain which are key to phenotyping pain in clinical trials. These measures are far superior to using nonspecific pain severity scales and would allow trials to use an enrichment enrolment design based on similar phenotypes when conducting exploratory interventional trials with new analgesics [1].

Before central sensitisation was proposed as a mechanism for chronic pain, two theories of pain were popular. The first proposed that pain pathways were continuously activated by a pain stimulus, with pain intensity proportional to sensory input. The second theory was a "gate theory" which centred nociceptive processing in the dorsal horn of the spinal cord. Pain intensity was thought to be the balance of inhibitory and facilitatory mechanisms. Central sensitisation is now an important concept. Central sensitisation involves early neuroplastic events which are heterosynaptic and homosynaptic, occurring within the CNS, which results in altered sensation, expanded receptive fields of pain, referral to somatic sites, and long-term potentiation [10, 11]. The concept of central sensitisation means that early and effective use of analgesics and adjuvant analgesics will be vital to preventing homosynaptic and heterosynaptic facilitation and long-term pain [12].

Opioid Receptor Dynamics and Novel Development

Mu, delta, and kappa opioid receptors are found in the peripheral and central nervous system. In animal models, there are interactions between mu receptors in the peripheral nerves, dorsal horn, and in various brainstem regions (principally the periaqueductal grey and the rostral ventromedial medulla) [13]. Intrathecal or intracerebroventricular morphine acts as a full mu receptor agonist in animal models. However, there is a 29–45-fold reduction in the dose needed for antinociception when morphine is given by both systematically and intrathecal [13]. Intracerebroventricular or intrathecal naloxone blocks systemic morphine analgesia [14]. Combinations of locally applied morphine and spinal morphine produce supra-

additive analgesia [15]. Tolerance to morphine antinociception develops quicker at peripheral sites compared with CNS sites. Analgesic tolerance develops to a greater extent with the coadministration of spinal and systemic morphine in CD-1 mice and results in a 12-fold right shift in dose-response curves. In contrast, supraspinal and systemic morphine produces only a twofold shift in dose-response curves over time [15]. Analgesic tolerance appears to be the result of a loss of peripheral analgesic responses to morphine and loss of supra-additive interactions between peripheral and CNS mu receptors [15]. Neuropathic injury leads to a loss of morphine analgesia. In the spinal nerve ligation animal model, there is a significant loss of topical morphine analgesia and a right shift in dose-response curves with intrathecal morphine, but there is no change in antinociception with intracerebroventricular morphine [16]. Ninety percent of dorsal horn mu receptors are lost in the spinal nerve ligation animal model which may account for the loss of antinociception [16].

One way to overcome peripheral mu receptor tolerance is to combine topical analgesics. Topical analgesia has been demonstrated with morphine, morphine-6-glucuronide, the enkephalin peptide DAMGO, meperidine, levorphanol, and buprenorphine [17]. Supra-additive analgesia is described with the combination of topical methadone and lidocaine. The combination of topical methadone plus topical morphine results in a 7.5-fold left shift in dose-response curves in animal models [17]. There is only additive antinociception when topical morphine is combined with topical meperidine as demonstrated by a 2.7-fold left shift in dose-response curves [17]. Hence supra-additive analgesia depends on the particular opioid combination. Topical meperidine minimises systemic toxicity resulting from conversion to normeperidine and potentially improves the meperidine therapeutic index.

Peripheral inflammation potentiates peripheral opioid analgesia [18]. Inflammation increases axonal transport of opioid receptors to the nerve terminal and increases opioid receptor synthesis [19, 20]. Inflammation disrupts the perineurium and facilitates opioid access to the receptors. Low pH found in inflamed tissues increases agonist efficacy by facilitating opioid receptor

G-protein interactions [21, 22]. Activation of the nerve by bradykinin released from mast cells and of TRPV-1 within inflamed nerves increases the trafficking of delta opioid receptors to membrane surfaces [23]. Nerve growth factor derived from inflammation upregulates certain kinases (MAP kinases) which, in turn, increase mu receptor axonal transport and expression. This results in increases topical opioids analgesia [24, 25]. In addition, analgesic tolerance does not develop in areas of inflammation. Opioid receptors undergo recycling and receptor signal transduction is preserved [26]. A large proportion of analgesia (50–80 %) may be mediated by systemic opioids binding to peripheral opioid receptors [27, 28]. In early stages of inflammation, analgesia is mediated by peripheral and central opioid receptors. However, after several days, peripheral opioid receptors will mediate most of the analgesia demonstrated in animal models [29].

Peripherally administered opioids are antinociception in animal models. Peripherally administered analgesics reduce pain as demonstrated by intra-articular opioids used after orthopaedic procedures and avoids problematic psychotomimetic side effects, withdrawal, and psychologic dependence. Novel arylacetamides (ADL10-0101), morphinan-based opioids (TRK-820), and peptide-based opioids (CR665) (FE200665) are in development [30]. Peripherally restricted opioid agonists are particularly attractive to use in the elderly who have an increased risk of gastrointestinal bleeding, renal failure, and fluid retention with NSAIDs as well as central side effects and increased falls risks with opioid analgesics [31].

In summary, regionally restricted or locally administered analgesics reduce toxicity but also reduces efficacy, since the supra-additive analgesia between supraspinal spinal and peripheral mu receptors does not occur. Another drawback to development of peripherally restricted opioids is that peripheral mu receptors develop analgesic tolerance quickly in non-inflammatory pain states or phenotypes. Analgesic tolerance to peripheral or topical opioid agonists is blunted by inflammation, so the pain mechanism will be important to topical opioid analgesia responses. Neuropathic pain reduces peripheral analgesia by reducing mu receptor expression, and alters transduction signals qualitative. Combinations of topical mu receptor agonists have some evidence for synergy in animal models, but are highly dependent on the particular mu agonist used in combination. Translational studies using animal models will be important in this regard. Combinations of peripherally restricted and topical mu agonists or systemic non-opioid analgesics such as tricyclic antidepressants, anticonvulsants, NSAIDs, or topical anaesthetics have not been explored in any great degree. This could potentially be an area of fruitful research.

Opioid Receptor Interactions and Dimers

Analgesic tolerance, side effects, physical dependence, and psychologic dependence associated with morphine are mediated through mu receptors. Morphine up-regulates delta receptor expression on presynaptic membranes [32–34]. Delta receptors interact with mu receptors to form receptor dimers. Mu-delta heterodimers initially are synergistic; inhibiting responses to neurotransmitter release. Neurotransmitter release is inhibited by delta receptors through activation of phospholipase A_2 and cyclic-AMP/protein kinase A pathways [33]. Delta receptor monomers when activated produce weak analgesia, probably due to low levels of expression on presynaptic membranes. However, when upregulated and combined with mu receptors, supra-additive antinociception occurs with mu/delta receptor agonist combinations [35, 36]. Delta agonists produce less analgesic tolerance and do not enhance opioid-related side effects [37, 38]. Mu receptors bound by a potent agonist are recycled and resensitised in endosomes. However, delta receptors, when activated, are downregulated and destroyed in lysosomes [39]. Activated delta receptors within a heterodimers drag mu receptors into lysosomes [39]. Delta receptors activated by endogenous peptides, such as enkephalin, cause morphine tolerance [40, 41]. Paradoxically, a combination of a delta receptor antagonist with mu receptor agonist enhances heterodimer expression [42]. Transduction which involves G-proteins coupled to the receptor (whether pertussis sensitive or insensitive), beta-2 arrestin interactions (which govern uncoupling of receptor G-protein interaction and receptor trafficking), and activation of various kinases are altered by heterodimer activation compared with monomers [42].

Heterodimers are demonstrated to occur naturally and have a distinctly different transduction pathway compared to monomers. Bivalent opioid ligands have been developed and tested in animal models and have an improved therapeutic index over monovalent potent mu receptor agonists. Bivalent opioids reduce psychologic dependence (as measured by reduced conditioned place preference in animal models), improve analgesia, and reduce side effects [43–47].

The combination of morphine with naltrindole (a low-dose delta receptor antagonist) augments and prolongs morphine antinociception in Sprague-Dawley rats and prevents and reverses antinociception tolerance [48]. These findings suggest that mu-delta receptor dimers exist and changes in dimer conformation by the mu agonists-delta antagonist alter mu receptor pharmacology to facilitate analgesia and reduce analgesic tolerance [49, 50].

Multiple Opioid Ligands

It is unlikely that the development of another potent mu agonist will have a significant impact on pain management. However, since it is now recognised that all three major opioid receptors interact either as closely located monomers or as dimers/oligomers, ligands with mixed opioid receptor activity may have a therapeutic advantage over potent mu agonists [51, 52]. Multivalent opioid ligands are merged, in that the same structure activates two separate receptors (merged pharmacophores). Conjugated pharmacophores have two separate structures, either directly attached to one another or separated by a linker or spacer. Finally, the two pharmacophores can be fused to one another. Certain peptide linkers or spacers between pharmacophores can be cleaved readily resulting in separate pharmacophores or can be made resistant to catabolism and facilitate interactions between binding sites within a dimer. Linkers can alter pharmacophore receptor affinity, depending on the length of the spacer. Linkers may also facilitate CNS penetration [51, 52]. Classes of multivalent ligands have been developed and include (1) peptide-peptide opioid pharmacophores, (2) peptide-non-peptide opioid pharmacophores, (3) opioid alkaloid double pharmacophores, and (4) opioid-non-opioid pharmacophores. The latter are characterised by two commercially available analgesics, tramadol and tapentadol, in which there is an opioid and mono-amine re-uptake inhibitor merged in a single structure.

The best-known peptide-peptide multivalent ligand is biphalin which links enkephalin monomers directly in a "tail-to-tail" coupling. Biphalin (H-Tyr-D-Ala-Gly-Phe-NH)$_2$ is 9,000 times more potent than native met-enkephalin. Biphalin produces less physical dependence than met-enkephalin in animal models [53, 54]. Increasing spacers between enkephalin pharmacophores reduces mu receptor affinity and retains delta receptor affinity [55].

The di-penta-dermorphin (dermorphin is derived from amphibian skin) has a 5-fold affinity for mu receptors and a 45-fold affinity for delta receptors relative to the monovalent peptide enkephalin derivative, DAMGO (D-Ala$_2$, NME Phe$_4$-Gly-ol^5) [56]. Replacing the tyrosine position line with 2,6-dimethyl-L-tyrosine improves binding to mu and delta receptors and results in the mu agonist/delta antagonist. By further modification of the pharmacophores using a pyrazone linker, catabolism of the peptide is blocked. This allows the modified bivalent pharmacophores to be given by mouth [57–59]. Other peptide-peptide and mu-delta receptor pharmacophores have been developed which have less analgesic tolerance and physical dependence, as well as less respiratory suppression and impaired gastrointestinal motility compared with potent mu agonists [51, 60, 61].

Opioid ligands have a "message" and an "address" structure. The "message" portion of the opioid peptide is in the N-terminus which is responsible for activating the receptor and transduction. The C-terminus contains the "address" which assists in binding to the receptor [51]. The opioid alkaloid ligand oxymorphone has been attached to the C-terminus of enkephalin to produce a delta receptor agonist and to the C-terminus of dynorphin to produce a kappa receptor agonist. By combining an opioid alkaloid to an opioid peptide, catabolism of the peptide is blocked [51]. Fentanyl has been combined with (D-Ala^2)-enkephalin as a mu-delta agonist which increases CNS penetration. Tolerance is reduced in animal models compared to monovalent mu agonists. The delta agonist reduces antinociception modestly but also potentially reduces psychologic dependence as measured by conditioned place preference [62–64].

Delta receptor antagonists reduce analgesic tolerance and physical dependence and improve analgesia with mu receptor agonists. Bivalent pharmacophores of delta receptor antagonist alkaloids and mu receptor agonist alkaloids have been developed [65]. Oxymorphone-naltrindole bivalent ligands have been produced with various linkers (MDAN series). The spacer is critical to activity. Bivalent ligands with spacers of 19–21 atoms produce antinociception 50-fold greater than that seen with morphine in animal models. The oxymorphone-naltrindole bivalent ligands are able to cross the CNS [66–68]. Oxymorphone-naltrindole is associated with reduced conditioned place preference suggesting that it would be clinically less addicting.

Bivalent opioid/non-opioid ligands have been produced. With chronic opioid exposure, cholecystokinin is upregulated in the brainstem and blocks analgesia. Enkephalin derivatives have been combined with cholecystokinin receptor blockers [69]. Endomorphin-2 agonists have been combined with NK1 receptor blockers (the receptor for the neuroexcitatory transmitter substance P) as a fused bivalent ligand [70]. This bivalent ligand produces analgesia without analgesic tolerance in animal models.

Multiple merged ligands have been developed. 14-alkoxy derivatives of epoxymorphinan have activity at the mu, kappa, and delta receptor.

These multivalent ligands have 60-fold greater antinociception than morphine but similar gastrointestinal adverse effects [71]. A naltrexone derivative (SORI-9409), is a 4-chlorophenyl substituted pyridomorphinan, and a delta receptor antagonist and moderate mu receptor agonist. This merged bivalent ligand is antinociceptive but does not produce physical tolerance in animal models [72, 73]. Hydromorphone has also been transformed into a pyridomorphinan derivative (SORI-20411 and SORI-20648). This merged multivalent ligand produces antinociception in animal models with reduced analgesic tolerance [74].

Designed multivalent ligands are potentially an approach to improving analgesia with reduced adverse effects, less analgesic tolerance, and reduced risk for addiction. Barriers to developing multivalent ligands include cost of production and the financial risk to pharmaceutical companies in developing a completely new line of analgesics. Priorities may be a third barrier. The development of disease modifying therapies rather than analgesics is, in general, the priority of most institutions and pharmaceutical companies. Reformulation of standard opioids is less of a risk. To meet the challenge of developing new analgesics, phase I–II studies should incorporate pharmacokinetic-pharmacodynamic studies in populations with well-characterised pain phenotypes. The phenotype should match the animal model in which the analgesic was tested. Adaptive designed studies could enrich the responsive phenotype to the analgesic in a Bayesian approach, followed by a "proof-of-concept" randomised phase III design which would compare standard treatment to the experimental arm in the same phenotype [1]. This would minimise the number of individuals required to study the drug, accelerate analgesic development, and minimise costs. This approach would avoid the need to treat large numbers of individuals with multiple pain phenotypes who are not likely to benefit from targeted analgesics. The present approach randomises individuals with multiple pain and uses relief alone as outcomes. This is cumbersome, costly and likely to miss important responses in subsets of responding individuals who have a particular pain phenotype.

Mu Receptor Genetics, G-Protein Interactions, and Opioid Responses

Opioid receptors modulate the affective component of pain and its severity without altering objective sensation or the ability to locate pain [75]. The three major receptors (mu, delta, and kappa) are activated by three endogenous opioid peptides (endorphin, enkephalin, and dynorphin, respectively). Mu receptors are most important for analgesia. Clinically, opioid responsiveness varies unpredictably between individuals, some responding to one opioid while not responding to another. Side effects also differ between individuals. Non-cross tolerance is well documented between opioids, such that switching opioids relieves pain when the first opioid is ineffective.

Genetic differences in response to opioids are well established in mice strains. BALB-C mice are highly responsive to morphine, while CxBK mice are insensitive [75]. Methadone retains full analgesic potency in CxBK mice which is blocked by naloxone, indicating that methadone analgesia in CxBK mice is mediated by different mu receptors than morphine [76]. The actions of methadone on the mu receptor are distinctly different from morphine. The same is true for the morphine metabolite morphine-6-glucuronide which retains analgesia in CxBK mice [76].

Genes contain both exons and introns. Exons are segments of transcribed mRNA translated into protein; introns are segments of DNA between exons which are not translated. Exons are processed and combined through spliced sequences [75]. The mu receptor is a 7 transmembrane, G-protein-coupled receptor (GPCR), with an extracellular N-terminus and intracellular C-terminus [75]. Mu receptor subtypes are formed from four different exons. The fourth exon encodes for the last 12 amino acids of the C-terminus. The C-terminus of the receptor is involved in transduction of signals through interactions with G-proteins and is responsible for receptor trafficking into endosomes for resensitisation or into lysosomes for downregulation and destruction [77, 78].

Single neurons produce one mu receptor subtype (variant) exclusively; there are regional variations in the expression of mu receptor subtypes.

Opioid affinity for mu receptor subtypes does not differ significantly, but transduction and intrinsic efficacy differ between opioids [75, 77, 79]. Each receptor subtype is activated by a particular opioid to a different extent. Analgesia is therefore the sum total of an opioid action at multiple mu receptor subtypes; the degree of analgesia depends on the subtype and the number of subtypes activated [75].

Signal transduction requires GTP-binding regulatory proteins (G-proteins). G-proteins are trimeric proteins which consist of an alpha, beta, and gamma subunit, G-alpha proteins are divided into various subtypes. Opioid ligands produce distinctly different conformational changes in mu receptors which, in turn, activate different sets of G-proteins [80]. In albino CD-1 mice, methadone antinociception is dependent upon Gi1, Gi3, Go1, and G11 proteins, whereas morphine antinociception is not dependent on these particular G-alpha proteins [80]. The same G-proteins are involved in delta receptor signalling. Different delta receptor agonists activate different sets of G-proteins which influence signal transduction and, ultimately, antinociception [81–83]. The clinical importance of these findings is that novel drugs could be designed based on relative G-protein activation profiles rather than receptor affinity. Secondly, this theoretically supports potential benefits to combination opioid agonists which activate complementary G-proteins.

Combinations of opioid agonists have been tested in animal models. In CD-1 mice, methadone and morphine have greater antinociception than the sum of the independent actions of morphine and methadone. This also occurs in the same model with methadone and morphine-6-glucuronide, codeine, or 6-acetyl morphine but not with fentanyl [84]. Oxycodone has a different signal transduction pattern than morphine. Oxycodone, unlike morphine, does not desensitise inward rectifying potassium channels [85]. Oxycodone interacts with different mu receptor subtypes and a different set of G-proteins than morphine doses [86, 87]. Oxycodone appears to be more effective in relieving visceral pain [88]. There is clinical evidence that the combination of oxycodone and morphine is better than morphine alone [89, 90]. In the same manner, buprenorphine and fentanyl have different analgesic efficacy in the same animal model, and is dependent on the pain mechanism and involved tissue [91]. Combinations of certain opioids may produce supra-additive, additive, or sub-additive analgesia. Opioid combinations with synergistic antinociception demonstrated in animal models should be tested prospectively in individuals with well-characterised pain phenotypes.

The type of G-protein interactions with mu receptors depends on the dose of opioid. Classically, morphine activates Go/i proteins resulting in inactivation of adenylyl cyclase and voltage-gated calcium channels. Neurotransmitter release from presynaptic neurons is blocked. At the postsynaptic level, morphine opens potassium channels and hyperpolarises neurons [92, 93]. However, at very low doses of morphine, adenylyl cyclase is activated and calcium influx is promoted [94]. This bimodal response is due to the activation of Gs proteins at very low morphine doses [95, 96]. Gs protein interactions with the receptor are blocked by ultra-low doses of naloxone [97]. In the Sprague-Dawley rat model, ultra-low doses of intrathecal naltrexone (0.05–0.1 ng) or systemic naltrexone (10 ng/kg) augment antinociception of submaximal doses of intrathecal morphine (5 mcg) and systemic morphine (7.5 mg/kg) [98]. The use of ultra-low-dose naltrexone and CTAP (selective mu receptor antagonist) with morphine reduces analgesic tolerance [48, 98]. Unfortunately, this combination also increases conditioned place preference, the rewarding effects of morphine, and potentially increases psychologic dependence [98]. Potentiation of morphine antinociception and inhibition of analgesic tolerance have been reported with a combination of morphine plus ultra-low doses of the delta receptor antagonist, naltrindole [48].

Intrathecal ultra-low-dose naloxone attenuates analgesic tolerance by preventing (1) the downregulation of glutamate transporters, (2) phosphorylation NMDA receptors, (3) upregulation of certain kinases, and (4) activation of glia [99]. Clinically low-dose naloxone infusions (0.25 mcg/kg/h) with PCA morphine for postoperative analgesia prevent opioid side effects and reduce opioid requirements [100, 101]. Nalbuphine, an opioid receptor agonist-antagonist, reduces side effects from intrathecal morphine without attenuating analgesia [102]. Intrathecal morphine or fentanyl (1.3 mg and 56 mcg, respectively) plus IV infusions of naloxone (5 mcg/kg/h) is used for postoperative analgesia. Reduces opioid side effects [103]. Oral naltrexone (100 mcg twice daily) in individuals on chronic intrathecal morphine improves pain scores compared with intrathecal morphine alone [104].

There is laboratory and clinical evidence that the combination of morphine plus ultra-low doses and mu or delta receptor antagonists improves the therapeutic index of morphine. Opioid receptor antagonists may act as chaperones to mu receptors and increase expression of mu receptors or change transduction after receptor activation [48, 105]. Most studies of ultra-low-dose mu receptor antagonists and morphine combinations involve patients in acute pain and short treatment intervals. Long-term safety data is not available. In light of animal studies which demonstrate increased conditioned place preference, there should be a concern about the potential increased risk for addiction with long-term use. However, the present development of opioid agonist-antagonist has been for other reasons. Prevention of illicit route conversion and opioid-related constipation have been the main reason [106–109].

Regulatory Proteins and Chaperones

Certain proteins regulate surface expressions of receptors and the degree of receptor coupling with G-proteins. Homer proteins regulate metabotropic glutamate receptors and influence glutamate receptor signalling [110]. Upregulation of Homer proteins uncouples glutamate receptor signalling and reduces chronic pain. Agents which upregulate Homer proteins could be a new therapy for chronic pain and potentially have supra-additive analgesic activity combined with morphine [111].

Chaperone proteins facilitate the cell surface expression of receptors. Receptor activity-modifying proteins (RAMPs) had been identified for calcitonin gene-related peptide (CGRP) receptors and kappa opioid receptors. Both CGRP receptor and the endogenous protein dynorphin are upregulated with morphine tolerance and morphine-induced hyperalgesia [112, 113]. Downregulation of RAMPs reduces the expression of CGRP receptors and reduces pain [114]. Combining RAMP down regulators with morphine may prevent morphine tolerance and morphine-related hyperalgesia.

Opioid-Induced Hyperalgesia and Morphine-Induced Inflammation

Repeated doses of morphine or fentanyl increase pain sensitivity, a syndrome known as opioid-induced hyperalgesia [115, 116]. Chronic morphine causes upregulation of proinflammatory cytokines such as tumour necrosis factor, interleukins, stromal-derived factor-1, and monocyte chemoattractant protein-1 and their respective receptors [117, 118]. In Sprague-Dawley mice, chronic morphine produces a constitutional expression of stromal-derived factor-1 and its receptor, CxCR4, in sensory nerves which is associated with tactile hyperalgesia. The CxCR4 receptor blocker, AMD3100, prevents morphine-related tactile hyperalgesia in animal models [119].

Microglia are activated by morphine. Suppression of glial proinflammatory responses improves opioid analgesia. Minocycline and AV411 (ibudilast) attenuates glial proinflammatory responses and reduces naloxone-precipitated withdrawal in animal models. AV411 does not simply attenuate physical dependence but causes a three- to fivefold increase in morphine and oxycodone potency [120].

These novel approaches to pain management have the potential of extending the therapeutic index of potent mu agonists by blocking counter-opioid responses and reducing opioid side effects.

Opioids and NSAIDs

Combinations of opioids and NSAIDs are frequently used. A popular choice is a cyclooxygenase-2 (Cox-2) inhibitor. Another common approach is to use combinations empirically, assuming that any combination of NSAID and opioid is equally effective. However, in animal models, hydrocodone and ibuprofen have supraadditive whereas hydrocodone has only additive analgesia with other NSAIDs [121]. Morphine has supra-additive analgesia with diclofenac, ketoprofen, meloxicam, metamizol, naproxen, nimesulide, parecoxib, and piroxicam in animal models [122]. Supra-additive analgesia is independent of selective Cox-1 or Cox-2 isoenzyme inhibition and appears to be a direct action of NSAIDS on nociceptive processing within the spinal cord, independent of prostaglandin synthesis [122]. Clinicians need to explore particular opioid/NSAIDs combinations in comparison trialsand in animal models.

What Needs to Be Done to Develop Analgesics in the Twenty-First Century?

It is not reasonable to expect a single analgesic to be suitable for all individuals and all pain phenotypes [1]. As a parallel development, targeted antitumour drugs are being developed in oncology, based on cancer phenotype with a Bayesian approach to trial design [123].

Personalised genomic markers may lead to rational analgesic choices which would improve responses and the drug therapeutic index [124–127]. Genetic markers potentially include mu receptor genotype, cytochrome genotype, and single-nucleotide polymorphisms involved in pain-processing pathways such as occurs with catecholamine-O-methyltransferase. Genotype may better predict analgesic pharmacodynamic-pharmacokinetic relationships in those who would respond to a particular analgesic epigenetic marker of mu receptor promoter site methylation may have clinical relevance.

Pain is a complex process which involves interactions between peripheral and central nervous system pathways. Multiple ion channels, opioid and non-opioid receptors, and a large number of neurotransmitters are involved in pain processing. It is unrealistic to anticipate an analgesic which interacts with a single receptor, transporter, or ion channel to significantly reduce pain in a large number of individuals. Bivalent opioid agonists, multivalent opioid/non-opioid receptor drugs, and opioid-monoamine transporter inhibitor bivalent analgesics have advantages, as demonstrated in animal models and clinically [128, 129].

At least ten different independent neurologic mechanisms may initiate or sustain pain [130]. Each mechanism involves many potential analgesic targets. Within each disease category (e.g., diabetic neuropathy or postherpetic neuralgia), distinctly different pain mechanisms are demonstrated [130]. Each distinct pain phenotype within a disease category could have a different response to an analgesic. If pain is due to the impaired activation of sodium channels, for example, it is unlikely that an NSAID will be effective [131]. The present regulatory trial design, as mentioned before, uses disease category and pain severity as the principal variable. These trials will, at best, have modest outcomes, and many who participate in studies will have pain which remains unrelieved. If a 33–50 % reduction in pain and an NNT of 3 define a good analgesia, then most patients will remain in pain.

In oncology, the term "oncogene addiction" has been used to refer to particular mutations in transduction pathways which are essential for the cancer to survive and which are presently successfully targeted [132–134]. In the same way, we should attempt to define "pain addiction" pathways which are essential to maintaining chronic maladaptive pain and target these pathways in translational studies. The first step would be to phenotype pain, which would involve not only detecting presence and severity but also the nature of pain [1, 135]. This would require redefining pain from the original classification of "malignant or nonmalignant pain" or "somatic, visceral or neuropathic pain" to "adaptive or maladaptive" pain, to phenotyping maladaptive pain based upon pain characteristics, genotype, and perhaps imaging through fMRI technologies.

Future trials should include not only pain response but also "disease" modification. Reducing the risk of developing maladaptive chronic pain is an important outcome but rarely included in analgesic trials [1, 136].

The use of fMRI is an important step forward in understanding pain mechanisms phenotypes and analgesic responses. Interventional studies which include fMRI will allow us to understand the relationship of phenotype and pain matrix responses [137–143].

Analgesic combination trials should be developed which are based on mechanistic paradigms. One analgesic may be inactive when given alone, but when given with a second analgesic, supra-additive analgesia may be observed. This may be due to pharmacokinetic or pharmacodynamic interactions [144]. Rather than studying each drug separately, a "proof-of-concept" phase II pain trial of the combination should be performed with pharmacokinetic-pharmacodynamic correlations to analgesic outcomes and pain phenotype. This would be followed by a phase III randomised control trial which compares the combination with "standard of care" in the same pain phenotype. This would be better than using a non-inferiority randomised control trial consisting of individuals who have pain arising from several different mechanisms. It is likely that several effective analgesics have been abandoned in the past because of the present trial design paradigm required for analgesic approval by regulatory agencies [1].

Placebo mechanisms obscure analgesic efficacy. Placebo effects are not additive to drug responses [1, 145–147]. The way to minimise placebo responses is to have a "run-in" pretrial before a randomised trial to eliminate placebo responders or use crossover trial designs which detect placebo responders without involving a large number of individuals. This is better than conducting large parallel randomised control trials that cannot seperrate placebo responders from analgesic responders [147–152].

Animal models which are used to screen analgesics, frequently involve pain mechanisms that differ from the population for whom the analgesic is being tested clinically. Pain mechanisms associated with the analgesic response may be well characterised in animal models, yet the analgesic is tested clinically in individuals with a wide variety of pain mechanisms or phenotypes. Responsive subsets of individuals may be obscured by the lack of response in most individuals when an analysis is based upon the change in the mean pain intensity scores. Clinical trials should require pain phenotypes matched to animal model [1]. Another barrier to analgesic development is the relative inability to study spontaneous pain in the laboratory animals; spontaneous pain is a common experience in patients with chronic pain. Most animal pain models involve evoked pain [153].

Receptor, ion channel, or transporter targets important to analgesic drug activity are often found after analgesic discovery and approval, as has occurred with ketamine, gabapentinoids, and NSAIDs [154]. In the past, there has been a long delay between identifying potential receptor targets (such as nerve growth factor and receptor) and the development of an analgesic to target that pathway [155, 156]. The development of techniques to explore genome-wide single-nucleotide polymorphisms associated with pain may shorten the gap between discovery of a pain pathway and the development of an analgesic which targets the pathway [1, 157, 158]. Genome-wide association studies using well characterised phenotype/genotype cohorts of pain patients and matched controls will help to identify future targets for analgesic development [1].

Stem cell biology techniques, in particular, have advanced pluripotential methodologies, making it possible to develop neurons from human fibroblasts [159]. This will allow investigators to detect differences in neuron structure and function in those with and without pain. Pluripotential methodologies will also provide a means of developing treatments [160].

Bench research in pain mechanisms and the human genome project should advance analgesic development into targeted therapies. A major barrier is the characterisation of pain phenotypes and "pain addiction" pathways so as to adequately test targeted agents. Multivalent analgesics have the potential of improving the therapeutic index of potent mu agonists. Present concerns over increasing opioid-related deaths and opioid abuse have diverted the attention of the pharmaceutical industry and drug regulatory agencies to develop abuse-resistant forms of opioids rather than safer targeted analgesics. The cost of drug development and the length of time to drug approval are significant barriers to analgesic development. Pharmaceutical companies are reluctant to take a significant financial risk in developing new targeted multivalent analgesics. The present trial procedures required for approval are probably not adequate for targeted analgesics. New trial designs which would mimic designs presently evolving in testing targeted anticancer drugs are needed [161].

References

1. Woolf CJ. Overcoming obstacles to developing new analgesics. Nat Med. 2010;16(11):1241–7.
2. Compton P, Charuvastra VC, Ling W. Pain intolerance in opioid-maintained former opiate addicts: effect of long-acting maintenance agent. Drug Alcohol Depend. 2001;63(2):139–46.
3. Basbaum AI et al. Cellular and molecular mechanisms of pain. Cell. 2009;139(2):267–84.
4. McMahon SB, Malcangio M. Current challenges in glia-pain biology. Neuron. 2009;64(1):46–54.
5. Latremoliere A, Woolf CJ. Central sensitization: a generator of pain hypersensitivity by central neural plasticity. J Pain. 2009;10(9):895–926.
6. Saito YA, Mitra N, Mayer EA. Genetic approaches to functional gastrointestinal disorders. Gastroenterology. 2010;138(4):1276–85.
7. Fischer TZ, Waxman SG. Familial pain syndromes from mutations of the NaV1.7 sodium channel. Ann N Y Acad Sci. 2010;1184:196–207.
8. Tegeder I, Lotsch J. Current evidence for a modulation of low back pain by human genetic variants. J Cell Mol Med. 2009;13(8B):1605–19.
9. Bouhassira D, Attal N. Diagnosis and assessment of neuropathic pain: the saga of clinical tools. Pain. 2011;152(3 Suppl):S74–83.
10. Woolf CJ, Salter MW. Neuronal plasticity: increasing the gain in pain. Science. 2000;288(5472):1765–9.
11. Woolf CJ. Central sensitization: implications for the diagnosis and treatment of pain. Pain. 2011;152(3 Suppl):S2–15.
12. Jaggi AS, Singh N. Role of different brain areas in peripheral nerve injury-induced neuropathic pain. Brain Res. 2011;1381:187–201.
13. Yeung JC, Rudy TA. Multiplicative interaction between narcotic agonisms expressed at spinal and supraspinal sites of antinociceptive action as revealed by concurrent intrathecal and intracerebroventricular injections of morphine. J Pharmacol Exp Ther. 1980;215(3):633–42.
14. Yeung JC, Rudy TA. Sites of antinociceptive action of systemically injected morphine: involvement of supraspinal loci as revealed by intracerebroventricular injection of naloxone. J Pharmacol Exp Ther. 1980;215(3):626–32.

15. Kolesnikov YA et al. Peripheral morphine analgesia: synergy with central sites and a target of morphine tolerance. J Pharmacol Exp Ther. 1996;279(2):502–6.

16. Rashid MH et al. Loss of peripheral morphine analgesia contributes to the reduced effectiveness of systemic morphine in neuropathic pain. J Pharmacol Exp Ther. 2004;309(1):380–7.

17. Kolesnikov YA, Oksman G, Pasternak GW. Topical methadone and meperidine analgesic synergy in the mouse. Eur J Pharmacol. 2010;638(1–3):61–4.

18. Stein C. Peripheral mechanisms of opioid analgesia. Anesth Analg. 1993;76(1):182–91.

19. Young 3rd WS et al. Opioid receptors undergo axonal flow. Science. 1980;210(4465):76–8.

20. Laduron PM. Axonal transport of opiate receptors in capsaicin-sensitive neurones. Brain Res. 1984;294(1):157–60.

21. Gendron L et al. Morphine priming in rats with chronic inflammation reveals a dichotomy between antihyperalgesic and antinociceptive properties of deltorphin. Neuroscience. 2007;144(1):263–74.

22. Vetter I et al. The effects of pH on beta-endorphin and morphine inhibition of calcium transients in dorsal root ganglion neurons. J Pain. 2006;7(7):488–99.

23. Zhang X, Bao L, Guan JS. Role of delivery and trafficking of delta-opioid peptide receptors in opioid analgesia and tolerance. Trends Pharmacol Sci. 2006;27(6):324–9.

24. Yamdeu RS et al. p38 Mitogen-activated protein kinase activation by nerve growth factor in primary sensory neurons upregulates mu-opioid receptors to enhance opioid responsiveness toward better pain control. Anesthesiology. 2011;114(1):150–61.

25. Stein C, Schafer M, Machelska H. Attacking pain at its source: new perspectives on opioids. Nat Med. 2003;9(8):1003–8.

26. Zollner C et al. Chronic morphine use does not induce peripheral tolerance in a rat model of inflammatory pain. J Clin Invest. 2008;118(3):1065–73.

27. Craft RM et al. Opioid antinociception in a rat model of visceral pain: systemic versus local drug administration. J Pharmacol Exp Ther. 1995;275(3):1535–42.

28. Shannon HE, Lutz EA. Comparison of the peripheral and central effects of the opioid agonists loperamide and morphine in the formalin test in rats. Neuropharmacology. 2002;42(2):253–61.

29. Machelska H et al. Different mechanisms of intrinsic pain inhibition in early and late inflammation. J Neuroimmunol. 2003;141(1–2):30–9.

30. DeHaven-Hudkins DL, Dolle RE. Peripherally restricted opioid agonists as novel analgesic agents. Curr Pharm Des. 2004;10(7):743–57.

31. Kindler LL et al. Drug response profiles to experimental pain are opioid and pain modality specific. J Pain. 2011;12(3):340–51.

32. Cahill CM et al. Prolonged morphine treatment targets delta opioid receptors to neuronal plasma membranes and enhances delta-mediated antinociception. J Neurosci. 2001;21(19):7598–607.

33. Zhang Z, Pan ZZ. Synaptic mechanism for functional synergism between delta- and mu-opioid receptors. J Neurosci. 2010;30(13):4735–45.

34. Wang HB et al. Coexpression of delta- and mu-opioid receptors in nociceptive sensory neurons. Proc Natl Acad Sci USA. 2010;107(29):13117–22.

35. Horan P et al. Antinociceptive interactions of opioid delta receptor agonists with morphine in mice: supra- and sub-additivity. Life Sci. 1992;50(20):1535–41.

36. Rossi GC, Pasternak GW, Bodnar RJ. Mu and delta opioid synergy between the periaqueductal gray and the rostro-ventral medulla. Brain Res. 1994;665(1):85–93.

37. Negus SS et al. Role of delta opioid efficacy as a determinant of mu/delta opioid interactions in rhesus monkeys. Eur J Pharmacol. 2009;602(1):92–100.

38. Stevenson GW et al. Interactions between delta and mu opioid agonists in assays of schedule-controlled responding, thermal nociception, drug self-administration, and drug versus food choice in rhesus monkeys: studies with SNC80 [(+)-4-[(alphaR)-alpha-((2S,5R)-4-allyl-2,5-dimethyl-1-piperazinyl)-3-methoxybenzyl]-N,N-diethylbenzamide] and heroin. J Pharmacol Exp Ther. 2005;314(1):221–31.

39. He SQ et al. Facilitation of mu-opioid receptor activity by preventing delta-opioid receptor-mediated codegradation. Neuron. 2011;69(1):120–31.

40. Tang J, Yang HY, Costa E. Inhibition of spontaneous and opiate-modified nociception by an endogenous neuropeptide with Phe-Met-Arg-Phe-NH2-like immunoreactivity. Proc Natl Acad Sci USA. 1984;81(15):5002–5.

41. Chefer VI, Shippenberg TS. Augmentation of morphine-induced sensitization but reduction in morphine tolerance and reward in delta-opioid receptor knockout mice. Neuropsychopharmacology. 2009;34(4):887–98.

42. Gupta A et al. Increased abundance of opioid receptor heteromers after chronic morphine administration. Sci Signal. 2010;3(131):ra54.

43. Jordan BA, Devi LA. G-protein-coupled receptor heterodimerization modulates receptor function. Nature. 1999;399(6737):697–700.

44. Gomes I et al. G protein coupled receptor dimerization: implications in modulating receptor function. J Mol Med. 2001;79(5–6):226–42.

45. Jordan BA et al. Oligomerization of opioid receptors with beta 2-adrenergic receptors: a role in trafficking and mitogen-activated protein kinase activation. Proc Natl Acad Sci USA. 2001;98(1):343–8.

46. Gomes I et al. Oligomerization of opioid receptors. Methods. 2002;27(4):358–65.

47. Rios CD et al. G-protein-coupled receptor dimerization: modulation of receptor function. Pharmacol Ther. 2001;92(2–3):71–87.

48. Abul-Husn NS et al. Augmentation of spinal morphine analgesia and inhibition of tolerance by low doses of mu- and delta-opioid receptor antagonists. Br J Pharmacol. 2007;151(6):877–87.

49. Gomes I et al. Heterodimerization of mu and delta opioid receptors: a role in opiate synergy. J Neurosci. 2000;20(22):RC110.

50. Gomes I et al. A role for heterodimerization of mu and delta opiate receptors in enhancing morphine analgesia. Proc Natl Acad Sci USA. 2004;101(14): 5135–9.

51. Ballet S, Pietsch M, Abell AD. Multiple ligands in opioid research. Protein Pept Lett. 2008;15(7): 668–82.

52. Schiller PW et al. The opioid mu agonist/delta antagonist DIPP-NH(2)[Psi] produces a potent analgesic effect, no physical dependence, and less tolerance than morphine in rats. J Med Chem. 1999;42(18): 3520–6.

53. Horan PJ et al. Antinociceptive profile of biphalin, a dimeric enkephalin analog. J Pharmacol Exp Ther. 1993;265(3):1446–54.

54. Lipkowski AW, Konecka AM, Sadowski B. Double enkephalins. Pol J Pharmacol Pharm. 1982;34(1–3): 69–71.

55. Costa T et al. Receptor binding and biological activity of bivalent enkephalins. Biochem Pharmacol. 1985;34(1):25–30.

56. Lazarus LH et al. Dimeric dermorphin analogues as mu-receptor probes on rat brain membranes. Correlation between central mu-receptor potency and suppression of gastric acid secretion. J Biol Chem. 1989;264(1):354–62.

57. Jinsmaa Y et al. Oral bioavailability of a new class of micro-opioid receptor agonists containing 3,6-bis[Dmt-NH(CH(2))(n)]-2(1H)-pyrazinone with central-mediated analgesia. J Med Chem. 2004;47(10): 2599–610.

58. Okada Y et al. Unique high-affinity synthetic mu-opioid receptor agonists with central- and systemic-mediated analgesia. J Med Chem. 2003;46(15):3201–9.

59. Bryant SD et al. Dmt and opioid peptides: a potent alliance. Biopolymers. 2003;71(2):86–102.

60. Freye E, Latasch L, Portoghese PS. The delta receptor is involved in sufentanil-induced respiratory depression – opioid subreceptors mediate different effects. Eur J Anaesthesiol. 1992;9(6):457–62.

61. Weltrowska G et al. A chimeric opioid peptide with mixed mu agonist/delta antagonist properties. J Pept Res. 2004;63(2):63–8.

62. Kalso E. Improving opioid effectiveness: from ideas to evidence. Eur J Pain. 2005;9(2):131–5.

63. Petrov RR et al. Synthesis and evaluation of 3-aminopropionyl substituted fentanyl analogues for opioid activity. Bioorg Med Chem Lett. 2006;16(18): 4946–50.

64. Gentilucci L. New trends in the development of opioid peptide analogues as advanced remedies for pain relief. Curr Top Med Chem. 2004;4(1):19–38.

65. Abdelhamid EE et al. Selective blockage of delta opioid receptors prevents the development of morphine tolerance and dependence in mice. J Pharmacol Exp Ther. 1991;258(1):299–303.

66. Daniels DJ et al. Opioid-induced tolerance and dependence in mice is modulated by the distance between pharmacophores in a bivalent ligand series. Proc Natl Acad Sci USA. 2005;102(52):19208–13.

67. Portoghese PS et al. Opioid agonist and antagonist bivalent ligands. The relationship between spacer length and selectivity at multiple opioid receptors. J Med Chem. 1986;29(10):1855–61.

68. Lenard NR, Roerig SC. Development of antinociceptive tolerance and physical dependence following morphine i.c.v. infusion in mice. Eur J Pharmacol. 2005;527(1–3):71–6.

69. Lee YS et al. Design and synthesis of novel hydrazide-linked bifunctional peptides as delta/mu opioid receptor agonists and CCK-1/CCK-2 receptor antagonists. J Med Chem. 2006;49(5):1773–80.

70. Foran SE et al. A substance P-opioid chimeric peptide as a unique nontolerance-forming analgesic. Proc Natl Acad Sci USA. 2000;97(13):7621–6.

71. Lattanzi R et al. Synthesis and biological evaluation of 14-alkoxymorphinans. 22.(1) Influence of the 14-alkoxy group and the substitution in position 5 in 14-alkoxymorphinan-6-ones on in vitro and in vivo activities. J Med Chem. 2005;48(9):3372–8.

72. Ananthan S et al. Synthesis, opioid receptor binding, and biological activities of naltrexone-derived pyrido- and pyrimidomorphinans. J Med Chem. 1999;42(18): 3527–38.

73. Wells JL et al. In vivo pharmacological characterization of SoRI 9409, a nonpeptidic opioid mu-agonist/delta-antagonist that produces limited antinociceptive tolerance and attenuates morphine physical dependence. J Pharmacol Exp Ther. 2001;297(2): 597–605.

74. Ananthan S et al. Identification of opioid ligands possessing mixed micro agonist/delta antagonist activity among pyridomorphinans derived from naloxone, oxymorphone, and hydromorphone [correction of hydropmorphone]. J Med Chem. 2004;47(6):1400–12.

75. Pasternak GW. Molecular insights into mu opioid pharmacology: from the clinic to the bench. Clin J Pain. 2010;26 Suppl 10:S3–9.

76. Chang A et al. Methadone analgesia in morphine-insensitive CXBK mice. Eur J Pharmacol. 1998;351(2): 189–91.

77. Abbadie C, Pasternak GW. Differential in vivo internalization of MOR-1 and MOR-1C by morphine. Neuroreport. 2001;12(14):3069–72.

78. Tanowitz M, Hislop JN, von Zastrow M. Alternative splicing determines the post-endocytic sorting fate of G-protein-coupled receptors. J Biol Chem. 2008;283(51):35614–21.

79. Abbadie C, Pan YX, Pasternak GW. Differential distribution in rat brain of mu opioid receptor carboxy terminal splice variants MOR-1C-like and MOR-1-like immunoreactivity: evidence for region-specific processing. J Comp Neurol. 2000;419(2):244–56.

80. Sanchez-Blazquez P, Gomez-Serranillos P, Garzon J. Agonists determine the pattern of G-protein activation

in mu-opioid receptor-mediated supraspinal analgesia. Brain Res Bull. 2001;54(2):229–35.

81. Sanchez-Blazquez P, Garzon J. Delta opioid receptor subtypes activate inositol-signalling pathways in the production of antinociception. J Pharmacol Exp Ther. 1998;285(2):820–7.

82. Garzon J, Martinez-Pena Y, Sanchez-Blazquez P. Gx/z is regulated by mu but not delta opioid receptors in the stimulation of the low Km GTPase activity in mouse periaqueductal grey matter. Eur J Neurosci. 1997;9(6):1194–200.

83. Garzon J, Garcia-Espana A, Sanchez-Blazquez P. Opioids binding mu and delta receptors exhibit diverse efficacy in the activation of Gi2 and G(x/z) transducer proteins in mouse periaqueductal gray matter. J Pharmacol Exp Ther. 1997;281(1):549–57.

84. Bolan EA, Tallarida RJ, Pasternak GW. Synergy between mu opioid ligands: evidence for functional interactions among mu opioid receptor subtypes. J Pharmacol Exp Ther. 2002;303(2):557–62.

85. Smith MT. Differences between and combinations of opioids re-visited. Curr Opin Anaesthesiol. 2008;21(5): 596–601.

86. Virk MS, Williams JT. Agonist-specific regulation of mu-opioid receptor desensitization and recovery from desensitization. Mol Pharmacol. 2008;73(4):1301–8.

87. Nielsen CK et al. Oxycodone and morphine have distinctly different pharmacological profiles: radioligand binding and behavioural studies in two rat models of neuropathic pain. Pain. 2007;132(3):289–300.

88. Staahl C et al. Differential effect of opioids in patients with chronic pancreatitis: an experimental pain study. Scand J Gastroenterol. 2007;42(3):383–90.

89. Blumenthal S et al. Postoperative intravenous morphine consumption, pain scores, and side effects with perioperative oral controlled-release oxycodone after lumbar discectomy. Anesth Analg. 2007;105(1): 233–7.

90. Sima L et al. Efficacy of oxycodone/paracetamol for patients with bone-cancer pain: a multicenter, randomized, double-blinded, placebo-controlled trial. J Clin Pharm Ther. 2012;37(1):27–31.

91. Andresen T et al. Effect of transdermal opioids in experimentally induced superficial, deep and hyperalgesic pain. Br J Pharmacol. 2011;164(3):934–45.

92. Uhl GR, Childers S, Pasternak G. An opiate-receptor gene family reunion. Trends Neurosci. 1994;17(3): 89–93.

93. North RA, Williams JT. Opiate activation of potassium conductance inhibits calcium action potentials in rat locus coeruleus neurones. Br J Pharmacol. 1983;80(2):225–8.

94. Smart D, Lambert DG. The stimulatory effects of opioids and their possible role in the development of tolerance. Trends Pharmacol Sci. 1996;17(7):264–9.

95. Crain SM, Shen K. Enhanced analgesic potency and reduced tolerance of morphine in 129/SvEv mice: evidence for a deficiency in GM1 ganglioside-regulated excitatory opioid receptor functions. Brain Res. 2000;856(1–2):227–35.

96. Crain SM, Shen KF. Ultra-low concentrations of naloxone selectively antagonize excitatory effects of morphine on sensory neurons, thereby increasing its antinociceptive potency and attenuating tolerance/dependence during chronic cotreatment. Proc Natl Acad Sci USA. 1995;92(23):10540–4.

97. Wang HY et al. Ultra-low-dose naloxone suppresses opioid tolerance, dependence and associated changes in mu opioid receptor-G protein coupling and Gbetagamma signalling. Neuroscience. 2005;135(1): 247–61.

98. Powell KJ et al. Paradoxical effects of the opioid antagonist naltrexone on morphine analgesia, tolerance, and reward in rats. J Pharmacol Exp Ther. 2002;300(2):588–96.

99. Lin SL et al. Co-administration of ultra-low dose naloxone attenuates morphine tolerance in rats via attenuation of NMDA receptor neurotransmission and suppression of neuroinflammation in the spinal cords. Pharmacol Biochem Behav. 2010;96(2): 236–45.

100. Gan TJ et al. Opioid-sparing effects of a low-dose infusion of naloxone in patient-administered morphine sulfate. Anesthesiology. 1997;87(5):1075–81.

101. Maxwell LG et al. The effects of a small-dose naloxone infusion on opioid-induced side effects and analgesia in children and adolescents treated with intravenous patient-controlled analgesia: a double-blind, prospective, randomized, controlled study. Anesth Analg. 2005;100(4):953–8.

102. Wang JJ, Ho ST, Tzeng JI. Comparison of intravenous nalbuphine infusion versus naloxone in the prevention of epidural morphine-related side effects. Reg Anesth Pain Med. 1998;23(5):479–84.

103. Rebel A, Sloan P, Andrykowski M. Postoperative analgesia after radical prostatectomy with high-dose intrathecal morphine and intravenous naloxone: a retrospective review. J Opioid Manag. 2009;5(6): 331–9.

104. Hamann S, Sloan P. Oral naltrexone to enhance analgesia in patients receiving continuous intrathecal morphine for chronic pain: a randomized, double-blind, prospective pilot study. J Opioid Manag. 2007;3(3):137–44.

105. Bernier V, Bichet DG, Bouvier M. Pharmacological chaperone action on G-protein-coupled receptors. Curr Opin Pharmacol. 2004;4(5):528–33.

106. Simpson K et al. Fixed-ratio combination oxycodone/naloxone compared with oxycodone alone for the relief of opioid-induced constipation in moderate-to-severe noncancer pain. Curr Med Res Opin. 2008;24(12):3503–12.

107. Vondrackova D et al. Analgesic efficacy and safety of oxycodone in combination with naloxone as prolonged release tablets in patients with moderate to severe chronic pain. J Pain. 2008;9(12):1144–54.

108. Katz N et al. Morphine sulfate and naltrexone hydrochloride extended release capsules in patients with chronic osteoarthritis pain. Postgrad Med. 2010;122(4):112–28.

109. Meissner W et al. A randomised controlled trial with prolonged-release oral oxycodone and naloxone to prevent and reverse opioid-induced constipation. Eur J Pain. 2009;13(1):56–64.

110. Brakeman PR et al. Homer: a protein that selectively binds metabotropic glutamate receptors. Nature. 1997;386(6622):284–8.

111. Tappe A et al. Synaptic scaffolding protein Homer1a protects against chronic inflammatory pain. Nat Med. 2006;12(6):677–81.

112. Xie JY et al. Cholecystokinin in the rostral ventromedial medulla mediates opioid-induced hyperalgesia and antinociceptive tolerance. J Neurosci. 2005;25(2):409–16.

113. Ossipov MH et al. Underlying mechanisms of pronociceptive consequences of prolonged morphine exposure. Biopolymers. 2005;80(2–3):319–24.

114. McLatchie LM et al. RAMPs regulate the transport and ligand specificity of the calcitonin-receptor-like receptor. Nature. 1998;393(6683):333–9.

115. Angst MS, Clark JD. Opioid-induced hyperalgesia: a qualitative systematic review. Anesthesiology. 2006;104(3):570–87.

116. Ossipov MH et al. Antinociceptive and nociceptive actions of opioids. J Neurobiol. 2004;61(1):126–48.

117. Johnston IN et al. A role for proinflammatory cytokines and fractalkine in analgesia, tolerance, and subsequent pain facilitation induced by chronic intrathecal morphine. J Neurosci. 2004;24(33):7353–65.

118. Hutchinson MR et al. Proinflammatory cytokines oppose opioid-induced acute and chronic analgesia. Brain Behav Immun. 2008;22(8):1178–89.

119. Wilson NM et al. CXCR4 signalling mediates morphine-induced tactile hyperalgesia. Brain Behav Immun. 2011;25(3):565–73.

120. Hutchinson MR et al. Reduction of opioid withdrawal and potentiation of acute opioid analgesia by systemic AV411 (ibudilast). Brain Behav Immun. 2009;23(2):240–50.

121. Kolesnikov YA, Wilson RS, Pasternak GW. The synergistic analgesic interactions between hydrocodone and ibuprofen. Anesth Analg. 2003;97(6):1721–3.

122. Miranda HF, Sierralta F, Prieto JC. Synergism between NSAIDs in the orofacial formalin test in mice. Pharmacol Biochem Behav. 2009;92(2):314–8.

123. Zhou X et al. Bayesian adaptive design for targeted therapy development in lung cancer – a step toward personalized medicine. Clin Trials. 2008;5(3): 181–93.

124. Lotsch J. Genetic variability of pain perception and treatment-clinical pharmacological implications. Eur J Clin Pharmacol. 2011;67(6):541–51.

125. Lotsch J, Geisslinger G. A critical appraisal of human genotyping for pain therapy. Trends Pharmacol Sci. 2010;31(7):312–7.

126. Lotsch J, Geisslinger G. Pharmacogenetics of new analgesics. Br J Pharmacol. 2011;163(3):447–60.

127. Oertel B, Lotsch J. Genetic mutations that prevent pain: implications for future pain medication. Pharmacogenomics. 2008;9(2):179–94.

128. Christoph T, De Vry J, Tzschentke TM. Tapentadol, but not morphine, selectively inhibits disease-related thermal hyperalgesia in a mouse model of diabetic neuropathic pain. Neurosci Lett. 2010;470(2):91–4.

129. Tzschentke TM et al. Tapentadol hydrochloride: a next-generation, centrally acting analgesic with two mechanisms of action in a single molecule. Drugs Today (Barc). 2009;45(7):483–96.

130. Costigan M, Scholz J, Woolf CJ. Neuropathic pain: a maladaptive response of the nervous system to damage. Annu Rev Neurosci. 2009;32:1–32.

131. Dib-Hajj SD et al. Sodium channels in normal and pathological pain. Annu Rev Neurosci. 2010;33: 325–47.

132. Weinstein IB, Joe AK. Mechanisms of disease: oncogene addiction – a rationale for molecular targeting in cancer therapy. Nat Clin Pract Oncol. 2006;3(8):448–57.

133. Hubner A, Jaeschke A, Davis RJ. Oncogene addiction: role of signal attenuation. Dev Cell. 2006;11(6): 752–4.

134. Rothenberg SM et al. Modeling oncogene addiction using RNA interference. Proc Natl Acad Sci USA. 2008;105(34):12480–4.

135. Hsieh AY et al. Comparisons of catastrophizing, pain attitudes, and cold-pressor pain experience between Chinese and European Canadian young adults. J Pain. 2010;11(11):1187–94.

136. Rappaport BA, Cerny I, Sanhai WR. ACTION on the prevention of chronic pain after surgery: public-private partnerships, the future of analgesic drug development. Anesthesiology. 2010;112(3):509–10.

137. Tracey I, Johns E. The pain matrix: reloaded or reborn as we image tonic pain using arterial spin labelling. Pain. 2010;148(3):359–60.

138. Davis KD et al. Event-related fMRI of pain: entering a new era in imaging pain. Neuroreport. 1998;9(13): 3019–23.

139. Schneider F et al. Subjective ratings of pain correlate with subcortical-limbic blood flow: an fMRI study. Neuropsychobiology. 2001;43(3):175–85.

140. Takemura Y et al. Effects of gabapentin on brain hyperactivity related to pain and sleep disturbance under a neuropathic pain-like state using fMRI and brain wave analysis. Synapse. 2011;65(7): 668–76.

141. Borsook D, Becerra L. CNS animal fMRI in pain and analgesia. Neurosci Biobehav Rev. 2011;35(5): 1125–43.

142. Scrivani S et al. A fMRI evaluation of lamotrigine for the treatment of trigeminal neuropathic pain: pilot study. Pain Med. 2010;11(6):920–41.

143. Burgmer M et al. Fibromyalgia unique temporal brain activation during experimental pain: a controlled fMRI Study. J Neural Transm. 2010;117(1): 123–31.

144. Binshtok AM, Bean BP, Woolf CJ. Inhibition of nociceptors by TRPV1-mediated entry of impermeant sodium channel blockers. Nature. 2007; 449(7162):607–10.

145. Lui F et al. Neural bases of conditioned placebo analgesia. Pain. 2010;151(3):816–24.

146. Lu HC et al. Neuronal correlates in the modulation of placebo analgesia in experimentally-induced esophageal pain: a 3T-fMRI study. Pain. 2010;148(1): 75–83.

147. Eippert F et al. Direct evidence for spinal cord involvement in placebo analgesia. Science. 2009;326(5951):404.

148. Petrovic P et al. A prefrontal non-opioid mechanism in placebo analgesia. Pain. 2010;150(1):59–65.

149. Quessy SN, Rowbotham MC. Placebo response in neuropathic pain trials. Pain. 2008;138(3):479–83.

150. Hrobjartsson A, Gotzsche PC. Unreliable analysis of placebo analgesia in trials of placebo pain mechanisms. Pain. 2003;104(3):714–5; author reply 715–6.

151. Hamunen K, Kalso E. A systematic review of trial methodology, using the placebo groups of randomized controlled trials in paediatric postoperative pain. Pain. 2005;116(1–2):146–58.

152. Dworkin RH, Katz J, Gitlin MJ. Placebo response in clinical trials of depression and its implications for research on chronic neuropathic pain. Neurology. 2005;65(12 Suppl 4):S7–19.

153. Mogil JS. Animal models of pain: progress and challenges. Nat Rev Neurosci. 2009;10(4):283–94.

154. Bauer CS et al. The anti-allodynic alpha(2)delta ligand pregabalin inhibits the trafficking of the calcium channel alpha(2)delta-1 subunit to presynaptic terminals in vivo. Biochem Soc Trans. 2010;38(2):525–8.

155. Woolf CJ et al. Nerve growth factor contributes to the generation of inflammatory sensory hypersensitivity. Neuroscience. 1994;62(2):327–31.

156. Cattaneo A. Tanezumab, a recombinant humanized mAb against nerve growth factor for the treatment of acute and chronic pain. Curr Opin Mol Ther. 2010;12(1):94–106.

157. Tegeder I et al. GTP cyclohydrolase and tetrahydrobiopterin regulate pain sensitivity and persistence. Nat Med. 2006;12(11):1269–77.

158. Reimann F et al. Pain perception is altered by a nucleotide polymorphism in SCN9A. Proc Natl Acad Sci USA. 2010;107(11):5148–53.

159. Braun SM, Jessberger S. Previews. Crossing boundaries: direct programming of fibroblasts into neurons. Cell Stem Cell. 2010;6(3):189–91.

160. Wernig M et al. Neurons derived from reprogrammed fibroblasts functionally integrate into the fetal brain and improve symptoms of rats with Parkinson's disease. Proc Natl Acad Sci USA. 2008;105(15): 5856–61.

161. Printz C. BATTLE to personalize lung cancer treatment. Novel clinical trial design and tissue gathering procedures drive biomarker discovery. Cancer. 2010;116(14):3307–8.

Index

A

Access to Controlled Medicines Programme
    (ACMP), 258
ACM. *See* Adequacy of Consumption Measure (ACM)
ACMP. *See* Access to Controlled Medicines
    Programme (ACMP)
Action potential stimulation (APS), 148
Acupuncture
    electroacupuncture technique, 145
    neurophysiological mechanisms, 144
    therapies classification, 144
    treatment, lumbar pain, 144–145
Adequacy of Consumption Measure (ACM), 252
American Society of Clinical Oncology
    (ASCO), 161
Anticancer therapy
    chemotherapy-related pain syndromes, 62–64
    pain syndromes, 60
    post-amputation pain, 62
    post-mastectomy pain, 61–62
    post-radiation therapy pain, 62
    postsurgical neuropathy, 60–61
    post-thoracotomy pain, 61
Anticonvulsants, 182–183
Antidepressants
    bupropion and duloxetine, 182
    description, 180
    SNRIs and SSRIs, 180, 182
    TCAs, 180–181
APS. *See* Action potential stimulation (APS)
ASCO. *See* American Society of Clinical Oncology
    (ASCO)

B

Bone pain
    acid-sensing ion channels, 53, 54
    causes, 52, 53
    description, 52
    mechanism, 54
    osteoclasts, 53–54
    prostaglandins, 54
    tumor growth, 52
Breakthrough pain (BTP)
    abdominal pain, 125–126
    anesthesiological techniques, 125

anesthetic, 125
axial pain, 122
characteristics (n = 41), 157
diagnosis and treatment, 123
entonox, 126
epidemiology, 122
evaluation, 122, 123
fentanyl drops, 124
ketamine, 124–125
management, 123, 157
median (IQR) number, 157
morphine, 124
movements, 125
neuropathic pain, 126
opioid combinations, 124
predictable and unpredictable, 121–122
procedure pain, 126
sytemic corticosteroids, 125
transmucosal fentanyls, 126–127
treatment, 128
BTP. *See* Breakthrough pain (BTP)

C

Cancer
    care (*see* Care)
    curative treatment and pain reduction, 222
    description, 221–222
    fundamental features, 222
    pain (*see* Pain)
    religious thoughts, 222, 223
    spirituality (*see* Spirituality)
    treatment
        breast mortality, 25, 26
        cytotoxic chemotherapy, 26–28
        epigenetic pathways, 31–32
        immunotherapy, 34
        metastatic breast cancer, 25, 26
        proteasome inhibitors, 31
Cancer-induced bone pain (CIBP), 156–157
Cancer-related neuropathic pain
    cranial nerve neuropathy, 173
    plexus neuropathy, 171–172
    PNN (*see* Paraneoplastic neuropathy (PNN))
    radiculopathy, leptomeningeal metastases/vertebral
        body, 172–173

Cancer-related plexus neuropathy
  brachial plexopathies, 172
  cervical plexopathies, 171–172
  description, 171
  imaging workups, 171
  lumbosacral plexopathies, 172
  plexopathy, 171
  qualities, pain, 172
  radiation-induced lumbosacral plexopathy, 172
  sensory change/motor weakness, 172
Cannabinoids
  acute and chronic pain models, 156
  description, 155
  endogenous, 156
  Nabiximols, 156
  THC and CBD, 156
Capsaicins
  local anesthetics, 196
  multiple neuropeptides, 196
  resiniferatoxin, 196
  topical NSAIDs, 196
  topical opioids, 197
  vanilloid receptors, 196
Care
  description, 224
  first level, attention, 225–226
  second level, accompaniment, 226–227
  spirituality and caregivers, 225
  third level, crisis intervention, 227–228
CBT. See Cognitive behavioral therapy (CBT)
Celiac plexus block, NCPB
  destruction, 234–235
  injection, neurolytic solution, 234, 235
  Ischia's technique, 236, 237
  transcrural CT-guided posterior technique, 236
Challenges, pain management
  absenteeism, production loss and insurance
      costs, 263–264
  amplification, sensory signals, 264
  analgesic benefits, 264
  central sensitization, chronic pain, 265
  diabetes, 264
  G-protein interactions, 269–270
  molecular structure, opioid receptor and signal
      transduction, 264
  morphine-induced inflammation, 271
  multiple opioid ligands, 267–268
  mu receptor genetics, 269
  Neuropathic Pain Syndrome Inventory and Pain
      Scale, 264–265
  nociceptive input, 264
  opioid-induced hyperalgesia, 271
  opioids
      and NSAIDs, 271
      receptor dynamics and novel development,
          265–266
      receptor interactions and dimers, 266–267
  pain assessment, 264
  pain-processing disorders, 264
  physicians, 264

regulatory proteins and chaperones, 270–271
responses, opioids, 270
in twenty-first century
    analgesic combination trials, 272
    animal models, 272–273
    Bayesian approach to trial design, 271
    "disease" modification, 272
    fMRI, 272
    neurologic mechanisms, 272
    "oncogene addiction", 272
    peripheral and central nervous system
        pathways, 271
    personalized genomic markers, 271
    Placebo effects, 272
    receptor, ion channel/transporter, 273
    stem cell biology techniques, 273
Chemotherapy-induced neuropathic pain
    (CINP), 166, 170
Chemotherapy-induced peripheral
    neuropathy (CIPN)
  agents, 176
  clinical manifestations, 176
  patients and physicians, 176
  peripheral sensory nerves, 176
  physical examination, 176
Chemotherapy-related pain syndromes
  bortezomib, 63
  cisplatin, 63
  pain, management, 64
  peripheral neuropathy, 62–63
  vincristine, 63
Chronic cancer pain syndromes
  description, 103–104
  multifocal bone pain, 103–105
  pelvis and hip, 105
Chronic intestinal obstruction, 106
CIBP. See Cancer-induced bone pain (CIBP)
CINP. See Chemotherapy-induced neuropathic
    pain (CINP)
CIPN. See Chemotherapy-induced peripheral
    neuropathy (CIPN)
CMN. See Compression (mono)neuropathies
    (CMN)
Cognitive behavioral therapy (CBT), 215
Complex regional pain syndrome (CRPS)
  clinical characteristics, 175
  description, 175
  development pathways, 175
  diagnostic criterias, 175
Compression (mono)neuropathies (CMN)
  "breakthrough" pains, 192
  clinical descriptions, 192
  defined, 192
  neuropathic pain, 192
  observed in patients with cancer, 193–194
  suprascapular nerve entrapment, 193
  symptoms, 192, 193
Cranial nerve neuropathy, 173
CRPS. See Complex regional pain syndrome
    (CRPS)

CYP. *See* Cytochrome P (CYP)
Cytochrome P (CYP), 39
Cytotoxic chemotherapy
    alkylating agents, 27
    antifolates, 28
    antimetabolites, 27
    cell cycle, 27
    chemotherapy, 26–27
    clinical indications, 27
    description, 26
    DNA function, 27
    heavy metals, 27
    mechanisms, 27

D
DDD. *See* Defined daily dose (DDD)
Defined daily dose (DDD), 251
Dexamethasone, noncancer-related pain, 198
Diffuse noxious inhibitory control
        (DNIC), 135
DNIC. *See* Diffuse noxious inhibitory
        control (DNIC)
Dorsal root ganglion (DRG), 51
DRG. *See* Dorsal root ganglion (DRG)
Drug elimination
    alfentanil, 117
    buprenorphine, 116
    codeine, 113, 114
    fentanyl, 116–117
    hydromorphone, 115
    methadone, 116
    morphine, 115
    opioid therapy, 113, 114
    oxycodone, 115
    pethidine, 117
    tapentadol, 117
    tramadol, 114–115
Drugs, pain management
    adjuvant analgesics, 153
    animal models, bone pain, 156–157
    antidepressants, 154, 155
    assessment, 154
    BTP (*see* Breakthrough pain (BTP))
    cannabinoids (*see* Cannabinoids)
    capsaicin, 156
    descending inhibitory control, 154, 155
    disease-oriented trials, 153
    duloxetine, 161
    gabapentinoids, 153
    interventional analgesia, 157–158
    multiple adjuvant analgesics, 153
    opioids, 154–155, 161
    single-agent analgesics, 153
    steroids, 158
    tapentadol, 159–160
    ziconotide, 158–159
Duloxetine, 161
DWB. *See* Dynamic weight bearing (DWB)
Dynamic weight bearing (DWB), 86

E
Electrical stimulation test, 136
Electroacupuncture technique, 145
Endocrine treatment
    breast cancer, 32
    prostate cancer, 34
    ubiquitin-proteasome pathway, 32–33
Epidemiology
    advanced cancer, 9
    advanced disease/end of life, 9, 14–16
    assessment methods, 7
    classification, 8
    definition, 6
    early/mixed-stage cancer, 9–13
    epidemiology, 17, 20
    evaluation, 6
    identification, study, 9
    meta-analysis, 9
    physician, 7–8
    population, 8–9
    prevalence, 8
    primary tumor site, 9, 18–19
    risk factor, 17
    severity, 17
    study population, 6
    tumor, 6
Epigenetic pathways, 31–32
Evidence-based therapy, 1

F
"Family disease", 216

G
GFAP. *See* Glial fibrillary acidic protein (GFAP)
Glial fibrillary acidic protein (GFAP), 80
Glossopharyngeal neuralgia, 173

H
Hepatic distension syndrome, 106
Hypogastric superior plexus block, 241

I
Immunotherapy, 34
Interventional analgesia
    spinal bolus levobupivacaine/sublingual
            ketamine, 158
    spinal opioids, 157
Interventional techniques
    cancer pain management, 232
    description, 232
    hypogastric superior plexus block, 241
    multimodal approach, 232
    NCPB (*see* Neurolytic celiac plexus block (NCPB))
    neuraxial infusions (*see* Neuraxial infusions)
    neuroablative techniques, 232
    PCC (*see* Percutaneous cervical cordotomy (PCC))

L

Liaison psychiatrist, patients with chronic pain
  biofeedback, 215–216
  CBT, 215
  communication skills, 217–218
  description, 214
  "family disease", 216
  medical hypnosis, 215–216
  palliative care units, 216
  psychodynamic approach, 215
  psychopharmacotherapy, 216–217
  psychosocial interventions, 214–215
  psychotherapeutic intervention, 215
  relaxation techniques, 215–216
Long-term survivors, rehabilitation, 207–208

M

Malignant perineal pain, 106
MAOIs. *See* Monoamine oxidase inhibitors
      (MAOIs)
Matrix metalloproteases (MMPs), 80
MDR. *See* Multidrug resistance (MDR)
Mechanisms
  anticancer therapy (*see* Anticancer therapy)
  central pain syndromes, 58
  classification, 48
  description, 48
  infections, 64
  intensity, 48
  leptomeningeal metastases, 59
  muscle-related pain, 64–65
  nociceptive, patient (*see* Nociceptive pain)
  osteoporosis, 65
  plexopathy, 59–60
  spinal cord compression, 59
  tumor-related mononeuropathy, 59
  wounds/pressure ulcers, 65
Metabolism, opioids
  cytochrome P450, 113
  glucuronidation, 113
Methadone maintenance
  cold pressor test, 135
  electrical stimulation test, 136
M3G. *See* Morphine-3-glucoronide (M3G)
M6G. *See* Morphine-6-glucoronide (M6G)
Midline retroperitoneal syndrome, 106
MMPs. *See* Matrix metalloproteases
      (MMPs)
Monoamine oxidase inhibitors
      (MAOIs), 160
Morphine, 1, 2, 124
Morphine-3-glucoronide (M3G), 138
Morphine-6-glucoronide (M6G), 38–39
Motor functions
  DWB, 86
  walking pattern, 86
Multidrug resistance (MDR)
  human genetic variability, 42
  transporters, 42

Multifocal bone pain
  radiotherapy, 103
  vertebral syndromes, 103, 105
Multiple opioid ligands, 267–268
Mu-opioid receptors
  description, 41
  genetic variability, 42
  polymorphism, 41–42
  SNP, 42

N

Neuraxial infusions
  description, 241
  intraventricular opioids, 242
  morphine, opioids, 241
  RCTs, spinal, 241
Neurolytic celiac plexus block (NCPB)
  acute/long-term analgesia, 237
  anatomical recalls, 233
  anteroposterior view of contrast dye,
        PPBS, 239, 240
  approach at T11–T10 level, PPBS technique,
        239, 240
  Boas's technique, 234, 235
  celiac plexus block, 234–237
  clinical efficacy, 238
  Cochrane Database Systematic Review, 241
  correlating X-ray images, 238
  destruction, splanchnic-celiac axis, 240
  diagnostic CT scan, 238
  effectiveness, long-lasting pain relief, 237
  EUS-NCPB, 233
  high abdomen pain pathways, 232
  instruments, 234
  laparoscopy, 236
  latero-lateral view of contrast dye, PPBS, 239, 240
  nerve neurolysis, 232–233
  opioids, 238
  pancreatic carcinoma, 232
  percutaneous techniques, 234
  plexus and adjacent vessels, 236
  PPBS, 240, 241
  side effects and complications, 236–237
  solutions, nervous structures, 233–234
  splanchnic and celiac denervation, 239
  and splanchnic nerves, 236
  transaortic technique, 236
Neuroma transposition model, 73
Neuropathic pain
  allodynia, 58
  assessment
    conventional electrophysiological
          techniques, 179
    diagnosis, 178
    EFNS, 178–179
    nociceptive pain, 179
    screening tools, 179
  bortezomib, 79
  cancer-related (*see* Cancer-related neuropathic pain)

central sensitization, 168–170
chemotherapy-induced, 76
cisplatin, 78–79
common symptoms and signs, 170, 171
definition, 166
description, 56
epidemiology, 166–167
etiology, 167
invasion-induced, 76
management, 165
mechanical destruction, neurons, 168
mechanisms, 57
motor and/or autonomic dysfunction, 171
neurotoxic chemotherapies, 166
oxaliplatin, 79
paclitaxel, 78
pathophysiologic mechanism, peripheral and
    central sensitization, 168
peripheral sensitization and spontaneous nerve
    activity
    chemical mediators, 168
    CINP, 170
    ion channels and receptors, 168
    nociceptors, high thresholds, 168, 169
    pathologic adrenergic coupling, 170
    TRPV1, 168
peripheral sensory nerve injury and regeneration,
    170–171
pharmacologic treatment (see Pharmacologic
    treatment, neuropathic pain)
PHN, 178
quality, 171
treatment, 179–180
treatment-related (see Treatment-related
    neuropathic pain)
types, chronic cancer, 165
vincristine, 78
N-methyl-D-aspartate (NMDA) receptors, 51–52,
    110, 136–137
Nociceptive pain
bone pain, cancer patient, 52–55
somatic pain, cancer patient (see Somatic pain)
visceral pain, cancer patient (see Visceral pain)
Noncancer-related pain, daily practice
capsaicin (see Capsaicins)
CMN (see Compression (mono)neuropathies
    (CMN))
description, 191
dexamethasone, 198
loss, tissue integrity and normal
    function, 192
muscle wasting and overuse, 195
osteoarthritis, 198
osteoporosis (see Osteoporosis, noncancer-related
    pain)
skin pain, 195–196
specific diagnosis and classification,
    pain, 192
Non-pharmacological treatment
acupuncture (see Acupuncture)

adjuvants, 143
APS, 148
external neuromodulation, 146, 147
local treatment, 143–144
pulse radio-frequency neuromodulation, 148
radio-frequency lesioning, 147–148
sensory nerves, 147
TENS (see Transcutaneous electrical nerve
    stimulation (TENS))
NSAIDs. See Topical nonsteroidal anti-inflammatory
    drugs (NSAIDs)

O
Opioid analgesics
ACM, 252
ACMP, 258
attitude barriers, 256–257
availability, accessibility and
    affordability, 253
barriers, 255
cancer patients, 250
DDD, 251
economic barriers, 257
global situation, 253
health-care professionals, 258
knowledge barriers, 256
legislative and policy barriers, 255–256
morphine, 251
per capita consumption, 251
PPSG, 251
treatment, 251
UNDP, 252
UN economic and social council, 258
WHO policy guidelines, 257–258
Opioid-induced hyperalgesia (OIH)
anecdotal reports, 134
cancer patients, 136
consumption, 132
diagnosis, 138
DNIC, 135
dynorphin, 137
fentanyl, 133
gabapentin, 140
glutamate transporter system, 137
heroin, 133
hyperalgesia, 132
ketamine, 138
methadone maintenance, 135–136
M3G, 138
morphine exposition, 137
naive individuals, 134
NMDA receptors, 136–137
noncancer pain patients, 135
opioid tolerance, 138
RVM, 137
subtypes, humans, 134
therapy, 132
tissue injury, 133
treatment, 139

Opioids
  drug absorption, 111
  enkephalins, 111
  metabolism, 113
  metabolites, 113
  NMDA, 110
  nociceptins, 111
  and NSAIDs, 271
  pharmacokinetics, 109, 112
  receptor dynamics and novel development
    ADL10-0101 and TRK-820, 266
    analgesic tolerance, 265
    drawbacks in development, 266
    inflammation, 265
    intracerebroventricular/intrathecal naloxone
        blocks, 265
    low pH, 265–266
    Mu, delta and kappa, 265
    nerve growth factor, 266
    neuropathic pain, 266
    peripheral mu receptor tolerance, 265
    systemic non-opioid analgesics, 266
    topical meperidine, 265
  receptor interactions and dimers
    bivalent opioid ligands, 267
    delta agonists, 266–267
    G-proteins, 267
    Mu-delta heterodimers, 266
    Sprague-Dawley rats, 267
  receptors, 110
  subtypes, 109, 110
  transmembrane structures, 110, 111
  WHO pain ladder, 117–118
Osteoarthritis, noncancer-related pain, 198
Osteoporosis, noncancer-related pain
  bisphosphonates, 197
  in cancer, 197
  cause, pain, 197–198
  fractionated heparin, 197

P
Pain and Policy Studies Group (PPSG), 251
Pain assessment
  acute, 100, 102–103
  bone pain, 100
  chemotherapy, 101
  description, 95
  disease, 100, 101
  evaluation, 96
  laboratory testing, 98
  lesions, 99
  opioids, 97
  oral mucositis, 101
  pain intensity, 97–98
  physical examination, 98
  PSA, 99
  radiological examination, 99
  radiotherapy, 101

symptoms and signs, 96
syndromes, 96
visceral pains, 100
Pain-related disability
  components, 205
  impairment, 204
  maximal physical efficiency, 204
  neurophysiology, 204
  person's body and features, 204
  puzzle, composed by clinician, 205, 206
  quality of life and functional autonomy, 204
  rehabilitation and occupational therapy, 205
  structure, processes and rehabilitation
      outcomes, 205
Palliative care units, 208, 216
PAM. See Pressure application measurement (PAM)
Paraneoplastic neurological syndromes (PNS), 58
Paraneoplastic neuropathy (PNN), 173
PBPS. See Posterior percutaneous splanchnicectomy
        (PBPS)
PCC. See Percutaneous cervical cordotomy (PCC)
Percutaneous cervical cordotomy (PCC)
  bilateral destruction, reticular spinal fibers, 245
  changes, respiratory function, 244
  description, 242
  destroy, lateral spinothalamic tract, 242
  electrode into spinal cord, 242, 243
  fluoroscopy, correct electrode position, 242, 243
  A 18 G needle, 242
  left cordotomy, with unilateral pain from C6 to T8,
      243, 244
  motor stimulations, 242
  myelography and neurophysiological stimulations,
      242
  neurosurgical procedures, 245
  pain contralaterally to cordotomy, 244
  pain ipsilaterally to cordotomy, 243–244
  percutaneous cordotomy, 244, 245
  results and complications, 244, 245
  spinal cord, dentate ligaments and dural sac,
      242, 243
  vertebroplasty, 245
Percutaneous techniques, NCPB, 234
Phantom limb pain (PLP)
  central and peripheral mechanisms, 174
  defined, 174
  pain characteristics, 174
  peripheral nerve system, 175
  somatosensory cortical areas, 174–175
Pharmacogenetics, cancer pain
  biological mechanisms, 39
  cellular response, 42–43
  CYP enzymes, 40
  drug therapy, 38
  genetic variability, 39
  MDR transporters, 42
  M6G, 38–39
  morphine, 38, 39, 43
  mu-opioid receptors, 41–42

opioids, 38
UGT2B7, 40–41
Pharmacological local treatments
botox, 149
capsaicin, 148–149
placebo analgesia, 149
Pharmacologic treatment, neuropathic pain
anticonvulsants, 182–183
antidepressants (*see* Antidepressants)
cannabinoids, 183–184
NMDA receptor, 183
opioids, 180
topical agents, 183
tramadol, 183
PHN. *See* Postherpetic neuralgia (PHN)
Physicians and cancer survivors, 1
PLP. *See* Phantom limb pain (PLP)
PMPS. *See* Postmastectomy pain syndrome (PMPS)
PNN. *See* Paraneoplastic neuropathy (PNN)
PNS. *See* Paraneoplastic neurological
syndromes (PNS)
Posterior percutaneous splanchnicectomy
(PBPS), 234, 235
Postherpetic neuralgia (PHN), 178
Postmastectomy pain syndrome (PMPS), 174
Post-thoracotomy pain syndrome (PTPS), 174
PPSG. *See* Pain and Policy Studies Group (PPSG)
Preclinical cancer pain models
bone cancer pain, 73–74
chemokines, 82
clinical implication, 82–83
cytokines, 80–81
description, 71–72
electrical stimulation, 83
GFAP, 80
immune factors, 79
inflammatory cells, 80
interleukins, 81–82
MATLyLu, 74–75
measurement, animal, 83
mechanical stimulation, 84
metastatic bone tumors, 72
MMPs, 80
MRMT-1, 76
orofacial, 73
pancreatic, 73
paw pressure test, 84
presentation, animal models, 86–87
R-3327 adenocarcinoma, 74
skin, 72
tail-pinch test, 84
TNF and INF, 81
tumors, 72
von frey apparatus, 84
WDR, 75
Pressure application measurement (PAM), 84
Prostate-specific antigen (PSA), 99
PSA. *See* Prostate-specific antigen (PSA)
Psychodynamic approach, 215

Psychopharmacotherapy, 216–217
Psychosocial problems
anxiety disorders, 213–214
brain, 212
concept, "quality of life", 212
and depression, 213
description, 212
Liaison psychiatrist (*see* Liaison psychiatrist,
patients with chronic pain)
medications, 212
progressive depression, patient, 213
psychiatric disorders, 213
psychiatrists, 213
and psychological aspects, 212
spiritual dimension, pain, 212
uncontrolled pain, 212
PTPS. *See* Post-thoracotomy pain
syndrome (PTPS)

R
Radiation-induced neuropathy (RNP), 175
Radical neck dissection (RND), 174
Regulatory proteins and chaperones, 270–271
Rehabilitation
description, 204
disorders, 204
in early stages, 205–206
in long-term survivors, 207–208
pain-related disability, 204–205
palliative care unit, 208
during relapses, 207
during remission phases, 206–207
Relapses, 207
Remission phases, 206–207
RND. *See* Radical neck dissection (RND)
RNP. *See* Radiation-induced neuropathy (RNP)
Rostral ventromedial medulla (RVM)
descending pathway, 138
lidocaine, 137
neurons, 137
RVM. *See* Rostral ventromedial medulla (RVM)

S
Single-nucleotide polymorphisms (SNP), 42
Skin cancer pain model, 72
Skull metastases, 105
SNP. *See* Single-nucleotide polymorphisms (SNP)
Somatic pain
cytokines, 52
DRG, 51
microglia and nerve cells, 52
NMDA, 51–52
structures, 49
sympathetic postganglionic fibers, 51
tissue damage, 49
transduction and sensitization, 49–50
trypsin, 49, 51

Spirituality
    defined, 222
    European working definition, 223
    existential challenges, 223
    reduction and research, 223
    religious considerations and foundations, 223
    transcendent and escape, 223
    value based considerations and attitudes, 223

T
Tapentadol
    CYP enzymes, 160
    inhibition, noradrenaline reuptake, 159
    isobolographic analysis, 160
    MAOIs, 160
    molecules, analgesia, 159
    μ-opioid and α2-adrenergic receptor
        agonists, 159
    treatment-emergent gastrointestinal adverse
        effects, 159
    UGT enzymes, 160
Targeted agents
    molecular biology techniques, 28–29
    signal transduction, 30
    tyrosine kinase inhibitors, 29
Targeting angiogenesis
    description, 30–31
    metastasis, 30
    VEGF system, 30
Taxanes (paclitaxel, docetaxel), 177
TCA. *See* Tricyclic antidepressants (TCA)
TENS. *See* Transcutaneous electrical nerve stimulation
        (TENS)
Tetrahydrocannabinol (THC)
    anxiogenic and psychoactive effects, 156
    and CBD, 156
Thalidomide, 178
THC. *See* Tetrahydrocannabinol (THC)
Thermal stimulation
    acetone tests, 86
    hargreaves plantar test, 85
    heat, 84
    hot/cold plate analgesia meter, 86
    tail-flick test, 85
TNF. *See* Tumor necrosis factor (TNF)
Topical nonsteroidal anti-inflammatory drugs
        (NSAIDs), 196
Topical opioids, capsaicins, 197
Transcutaneous electrical nerve stimulation (TENS)
    acupuncture, 145
    cancer patients, 146
    treatment, lumbar pain, 146, 147
Treatment-related neuropathic pain
    bortezomib, 178
    CIPN (*see* Chemotherapy-induced peripheral
        neuropathy (CIPN))
    CRPS (*see* Complex regional pain
        syndrome (CRPS))

    description, 173–174
    platinum agents, 176–177
    PLP, 174–175
    PMPS, 174
    post-RND pain (*see* Radical neck
        dissection (RND))
    PTPS, 174
    RNP, 175
    taxanes (paclitaxel, docetaxel), 177
    thalidomide, 178
    vinca alkaloid, 177–178
Tricyclic antidepressants (TCA), 217
Trigeminal neuralgia, 173
Tumor necrosis factor (TNF), 81

U
Ubiquitin-proteasome pathway, 32–33
UDP-glucuronosyltransferase 2B7
        (UGT2B7), 40–41
United Nations Development Programme
        (UNDP), 252
Uridine diphosphate-glucuronosyltransferase (UGT)
        enzymes, 160

V
VASPI. *See* Visual analogue scale of pain intensity
        (VASPI) scores
Vertebral syndromes
    funicular and radicular pains, 105
    metastases, 103
Vertebroplasty, PCC, 245
Vinca alkaloids, 177–178
Visceral pain
    mechanisms, 55
    pancreatic cancer, 56
    tumor tissue growth, 55
Visual analogue scale of pain intensity
        (VASPI) scores
    baseline in patients, 158
    mean percentage change, 159

W
WDR. *See* Wide dynamic range (WDR)
Wide dynamic range (WDR), 75

Z
Ziconotide
    disadvantages, 158
    and morphine, 158
    non-opioid intrathecal (IT) drugs, 158
    safety and efficacy, IT combination, 159
    systemic opioids and appropriate adjuvants, 159
    VASPI scores, 158, 159

Lightning Source UK Ltd.
Milton Keynes UK
UKOW07n0147030316

269472UK00005B/39/P

9 780857 292292